Praise for *aah...* The Pleasure Book

"This is one of the most important books you will ever read. Panoramic in scope and deep in wisdom, it is nothing less than a blueprint for a great life and our collective survival. In plain language, physician Jia Gottlieb plumbs the meaning of pleasure and pain to reach a vision of interdependence among all living things and their environment, where love, compassion, and balance are key. This book is a testament to excellent science, psychology, and ancient wisdom, mingled with inspiration and hope: a crucial message for our time."
— Larry Dossey, MD, author of *ONE MIND: How Our Individual Mind Is Part of a Greater Consciousness and Why It Matters*

"*aah...* exhale when you say it and dive into the mystery of the present moment with our longtime friend, Dr. Jia. This rich offering of yogic wisdom, contemplative thought, science, and practical philosophy is presented in a refreshingly personal and effective way. He starts us over and over again looking honestly at our present experience, at sensations, breath, patterns of mind, and the pleasure of being in true relationship with others. Please study this book again and again. Please research and study all the teachers and books that are referenced within."
— Richard Freeman, author of *The Mirror of Yoga* and co-author, with Mary Taylor, of *The Art of Vinyasa*

"Dr. Gottlieb dispels the biggest deception perpetuated on humankind: that we are flawed and our suffering is noble. This masterpiece is a clarion call to reinstate Pleasure—and her various faces of Beauty, Truth, and Freedom—as our essential compass, not just for achieving our own excellence and enlightenment, but for navigating the next stage of our human evolution."
— Lorraine Moller, winner of sixteen international marathons, Olympic medalist, and author of *On the Wings of Mercury*

"A work of penetrating insight, at once poetic and scientific, on what it means to be human in a unitary world fully embodied yet simultaneously transcendent. Destined to be a classic, **aah...** *The Pleasure Book* opens new horizons for human consciousness, unifying life and death and all that lies between—a must read."

— JEAN WATSON, PHD, RN, University of Colorado College of Nursing distinguished professor dean emerita, founder of the Watson Caring Science Institute

"I love this book! It is both profound and enjoyable. Dr. Gottlieb has created a brilliant synthesis that spans the molecular and spiritual levels of human experience and shows how each of us can master the art of truly enjoying life."

— REUBEN WIENINGER, MD, psychiatrist, musician, and yogi

"**aah...** is not your typical 'how to' book. Approach it as a lesson in living a healthy, environmentally conscious life. As a scholarly book, it invites you to delve deeply into the experience of feeling good and gently guides you through the complexities and confusion of pleasure-seeking and its pitfalls. It has something important to say to those with a puritanical streak as well as the hedonist."

— ROBERT DAVIS, PHD, Harvard environmental/natural resource economist

"This beautifully crafted book provides a comprehensive scaffolding for emerging theories and practices of consciousness that will help many people find their place and their pleasure."

— DARRELL LAHAM, PHD, neurocognitive psychologist, cognitive systems engineer, and consciousness researcher *aah...*

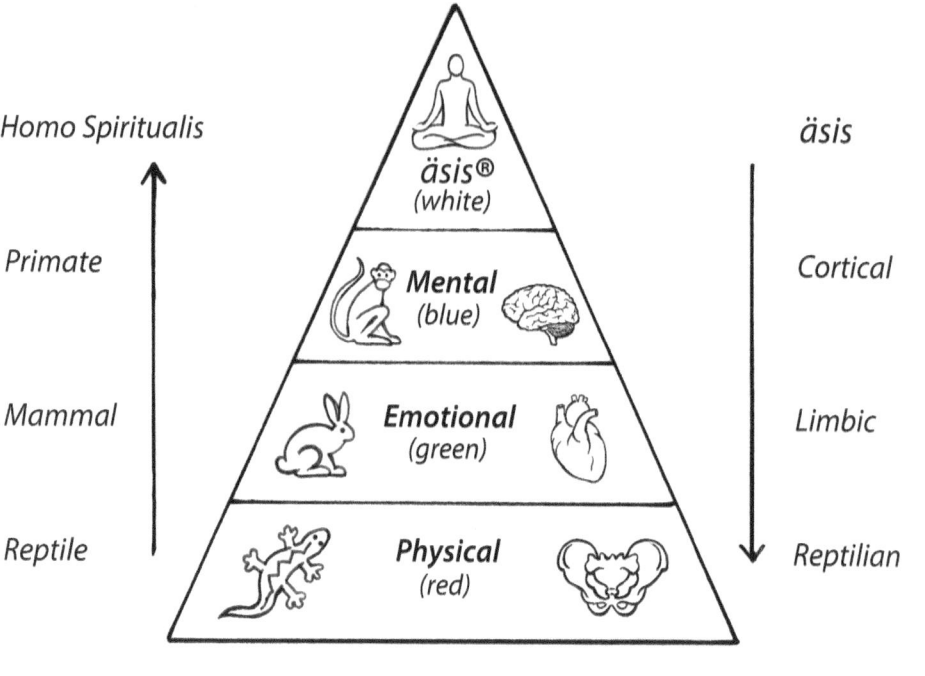

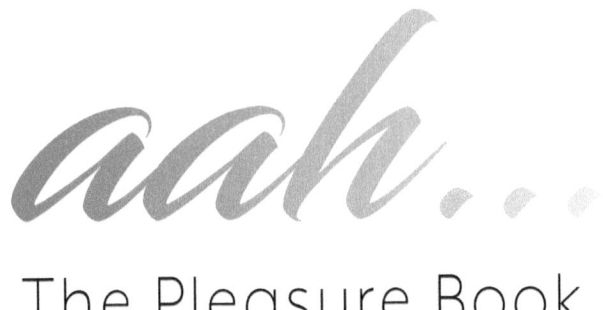

aah...
The Pleasure Book

JIA GOTTLIEB MD

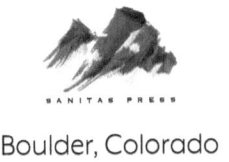

SANITAS PRESS

Boulder, Colorado

aah ... The Pleasure Book
©2020 by Jia Gottlieb, MD
Published by Sanitas Press
P.O. Box 3732
Boulder, Colorado 80307

All rights reserved under International and Pan-American Copyright Conventions. No part of this book may be used or reproduced in any manner whatsoever without written permission from the publisher, except in the case of brief quotations used in critical articles and reviews.

ISBN: 978-1-7343769-0-6 (print)
Also available in ebook, and audiobook

Edited by Jennifer Phelps
Front cover design by Mark Mitchell
Book design and composition by Sue Campbell Book Design
Author photo by Jeff Warnock
Part divider art by Amy Clay; www.amyclay.com
Figure Illustrations by Kersti Frigell; except as noted on pages 349–350
Typeset in Adobe Garamond

äsis is a registered trademark of Jia Gottlieb, MD

For further information please visit:
jiagottliebmd.com

The Source

*Just as the sun illumines the air and shines through it,
but keeps its source for itself, so You pour all pleasure*

*and every delight into every one of your creatures—
and into me—and yet You keep the root of pleasure*

*and guard delight's essence in Yourself so that
I might seek You as the ever giving source of*

what gives true pleasure and lasting delight.
—Meister Eckhardt

CONTENTS

Dedication 9

Part 1: Assumptions

Chapter 1   Why Pleasure. 15
Chapter 2   Welcome to the Pleasure Matrix 27
Chapter 3   The Origin of Original Sin 37
Chapter 4   The Ethics of Pleasure. 49
Chapter 5   An Epicurean Conspiracy 59
▲ 1. The Law of Original Wholeness

Part 2: The Science

Chapter 6   The Anatomy of Pleasure 75
Chapter 7   Your Sphinx Brain. 87
Chapter 8   The Pleasure Prism and Light-body. 95
▲ 2. The Law of Colors

Part 3: The Natural History

Chapter 9   Real Compared to What. 111
▲ 3. The Law of Contrast and Comparison
Chapter 10   Increasing Your Pleasure Capacity 121
Chapter 11   The Sensual Continuum 127
▲ 4. The Law of Thresholds
Chapter 12   Go with the Flow. 133
Chapter 13   The Evolution of Desire. 143
Chapter 14   Supersize Me 157
Chapter 15   The Pleasure Cycle. 165
▲ 5. The Law of Cycles

    Chapter 16   Surrender: The Artless Art 183

Part 4: **The Mystery**
    Chapter 17   Paradise Now 195
    Chapter 18   The 3 Gateways to Paradise 207
                ▲ 6. The Law of Desire and Surrender
    Chapter 19   It's a Fractal Thing 223

Part 5: **The Art and Practice**
    Chapter 20   Make Relationship 237
    Chapter 21   The Myth of Discipline. 247
    Chapter 22   For the Love of It 253
    Chapter 23   Freedom from Addiction 261
    Chapter 24   Erotica 271
    Chapter 25   Orgasm 1.0 281
    Chapter 26   Orgasm 2.0 287
    Chapter 27   Living in the Sweet Spot. 295
    Chapter 28   Renewable Pleasure for a Sustainable World. . . 311
                ▲ 7. The Law of Renewable Pleasure

Afterword 324
Appendix. 325
Acknowledgments. 327
Chapter Notes 328
Glossary. 342
Image credits 349
Index 351

Dedication

To My *Katanas*: Ashani, Jhana, and Satya,

In ancient China, there was a tradition of the family book where secret teachings were handed down through the generations. An accomplished acupuncturist recorded their most effective treatments and a martial artist their training methods and techniques. It is in this spirit that I offer you the beginnings of our family book, a distillation of the wisdom passed on to me and insights gained along the way. It is inspired by you and written for you, but for reasons that will become clear, the secrets I wish to impart need to be open-source. My hope is it will help you, and someday your offspring, avoid unnecessary suffering and enjoy the pleasures of a long and *aah*some life.

I must confess, like many men, being a father didn't come easy to me. I can remember wanting to be a father as far back as medical school and dreaming that someday I'd deliver my own child. Fortunately, I had the privilege of delivering all three of you girls at home, although your mother would remind me that she obviously delivered you.

A couple weeks after Ashani was born, I was walking down the long dirt driveway, feeling awkwardly left out of the loop. A mother's relationship is a given; the baby comes from her body and nourishes at her breast, but what was my role as a father? When a baby's born, so is a mother and a father. By the time I reached the end of the driveway, I decided that while your mother tended to your inner world—a task for which she was naturally endowed and gifted at doing—my job would be to guard the hive, buzz around, and bring home the nectar. I would teach you how to make it in the outer world, as my father had taught me. This meant giving you a philosophical education and instructing you, as best I could, how to live a good life.

Do you remember the question-and-answer game we used to play when you were kids? It began one morning while rushing across town to drop you off at day care. Jhana, you were in your car seat in front and Satya was in the back. Ashani, I think you were already in kindergarten. I had just cut through four lanes of busy traffic, re-living my halfback football days, only to get stuck in a long line of cars turning left. While waiting, I decided to strike up a conversation. Turning around, I said, "Girls! I have a question for you: What's the greatest pleasure in the whole wide world?" Of course, being four and two years old, you didn't understand the question, let alone the answer, so I answered for you, "B-R-E-A-T-H-I-N-G!" Then, by way of illustration, I took a long, deep breath.

The words weren't important. It was, after all, a make-believe conversation. What mattered was the emotional engagement, the energy exchange. I repeated the question and answer several times, and when you caught on and answered, "Breathing," I got excited.

"Yes! That's right! You got it! Breathing!" and I dramatically sucked in another big breath. The answer was familiar to you because I had begun training you in breathing from an early age. When you fell and skinned a knee, we would breathe together into the pain. When you were having an emotional meltdown and crying uncontrollably, I would sit you on my lap with your legs around my waist, one hand supporting your back and the other hand your head. As you exhaled with a cry, I gently lowered you into a supported backbend, and as you breathed in, lifted you up. Backbends are a powerful way to discharge energy. After two or three cycles of deep breathing together, I'd hold you close to me as you sobbed with relief. I raised you like a bear raises its cubs, trusting my instincts and not overthinking it.

We had fun playing our game in the car that morning, you delighting in my joy, and I enjoying yours. As time went on, it evolved into a series of questions and answers and became our own personal catechism.

"What's the greatest drink in the whole world?"

"Water!" you'd sing out in unison.

"And now a really tough one: What's the best flavor of ice cream in the whole world?"

"Vanilla!"

"What does Papa always say about money?"

"You can't buy happiness!"

One day, out of curiosity I asked, "So, Jhana, why can't you buy happiness?"

You thought for a moment and then to my surprise answered, "Because it's not in the store!"

"Where is it then?"

"It's in your body!"

"R-i-g-h-t!" I said, as you beamed with satisfaction.

And from that day, your answer became part of our catechism. As you all got older, I added more complicated questions, one of which referred to a personal language style I had developed where I ended words and sentences with "action" as in "Girls, time to get in the car-action," "Let's watch a movie-action," and "Are you ready for a big girl-action today?"

"So, why do I always call you my 'action-girls'?"

"Because we are a living process!"

Then the questions became more abstract: "What is the most important question in the whole wide world?"

"How do you know what you know?!" you'd exclaim.

"What kind of question is that?"

"Epistemological!" This was the first big word I taught you, and you loved to say it because it gave you a sense of power to use a word most adults didn't know.

Finally, in my most dramatic voice, I always ended with:

"What is the most powerful number in the w-h-o-l-e universe?"

"Zero!"

"And why is zero so powerful?"

"Because it's empty!"

We never tired of our call-and-response game and sometimes performed it for friends and family to everyone's amusement. I was proud of you and took pride in giving you a philosophical education, hoping someday you would recall your childhood catechism and understand what I had taught you. That day has arrived. You have grown up to be beautiful, intelligent, exceptional women. I dedicate this book to you, my beloved daughters, as an expression of the great honor it has been to be your father and in humble gratitude for all that you have taught me, which has informed every word of it. I offer it to you with all my heart.

… And when the time is ripe, please add your own insights—and pass it on.

Part 1: **Assumptions**

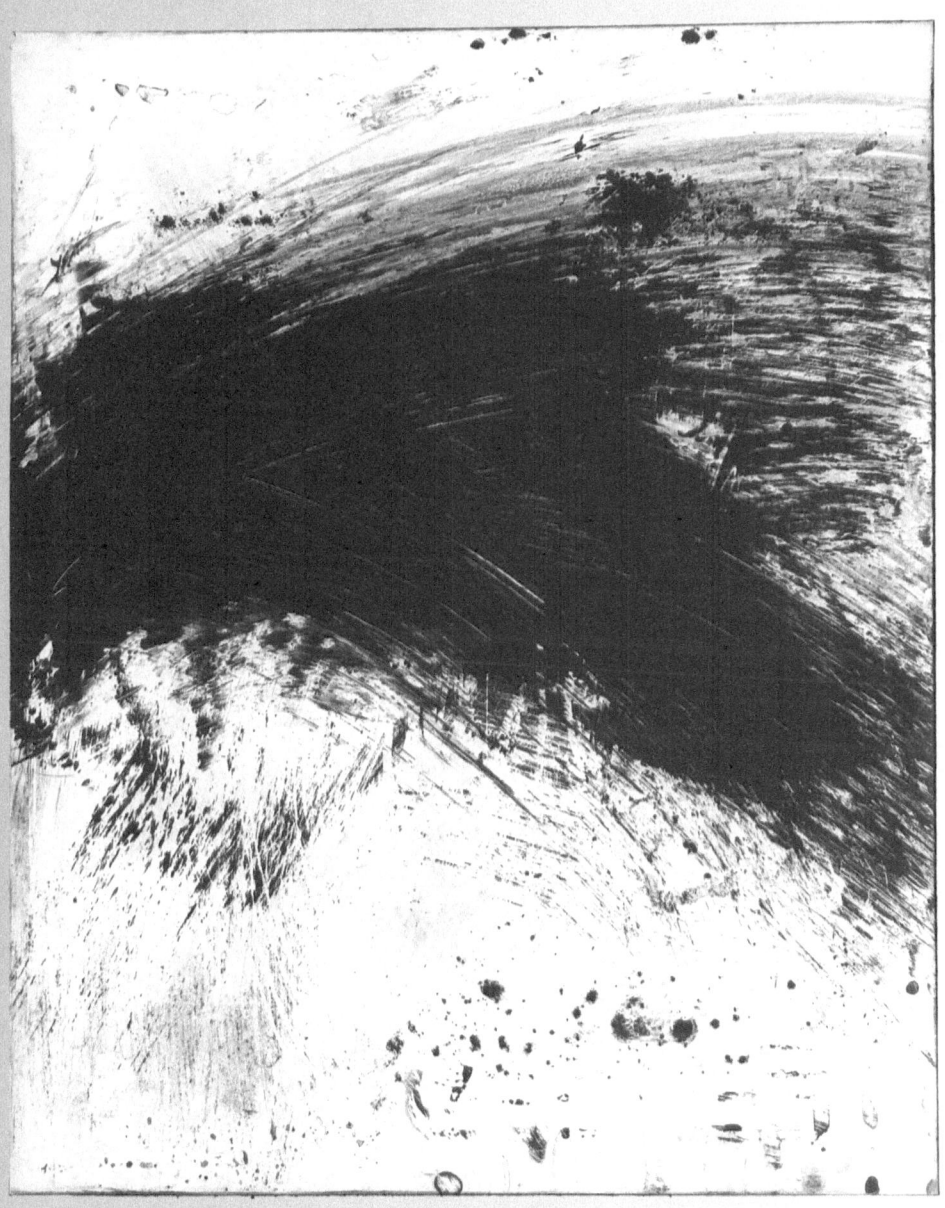

CHAPTER 1

Why Pleasure

*You were born from pleasure and
you are born for pleasure.
It is your origin, source,
and birthright.*
—JG

THIS IS A BOOK ABOUT PLEASURE, ONE OF LIFE'S MOST IMPORTANT AND MOST misunderstood experiences. Important, because it will likely determine the kinds of people you will meet, the quality of your life, your health, and even how long you live. Misunderstood, because in your search for pleasure, it's easy to get lost and end up in pain and suffering. Our current state of knowledge about pleasure is similar to our understanding of human sexuality before the Kinsey report of the 1940s or death and dying before Elisabeth Kübler-Ross wrote her book of the same title in 1969. Everyone's doing it. It's an important part of life. But no one's talking about it. The subject is taboo. Chances are you know more about how your car works than how pleasure does.

I know because when people would ask me, "What are you writing about?" I took the opportunity to conduct a little informal survey and have some fun.

"I'll tell you the topic if you promise to give me your very first association—the first thought that pops into your mind, okay?" Then in a neutral voice I'd say, "It's a book about pleasure."

Easily three out of five people answered "sex." How they answered was even more revealing: some responded in the same "matter-of-fact" way as I posed the question; others leaned in with a devilish smile as if to say, "Tell me more." The most interesting were those who hesitated awkwardly with an "Aah, um … pleasure, huh?" as though they had been caught in an indecent act of thinking about sex and then had to scramble to come up with a socially acceptable answer.

Obviously, there's more to pleasure than sex. Food was a close second, followed by an assortment of responses. Still, most people associated pleasure with the five senses—a fleeting sensual experience and nothing more. This common misunderstanding has led to a great deal of confusion. Take, for example, the recent explosion of happiness research. We're perfectly comfortable talking about happiness in public, but when it comes to pleasure, we feel uneasy. The irony of feeling uncomfortable about pleasure is a clue that something is terribly twisted. The topic touches sensitive, erogenous no-fly zones in our collective consciousness made forbidden by shame and guilt, as though parts of our body, and by extension parts of our lives, are "dirty," reflecting a moral disdain and distrust of the body in general.

Positive psychology researchers, bloggers, and even Buddhist monks go to great lengths to convince us that pleasure and happiness are different things. Pleasure, we're told, is a sensory gratification that depends upon external conditions—a good meal, listening to music, slipping into a hot bath—but soon passes and is therefore unreliable.

Happiness, in contrast, may be influenced by external circumstances but does not depend on them. It is not something you can buy like a new smartphone but an inner state of fulfillment that requires cultivation and endures beyond the momentary ups and downs of life. The implications are clear: chasing after pleasure is foolish; pursue happiness instead.

While this sounds good, the distinction between pleasure and happiness turns out to be a false dichotomy that only adds to our confusion. You may have heard about the World Happiness Report, which ranks 155 countries by their happiness level. The report is based on a single data point. Respondents are asked to evaluate their current lives on a visual ladder where 0 represents the worst possible life and 10, the best possible life.[1]

The word "happy" comes from the Middle English root *hap*, meaning "luck" or "fortune," as in happy birthday, happy-go-lucky, happenstance, and hapless. To equate something as profound as the best possible life—the "good life"—with something as lightweight as happiness is confusing. Martin Seligman, past president of the American Psychological Association and author of the 2002 national best-seller *Authentic Happiness*, has come to regret his choice of title. A decade later on his University of Pennsylvania "Authentic Happiness" website, Seligman confessed, "I actually detest the word 'happiness', which is so overused that it has become almost meaningless .... To understand what 'happiness' is really about, the first step is to dissolve 'happiness' into more workable terms."[2] In the chapters ahead, we'll do just that.

Why pleasure matters

It is important to understand that our desire for pleasure is not a choice we make, moral or otherwise. It is woven into the very fiber of our being and is fundamental to our human existence. We are biologically hard-wired to seek pleasure in the same way a single-celled amoeba extends a pseudopod (a stream of cytoplasm) toward nutrients and away from a sharp probe. Every organism moves toward what supports its existence and away from what threatens it simply because those that didn't were quickly eliminated from the gene pool. In primitive life forms, we refer to these survival responses as instinct. In more complex animals, like ourselves, these survival instincts have evolved into what we call pleasure and pain—the twin cardinal coordinates by which we take our bearings and navigate through life. Obviously, if your onboard GPS is out of whack, it's easy to get lost. It happens all the time.

The pursuit of pleasure is a given, but when we ask ourselves what kind of pleasures we should pursue, things get complicated. Unlike other organisms whose instincts evolved to adapt to the demands of a relatively static, natural environment, we humans create our own physical and psychological environments in the form of cities, houses, possessions, language, myths, beliefs, fashion, customs, laws, religion, and other cultural institutions. Navigating these complex urban and cultural landscapes is much more difficult, and to confound matters, they are continually shifting at an increasingly accelerating pace, spurred on by technology.

As humans we face countless dilemmas such as: Would it be better to live in the city or the countryside? Should I buy a house or rent? Am I religious? Should I own a gun? How do I feel about gay marriage? Abortion? What should I wear to the party? Our answers depend on what we prefer, which reflect our values. How you answer is just another way of saying what pleases you.

What pleases you turns out to be an extremely important question. As I noted at the outset, your answer will likely determine the kinds of people you meet, the quality of your life, your health, and how long you live. This is because the pleasures you seek become habits, habits become a lifestyle, and *in medicine, lifestyle is destiny.* According to a 2009 landmark study, 80 percent of the most common life-threatening diseases—diabetes, heart attack, stroke, and cancer—can be prevented through healthy lifestyle choices alone.[3] So, why aren't we making those healthy choices? Or to restate it more precisely: Why is it, that in our pursuit of pleasure, we often end up in pain and suffering?

This is a question of the utmost importance, and as a doctor, a question that has haunted me for decades. I see patients every day who know how much better they feel when they eat healthy foods, exercise regularly, and so on, but then don't do it. If we are pleasure seeking organisms, why would we not do the very things that make us feel good? The answer may surprise you.

Barking up the right tree

When I was sixteen, I thought smoking was cool and soon became addicted to cigarettes. Had I not kicked the habit (after eight years and countless failed attempts), I might easily have ended up with emphysema and on portable oxygen gasping for breath, or like my friend Scott, who recently died of lung cancer. Our poor choices are usually not for lack of information. I knew smoking was bad for me long before they started putting warning labels on cigarette packages, but I kept smoking anyhow. Everyone knows overeating is not healthy, but that hasn't stopped two out of three Americans from being overweight. We like to explain poor choices in moral terms, blaming ourselves or others for being weak and lacking discipline, or we medicalize it and call it an addiction. But such pronouncements do little to solve the problem. There's a reason.

In medical school, I learned that before you can prescribe an effective treatment, you first need an accurate diagnosis; you have to understand the underlying disease process, the pathophysiology. If you're barking up the wrong tree, it doesn't matter how loud you bark; it's the wrong tree. The problem is not lack of moral character or dopamine pathways run amok. These are merely the "symptoms" of a deeper cause. The real problem—the reason we aren't making healthy choices—is that we are deeply confused about pleasure—so confused, in fact, that we don't even know it.

Consider the following question: What would you say is the opposite of pain? Before reflexively answering, "pleasure," take a moment to think it over. Is pleasure really the opposite of pain? It's true, they point in opposite directions—pleasure moves us toward something, and pain moves us away—so you might assume our innate guidance system operates like a compass needle, orienting along the north and south poles. But as with a number of other common assumptions about pleasure, the compass needle analogy turns out to be wrong. The opposite of pain and the opposite of pleasure is the same thing!

Mull this over for yourself, and you'll understand why pleasure and pain often commingle in everything from a love-hate romantic relationship to marathon runners staggering across the finish line in ecstatic exhaustion. At the very least, getting your cardinal coordinates and bearings straight is worth the price of admission.

If you find this a bit confusing, or perhaps even disorienting, you're in good company. I was too. When I started writing this book over fifteen years ago, I knew pleasure felt good and pain didn't, but I couldn't tell you why. The more I investigated, the more questions I had. For instance, I learned that we have three kinds of pain receptors—mechanical, thermal, and chemical—but no one has ever found any pleasure receptors. So how do we "sense" pleasure and, for that matter, what makes an erogenous zone erotic? What about ecstasy and bliss? Are they the same thing? And where does peace of mind fit in? Why do some women have multiple orgasms and others do not? Can men have multiple orgasms too? What about the satisfaction of winning an award or completing a project? And what does all of this have to do with fulfillment and living a good life?

What is pleasure?

To begin unwinding our confusion about pleasure and to give you an idea of where this book is headed, let's begin with a simple working definition: *Pleasure is any experience that feels good.*

> If it fills your body with delightful sensations, evokes warm feelings in your heart and positive thoughts in your mind, brings a smile to your lips, excites, amuses or satisfies, lifts your spirits or inspires a sense of well-being, meaning, and purpose, then it's a pleasure.

This common-sense definition reveals the true nature of pleasure much in the same way as a glass prism reveals the true nature of light. Pleasure is a spectrum, and just as every color on your cell phone or computer screen is made up of three primary colors: red, green, and blue. Every pleasure you enjoy is made up of a spectrum of three primary experiences: physical, emotional, and mental. Think of it as a "Pleasure Prism" with four levels:

- Physical pleasures that are essential for our survival—food, sex, shelter, and associated creature comforts—form the foundation.[4] These are the elemental pleasures of the flesh, the raw datum of our senses, and are grounded in the present moment. Think red.

- Emotional pleasures of love, happiness, joy, excitement, and fun are at the second level. These are the feelings that make us human and mediate the social relationships necessary for rearing children and living within a herd. Think green.

- Mental pleasures are at the third level and include the delight of learning new ideas, recalling fond memories, and believing that our life has meaning and purpose, and the many other mental constructs that make us feel good. Think blue.

- Spiritual pleasures reside at the fourth and highest level—the sublime pleasures of ecstasy and bliss, as well as the rapture of communing with nature and coming to peace with how we fit into the big picture. Think white.

The levels of the Pleasure Prism are not arbitrary. They reflect the evolutionary developmental stages of the human forebrain—reptilian, early mammalian, primate—and their corresponding anatomical structures. Spiritual pleasure, however, has no specific anatomical correlate. It arises from the thorough cultivation and integration of the lower three levels and points to our future evolution, which I will call *Homo spiritualis*. (See Figure 7.)

Renewable pleasure

When it comes to feeling good, there's much more at stake than just getting a leg up on life. Our very survival as a species dangles precariously in the balance. I say this because the single greatest existential threat that faces us is not overpopulation, global warming, environmental pollution, nuclear annihilation, or being overtaken by silicon-based life forms. It is something much closer to home that underlies and gives rise to these threats: our human appetite!

Our rapacious appetite for energy is depleting our oil reserves, warming our atmosphere, and destroying the very life systems we depend upon. It is our appetite for stuff, all sorts of unnecessary stuff, that is "stuffocating" our lives and polluting our rivers and oceans. It is our appetite for political and economic domination that is squandering precious resources to build ever more ingenious weapons to destroy life. To a casual observer, it would appear that we are hell-bent on committing collective suicide and it is our uncontrollable hunger for pleasure that is killing us.

We have created a perverse world where the few suffer from too much and the many suffer from too little. We shrug off these disparities, pretending that's just the way life is—the old sperm-and-egg Darwinian competition—where the fastest and fittest get the prize and the winner takes all. If the fabulously wealthy were indeed happier and more fulfilled, perhaps the race to the top would be worth it. But the truth is even the rich and famous suffer the same basic emotional struggles and human dissatisfactions as the rest of us, only with more money. We are reminded of this every week by tabloid headlines that shock us with a seductive mixture of envy, pity, and *schadenfreude*, as we take solace that the American Dream isn't working for anyone.

Fortunately, there is a way out of this collective nightmare, a very simple and effective solution. It starts with learning how to control your own appetite, not by denying your pleasure-seeking nature, but by embracing it. Consciously turning toward pleasure with an open curiosity will allow you to learn how it works. With this knowledge, you will be able to harness your desire rather than be manipulated by it. As I will argue, *the only way to control the human appetite is to satisfy it, and the only thing capable of truly satisfying our appetite is high-quality renewable pleasure.* Happily, it's not hard to do. As Dr. Seuss reminds us in *The Cat in the Hat*, "It is fun to have fun. But you have to know how."

Pleasure is much more than just a personal experience. *Pleasure is a natural resource, as essential to our health and well-being as fresh air and clean water.* The difference is that air and water must be sourced externally, while the highest quality pleasure is sourced from within. Each one of us is a potential wellspring of pleasure for ourselves and for each other. We hold the key to our own collective happiness and salvation.

Learning how to cultivate and tap this vast and vital renewable resource is what this book is all about and is, I believe, the critical path to human flourishing and a sustainable future. It starts with understanding:

The Seven Immutable Laws of Pleasure

▲ 1. **Original Wholeness**—*You were born from pleasure and you are born for pleasure. It is your origin, source, and birthright.*

▲ 2. **Colors**—*Pleasure comes in four colors: red (physical), green (emotional), blue (mental), and white (spiritual).*

▲ 3. **Contrast and Comparison**—*Pleasure is relative and continually changes.*

▲ 4. **Thresholds**—*Pleasure is separated from pain by a threshold of intensity.*

▲ 5. **Cycles**—*Pleasure comes in waves.*

▲ 6. **Desire and Surrender**—*Pleasure is an inner dance of effort and relaxation.*

▲ 7. **Renewable Pleasure**—*The highest quality pleasure is that which you exchange with another being.*

What you will learn

Before we can discuss pleasure objectively, we need to first set aside our cultural biases or at least become aware of them.

Part 1: Assumptions begins with examining the origin of our cultural beliefs about pleasure. We explore the foundational story of Adam and Eve and discuss how Saint Augustine radically reinterpreted this story to create the bizarre concept of Original Sin. The section concludes with a brief review of what the Greeks—principally Epicurus and Aristotle—had to say about the ethics of pleasure, happiness, and the good life.

Part 2: The Science reviews how the neurobiology of pleasure evolved from our early reptilian, mammalian, and primate ancestors and formed the three divisions of the human forebrain. Utilizing the Pleasure Prism, we then examine how the triune brain is expressed through the three segments of our body—the pelvis, heart, and head—and their relationship to the three primary colors of pleasure.

Part 3: The Natural History takes an in-depth look at the phenomenology of pleasure and the close relationship between pleasure and pain. Other concepts include the relativity of pleasure, the role of habituation, and the essential nature of desire and surrender.

Part 4: The Mystery explores extreme states of pleasure—ecstasy, bliss, and equanimity—not only as sublime states of being, but as subtle energy centers in the body. You will learn how to anatomically locate these vital centers in your body and align them so that you can access these extraordinary flow states at will.

Part 5: The Art and Practice discusses how to apply what you've learned in real life. We begin with practical issues, such as relationships, discipline, addiction, sexuality, and the six essentials of a good life, and conclude by examining the key role renewable pleasure plays in living sustainably on the planet.

To help us in our inquiry, we will use two different approaches. The objective, scientific approach is analytical, from the Greek *ana*, "up," and *luein*, "loosen," like separating and loosening the strands of a knot. As with all scientific knowledge, what we now deem "factual" is only provisional—tentative threads that lead to more fundamental truths, which will be unraveled and revised as we learn more.

The second approach is subjective or phenomenological, from the Greek *phainomenon*, "that which appears," and *logos*, "study." It is the study of our personal experience based on what appears to our five senses at the ordinary level of reality in which we live. It is, technically, a synthetic approach. Unlike analysis, which breaks things apart, synthesis puts things together. It is a method of collecting data points like colored push pins in a cork board, and then stepping back and looking for an overall pattern.

Being subjective, it is more poetic and intuitive.

My job is like being a mountain guide, who's familiar with the terrain, having traversed these parts many times on my own and in the company of friends, family, and patients. I will make suggestions, give you a little history, point out some interesting sights, and share a few stories around the campfire, but you will have to carry your own pack. Which is to say, I encourage you to have your own experiences and come to your own conclusions. Ultimately, it is an exploration of a very personal nature, specifically *your* nature.

At the start of our adventure, it seems fitting to recite the cautionary words of Alexander Pope:

> A little learning is a dangerous thing;
> Drink deep, or taste not the Pierian spring:
> There shallow draughts intoxicate the brain,
> And drinking largely sobers us again.[5]

I should caution you that what you are about to read could transform your life, or at the very least, change your perception of it. It certainly has changed mine. Such an undertaking is not without hazard. Any time you stray from the herd, you run the risk of being criticized and misunderstood, as well as challenged by your own assumptions and upbringing. If you do choose to pursue pleasure wholeheartedly, as I am suggesting, it is crucial to keep your wits about you, go for the genuine article, and not settle for any cheap imitations.

Are you in? Okay then, grab your pack and let's head for those Pierian springs.

Chapter 2

Welcome to the Pleasure Matrix

You take the blue pill—the story ends, you wake up in your bed and believe whatever you want to believe. You take the red pill—you stay in Wonderland, and I show you how deep the rabbit hole goes. Remember: all I'm offering is the truth. Nothing more.
—The Matrix

Like the sci-fi classic *The Matrix*, we are living in a collective simulation created not by machines, but by the human imagination. We call it culture—a virtual web of beliefs, customs, and taboos, encoded in language and communicated through myths, stories, songs, and images—which we overlay on the natural world to understand and make sense of it. It is so familiar to us that we are hardly aware of the simulation and assume it's just the way life is. The power of this virtual reality—that I will refer to at times as our "cultural operating system" or simply the "matrix"—is very significant. It defines who we are, where we belong, what is expected of us, and even the purpose of our existence. It is what gives meaning to statements such as "I am an American," "I am a man," "I am a father," "I am a woman," "I am a mother," "I am a good person," and so on. It defines our relationship to the world, to each other, and to ourselves. It is life as we know it.

Pleasure plays an essential role in the simulation because it is largely through our desire for pleasure (and fear of pain) that our energies are harnessed and used to maintain the matrix. For this reason, examining our life through the prismatic lens of pleasure can provide profound insight into how our cultural operating system actually works, which may be more than you want to know. Because with knowledge comes choice, and with choice comes freedom and with freedom comes responsibility—for *what has been created by the human mind can be changed by the human mind.*

In the beginning

I have often found that the best way to understand something is to start at the beginning, at the source where the water runs purest, which is why I am fascinated with origins. Throughout this book, we will be looking at where things came from and how they got to be the way they are today. However, the goal is not to merely understand, but to comprehend from the Latin *com,* "with" and *prehendere,* "to grasp." That is, to take in hand what you learn and apply it in your daily life.

History is the study of the origins of human culture; science is the study of the origins of the material world. We will begin with history because our cultural assumptions, particularly about pleasure, strongly color all that follows. As Princeton psychologist Emily Pronin notes, "It's not that we're blind to the concept of bias, or to the fact that it exists. We're just blind to it in our own case."[1] Ironically, we are color blind to our own prejudice, or as I like to say, *the hardest dogma to escape is always our own.*[2]

The origins of our Western civilization can be traced to two very different sources—one located on the eastern shores of the Mediterranean centered around Jerusalem and the other in Athens, Greece. From Jerusalem came our creation myths and religious beliefs as recorded in the Hebrew Bible. From Athens came Greek philosophy, ethics, logic, and the beginnings of natural science. The dynamic tension between these two divergent streams gave birth to Western culture. We can date this birth to a historical period that German psychiatrist and philosopher Karl Jaspers called the *Achsenzeit,* Axial Age, roughly 800 to 200 BCE.

During this pivotal age, people across the globe began to migrate in large numbers into urban centers, bringing them into contact with new ideas and unfamiliar customs. Out of this tumultuous cross-fertilization of cultures sprang forth virtually all the world's major religions, such as Zoroastrianism and Judaism in the West and Hinduism, Buddhism, Confucianism, and Taoism in the East. We continue to live under the influences of these religions to this day.

We are now entering, I believe, a second Axial Age as disparate people of the world are once again thrown into close contact through mass media, the internet, and globalization. Every day on television screens and in the news, we are witnessing the clash of cultures around the world and within our own country, as traditional beliefs are crumbling and new ideas struggle to take root. Not surprisingly, our ideas about pleasure are also changing. It is an exciting and challenging time to be alive.

Let's begin our cultural exploration in and around the rock-strewn hills of Jerusalem where nomadic tribes of Semitic desert people scratched out a tenuous existence in a harsh land. They called themselves Jews and were flanked by the massive river civilizations of Egypt and Babylonia, who at one time or another would enslave them. Their survival was precarious, much as it is today.

As desert people, they stood out in bold relief to their windswept, arid surroundings. Perhaps, because of their insecurity or as a psychological defense against it, the Jews had the *chutzpah* (audacity) to claim that their God, with a capital "G," was the one and only all-powerful God. Moreover, their God created them in "His own image" and chose them as His special people with whom He entered into a sacred covenant, as Deuteronomy 14:2 states: "For you are a holy people to YHWH your God, and God has chosen you to be his treasured people from all the nations that are on the face of the earth."

This self-referential specialness of the desert people stands in sharp contrast to the humbler experience of the forest dweller. Those who grew up in a forest surrounded by the rich diversity of life naturally saw themselves as merely one living creature among many and part of the greater whole. Accordingly, forest dwellers developed a polytheistic concept of many gods, as was common among the ancient Greeks and most indigenous people of the world.[3]

A monotheistic cultural operating system is by definition exclusive. If you believe in one God, then there is one Truth, and you are either with the truth or "ag'in it." This dualistic thinking leads to a black-and-white, dogmatic inflexibility. Add to this the notion of specialness, and it's no surprise that in the world today it is the monotheists, the "People of the Book"—Jews, Christians, and Muslims—who are most aggressively and self-righteously at each other's throats.

However, monotheism gave us something even more toxic: a *des-ert-ed*, dead cosmos where only God, angels, and humans are fully imbued with spirit and therefore worthy of respect. In comparison, polytheistic indigenous people respect the whole of the natural world because everything—animals, plants, forests, rivers, caves, rocks, and mountains—are alive with spirit. They are our Mother Earth and Ocean, Father Sky and Mountain, Brother Fire and Buffalo, Sister Wind and Willow.

There is one more problem with monotheism I should mention because it has sown so much strife between men and women and has a major influence on how we experience pleasure. It is something that would be immediately obvious to any polytheist: There is no representation of the Divine Feminine. No Isis, Gaia, Demeter, nor Juno. The veneration of the Virgin Mother Mary is but a pale, neutered surrogate who is explicitly not divine despite her miraculous ability to maintain her virginity while giving birth to Jesus. The very notion of an immaculate conception denies nature and the body. As we shall see, the lack of a Divine Feminine and our historical embrace of a monopolar, male-centric matrix directly impacts our experience of pleasure.

These cultural assumptions are spelled out in the Book of Genesis, which describes the origin of the universe, life, man, woman, the status of pleasure, and our position within the natural order. It doesn't matter whether you believe that Genesis is the word of God or simply a reworking of older Babylonian creation myths because we are still under its cultural spell, which operates far below rational thought at a deep limbic, emotional level of our collective unconscious.

The story opens with an all-powerful God who creates the universe, bringing order out of chaos. He fashions Adam in his own image and likeness from clay and then breathes life (the Holy Spirit) into his nostrils. This establishes God as the lord and master of the eternal, mythic world and man as the lord and master of the temporal, earthly world who has "dominion over the fish of the sea, and over the fowl of the air, and over the cattle, and over all the earth, and over every creeping thing that creepeth upon the earth."[4] Note that "dominion" from the Latin *dominus* (lord, master) is the very definition of patriarchy.

This top-down, hierarchical perspective sounds self-centered and childish compared to the words of Chief Seattle, whose "primitive" animist ideas anticipated modern ecology: "Humankind has not woven the web of life. We are but one thread within it. Whatever we do to the web, we do to ourselves. All things are bound together. All things connect."[5]

In the Book of Genesis, Eve is created as an afterthought plucked from Adam's rib to provide him with a companion. This is the first clue that something has gone terribly wrong with this narrative, particularly as it relates to women. Everyone knows that "even the smartest man is born from a woman," as my father used to say.

It is no accident that Eve is the one who is beguiled by the serpent in the Garden of Eden to eat of the forbidden fruit from the Tree of Knowledge of Good and Evil. As a woman who sheds blood with the cycles of the moon and brings forth life, Eve is more closely connected to the natural world represented by the serpent. Her eating the fruit is a clear reference to pleasure, and that it is "forbidden" sets us against the truth of our biology. Had it simply been the "Tree of Knowledge," we would have a universal story of the lost innocence that every child undergoes, but adding "of Good and Evil" gives the narrative a perverse, moral twist.

Since it is Eve who convinces Adam to partake of the forbidden fruit, she is the temptress who caused the "Fall of Man" and introduced evil into the world. (This misogynistic narrative continues to this day, for instance, in the blaming of women for their own rape.)

It is also no accident that the first thing Adam and Eve gain knowledge of is their nakedness, which causes them to immediately cover their loins with fig leaves. It is at this precise instant—at the very birth of Western civilization—that sex became bound up with shame, guilt, and evil. And simultaneously, our psyche became ensnared in a double bind from which we have yet to escape. On the one hand, Adam and Eve were encouraged

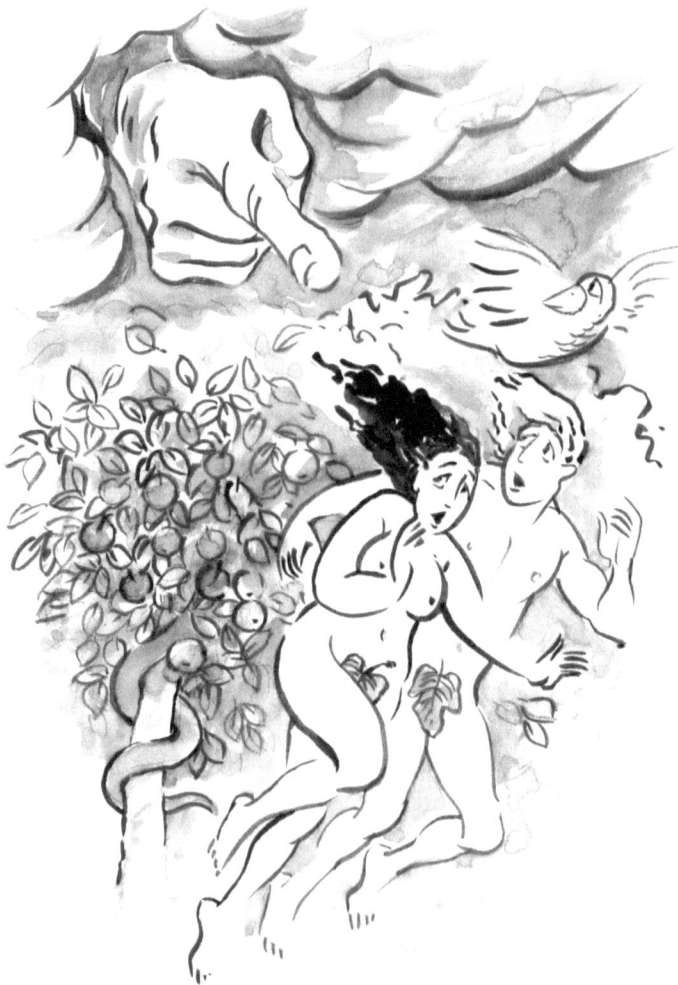

Figure 1: Adam and Eve expelled from the Garden of Eden.

to go forth and "be fruitful and multiply." On the other, sexual pleasure is forbidden fruit and sinful. Centuries later, Saint Augustine would twist this double bind tighter with his theory of Original Sin.

The Genesis narrative established a masculine god as the sole creative force in the cosmos and put man in charge of earthly concerns. At the same time, by making sex dirty with slurs like "slut" and "whore," it stripped a woman of her greatest power, the divine power to bring forth new life, and reduced her to an object of carnal pleasure—a "thing" that could be used and abused. Perhaps the institutionalization of absolute male dominion was a jealous response to prior eons of matriarchy or a global sea-change in human consciousness as Leonard Shlain argues in *The Alphabet Versus the Goddess*. Regardless of the cause, the result deprived a woman of her ontological status of being fully ensouled, sexually embodied, and a coequal with man. (*Ontology* is a useful Greek term from *ont*, "being" and *ology*, "the study of"—a branch of metaphysics dealing with the nature of being that describes its properties and relationships.)

It is no coincidence that mother in Latin is *mater* (matter). The feminine has always been closely associated with "matter" (earth) and with what we can touch, feel, see, hear, smell. The masculine has been associated with "spirit" (heaven), the abstract/transcendent (God the Father). Certainly as patriarchy gained power and the feminine was relegated to something lower, the split—the dualism between spirit and matter—became larger along with the denigration of anything to do with the senses. In this way, the feminine and its association to the body and sensuality was demonized.

The implications of this are staggering: exclusive male priesthoods, rape, chastity belts, stoning, witch hunts, burnings at the stake, genital mutilation, honor killings, denial of voting rights, anti-abortion, glass ceilings, destitute unwed mothers, matrimonial strife, and broken families, to name but a few. Men also suffer, though less obviously. They are denied their own feminine aspects of sensitivity, tenderness, intimacy, and vulnerability. Saddest of all, countless children are deprived of their mother's nurturing love and shuttled off to daycare before they are even old enough to walk.

The dark side of pleasure

The dark side of pleasure is bondage and arises from the misuse of power. Pleasure and power are intimately entwined in a number of ways. To begin with, power itself is pleasurable. It feels good to be strong, confident, in control of our lives, and able to get what we want. It gives us a sense of importance and self-esteem. But power can be intoxicating, and when the ego becomes overinflated, power can turn into a tyranny of egotistical self-indulgence. This unfortunately is our story, the story in which God gave "Western man" dominion over nature, and, like his Father before him, he shall bring order out of chaos and bend nature to his will. Translation: the world and everything in it (including women) exists for man's benefit and can be exploited as he sees fit. The consequences of this master-slave matrix are evident in the environmental abuse and destruction happening all around us.

It also plays out in the power relationship between sex and pleasure in everything from human trafficking and sex slaves to erotic, sadomasochistic fantasies. Sexual energy is like any other energy resource and can be used for good or harm. It is bought and sold in the boardrooms of Madison Avenue marketing firms and backstreet brothels every day. It can be effectively leveraged to get what one wants, as in the Stormy Daniels and Donald Trump imbroglio, or the Harvey Weinstein, #MeToo revelations. There is a saying, "Men exchange power for sex, and women exchange sex for power." The conflating of financial and political power with reproductive fitness may explain why the powerful are so susceptible to sexual promiscuity.

The power relationship of sex and pleasure is made explicit in BDSM (Bondage and Discipline, Sadism and Masochism) culture where a person's role is assigned as either "a top" (Dominant) or "a bottom" (Submissive). The excitement of BDSM comes from playing at the edge of pleasure and pain and being in or out of control. Such master-slave simulations of domination and humiliation are sexualized fantasies that reflect the top-down, hierarchical operating system that spawned them.

Ultimately, the real bondage is the human spirit has been cut off and alienated from its organic roots in the natural world, for *it is through the primal connection to our physical bodies that we source our natural intelligence and spiritual power.* Until we are willing to openly discuss the crippling darkness of our cultural assumptions in the light of day, we will continue to be enslaved by them. The task before us is to awaken from the hypnotic trance of the matrix and replace the old simulation with a healthier, more sustainable relationship with ourselves and Mother Earth. As with any meaningful change, it begins with an open awareness and willingness to consider new possibilities.

▲▲▲▲▲▲▲

In brief:

We live within a cultural matrix that colors all that we think and perceive. Our origin myth describes a distinctly male-dominated hierarchy with God at the top followed by man, woman, animals, and the rest of nature—in that order. Abuse runs downhill, which explains the inferior status of women, our ambivalence toward sex, and the devaluation of other living creatures and nature in general. It is admittedly a dark narrative that has held sway since the first Axial Age (800-200 BCE), but don't be disheartened. It is being challenged at the dawn of a second Axial Age that promises to be a more open-source, equitable approach.

Considerations:

Here are some suggestions to help you explore and embody the ideas presented. Notice how you feel as you read them. Certain words or images that catch your attention may indicate "glitches" in the matrix—hot button items that no longer serve you. I invite you to consider these suggestions as you go about your day. There are no right or wrong answers, only habits of thought and body to observe. (For further self-help resources, please see the Afterword.)

- When you go to the bathroom, have sex, or perform other bodily functions, is there a fig-leaf moment when you feel shame?

- How do you feel when you see yourself naked in the mirror?

- Do you have a spiritual connection with a favorite rock, tree, or special place?

- Do you believe in evil? If so, where does it exist?

- When you are in the presence of a sexually attractive person, notice the sensations that arise in your body.

- Do you take pleasure in having power over animals or people?

- In general, are you a red pill or blue pill kind of person?

CHAPTER 3

The Origin of Original Sin

> *But for this mystery [of original sin],*
> *the most incomprehensible of all, we*
> *remain incomprehensible to ourselves.*
> —Blaise Pascal

I GREW UP IN LA GRANGE JUST OUTSIDE CHICAGO, A TYPICAL WHITE MIDDLE-CLASS suburb with its share of imposing stone churches on prominent corners. The black kids lived on the other side of the tracks, and the one Asian family ran the local dry cleaners. What was not so typical was that my father was an Austrian Jew who met my mother during World War II in Southwest China when he worked for the U.S. Army, keeping the military trucks rolling over the Burma Road. He liked mechanical things and always had a Leica camera with him. As the story goes, he saw a picture of my mother in the window of a camera shop in Guiyang and after making some inquiries, followed her home one day in his jeep as she walked alongside the road.

After the war, my mother and two older siblings traveled to *Jinshan* (the Gold Mountain, as San Francisco was known) to await my father. Fresh off the boat, she would watch the traffic light changing colors for hours from her second-floor apartment window as the cars came and went. When my father arrived, they relocated to Chicago where he had been offered a job at a company run by an army buddy also named Gottlieb, whose mail they often mixed up.

We lived in a large three-story brick house on the corner of a busy thoroughfare. Built in 1899 in the southern colonial style, it had an imposing front porch with wooden columns and a carriage house at the back, which had a small room for servant's quarters. The lawn wrapped around on three sides with a sidewalk to match, making cutting the grass and winter shoveling a chore. To make ends meet, my mother rented rooms to men who came from southern Illinois to build railroad locomotives at the General Motors plant.

My father was a devout atheist who expressed his spirituality through the ethical principles by which he lived. "A child is a book of plain pages," he used to say. "You can write whatever you want on them." He took pride in not marking us with a religion, which allowed me to sort things out for myself. I remember a warm autumn morning when I was about eight years old, raking leaves in the yard as a family dressed in their Sunday finery walked by on their way to church. The parents tried to keep their children from staring at me, and I pretended not to notice, but it was awkward. The cognitive dissonance caused me to question things. When I asked my father who God was, he simply answered, "Nature."

At the age of twelve, I decided I was an agnostic. On several occasions when the topic of religion came up in homeroom discussions at school, I found myself arguing the agnostic position with my Christian classmates, as each of them tried to outdo the other with pious enthusiasm and Sunday school logic. In defense, I committed to memory a quote from the brilliant trial lawyer Clarence Darrow, who defended John Scopes for the right to teach the theory of evolution in public school in the famous Monkey Trial against the State of Tennessee. During the trial, a newspaper reporter asked, "Mr. Darrow, is it true that you don't believe in God?" To which he replied in a gravelly Ohio drawl, "Sir, I don't claim to know where so many foolish men are sure."[1]

Years later, I was shocked to discover how much my own relationship to pleasure had been corrupted by a religion I never professed. Such is the power of culture. If you swim in polluted waters, you can't help but get stained—which brings us to the story of St. Augustine.

Augustine's Original Sin

Culture is what happens when biology is expressed through the human mind. In the case of Augustine, his was a mind tormented with sexual lust and spiritual longing. Unfortunately, his personal inner battle would come to be embedded in our cultural DNA as the perverse doctrine of Original Sin.

Born in a provincial town of North Africa in present day Algeria to a pagan father and Christian mother in 354 CE, Augustine was destined to become one of Christendom's most seminal church fathers in every sense of the word. His intellectual gifts were recognized from an early age, and at seventeen he was sent to Carthage to study rhetoric. There, in the bloom of his youth, he had his first of many encounters with carnal temptation, which would obsess him for the rest of his life. Years later in his autobiography *Confessions*, he described his sexual awakening: "I came to Carthage, where a cauldron of illicit loves leapt and boiled about me. I was not yet in love, but I was in love with love."[2]

Driven by his carnal desire, he took up with a concubine who bore him a son. He stayed with them for thirteen years, bonded by what he would later call a "lustful love." At age thirty-two, still tormented by the flesh, he confessed: "I, in my great worthlessness had begged You [God] for chastity, saying, *'Grant me chastity and continence, but not yet.'* For I was afraid that You would hear my prayer too soon, and too soon would heal me from disease of which I wanted satisfied rather than extinguished."[3] We see here his struggle to reconcile his biology with the demands of the matrix—his red pill/blue pill dilemma.

After he moved to Milan, his devout Catholic mother arranged a proper society marriage for him, at which point he broke off his relationship with his concubine and illegitimate son. But while waiting for his betrothed eleven-year-old fiancée to come of age, he took up with another woman, derailing his mother's marriage plans. Eventually, he would abandon his second lover as well.

At the age of thirty-three, Augustine underwent a powerful spiritual conversion. Torn between his sexual lust and desire for spiritual salvation, he withdrew to a garden and wept bitterly beneath a fig tree, overwhelmed with a "terrible kind of shame" and self-condemnation. In the depth of his torment, he heard a sing-song child's voice wafting through the air, urging him to read a book of the Apostle that he had set aside earlier. He rushed back and picked up the book, which fell open to the following passage: "Not in riots and drunken parties, not in eroticism and indecencies, not in strife and rivalry, but put on the Lord Jesus Christ and make no provision for the flesh in its lusts."[4]

After reading those words, Augustine's turmoil was lifted, and he wrote, "I neither wished nor needed to read further. At once, with the last words of this sentence, it was as if a light of relief from all anxiety flooded into my heart. All the shadows of doubt were dispelled."[5] He had at last been saved by the power of the Lord's words.

We find in Augustine a man of profound passion who, despite his piety, continued to be haunted by a small biological problem: he couldn't control his spontaneous erections. This troubled him deeply. He had no doubt as to the purity of his faith, and yet his penis seemed to have a wicked mind of its own: "Sometimes it refuses to act when the mind wills, while often it acts against its will … wherein could be found a more fitting demonstration of the just deprivation of human nature by reason of its disobedience?"[6]

To a lesser man, these problems would have been shrugged off with a pint of ale and a roll in the sack, but for a deep thinker like Augustine, it was a problem of the utmost importance that demanded a theological explanation. In time, this explanation would become known as the doctrine of *Originale Peccatum,* Original Sin.

Augustine claimed that as the result of Adam having chosen to eat of the forbidden fruit (which had a distinctly sexual taste) against God's dictate, Adam committed an irreparable sin, the Original Sin, which would be transmitted to all future human beings through his semen. Yes, you heard me right. Although odd to a modern reader, the obsession with semen was commonplace at the time. Christianity, like other religions, grew out of ancient fertility cults. Just as semen was believed to mix with menstrual blood to bring forth human life, god's semen in the form of rain was believed to fertilize the earth-womb to bring forth crops. The ritual rain-dance was essentially a way to induce god to ejaculate and fertilize the earth. The title Christ, from the Greek *Khristos,* means "the anointed one." Originally the *Khristos* was smeared, not with frankincense and myrrh, but semen as a mark of his fertile potency.[7]

Clearly, we are not dealing with logic here. What we are dealing with is one man's attempt to reconcile the conflict between his head and the head of his penis, the conflict between reason and nature in the flesh, you might say. Augustine invented the concept of Original Sin to explain his lack of control and to absolve himself of his concupiscence and guilt, which in his brilliant mind became mixed up with lofty ideas of free will, or more precisely, the lack thereof. The only problem was that he managed to theologically project his sexual guilt onto the rest of us.

The power of Original Sin rests not in its logic, which is patently absurd, but in its emotional appeal that grabs us below the belt—akin to the feeling of shame at having your pants pulled down. (I used to have a recurrent dream of being in public, at a store or on the street, and suddenly, realizing I forgot to wear pants, I'd try to pull down my shirt to avoid exposing myself as I shamefully made my way home.) It is the emotional intensity of Original Sin that makes sex "dirty" and gives words like "fuck" their dark, aggressive power.

Interestingly, Augustine's reinterpretation of the "Fall of Man" was not immediately accepted by the Church Fathers in Rome. Early Christians were not obsessed with the idea of sin; neither, for that matter, were the Jews, who enjoyed sex, practiced polygamy, and believed they were born perfect in God's image. Augustine's ideas were strange and unorthodox for the times. But this did not deter him. He spent the last ten years of his life lobbying Rome to accept his radical doctrine and wrote numerous letters making his case. He apparently even engaged in some back-room, political horse-swapping and attempted to bribe the Pope with a gift of prized African Nubian horses.

Why did the Catholic church eventually embrace Augustine's concept of Original Sin as the gospel truth? Clearly, they understood that the very soul of humankind hung in the balance. Were we born innocent with the free will to discern between good and evil as his Christian Pelagian opponents maintained? Or were we, as Augustine argued, born wounded, stained with Original Sin and incapable of making moral discernments without the purifying salvation of Jesus Christ? The implications were immense and raised a number of thorny theological issues. What, for example, would be the fate of innocent babes who die unbaptized? Are they sinners who therefore would burn in hell, as Augustine claimed?

After a decade of vigorous debate and contemplation, the Church Fathers eventually realized Original Sin could be useful. Baptism would now serve two functions: initiation into the Church and cleansing Adam's semen-stain of Original Sin from one's soul as a prerequisite to entering heaven. In my line of work, we have a name for this sort of business model. It's called quackery—diagnosing a person with a disease they don't have and then curing them of it—and it's considered a criminal act by the medical board. We might dismiss this sort of spiritual quackery as *caveat emptor*, let the buyer beware, but Original Sin is much more than just a clever con; it is a heinous concept that cripples the human psyche.

A basic principle of martial arts is that to control an opponent, you must first break their balance to weaken them. Now, if your ambition were to unbalance and disable a person with a single blow, where would you strike? What vital point would you attack? Augustine, in an attempt to assuage his neurotic, carnal guilt and find salvation, was pitted against his own dark side. Instinctively, he attacked that most vulnerable fault line in the human psyche—a fault line he knew all too well—where a person's biology intersects with their cultural beliefs. In a single blow, he cleaved a person from what the Greeks called the *daemon* (one's instinctual natural intelligence) by proclaiming pleasure, especially sexual pleasure, a sin. The *daemon* had become a demon.

To tell a person whose entire biology is hardwired to seek pleasure that pleasure is morally wrong is to turn a person against themselves and cripple them with self-conflict at the very core of their being, making them incomprehensible even to themselves, as Pascal noted above. It's like embedding a piece of malware at the root level of one's operating system. With a fractured and unbalanced psyche, a person can easily be made into a compliant foot soldier in God's army and an obedient citizen of the state. This moralistic sleight of hand has led to a kind of crazy-making doublethink and self-doubt, which Saint Paul described most eloquently: "For the good that I would, I do not, but the evil which I would not, that I do."[8] I once saw a T-shirt that said: "Religion, the Devil's greatest invention." Surely, his second greatest invention was Original Sin.

What makes Original Sin so diabolical is that it is nearly impossible to escape. Whether you are a recovering Catholic, a confirmed atheist, or a fully realized libertine, your very liberation is in reaction to Original Sin, and therefore defined by it in the same way as a mold and the molded object define each other.

I once attended Burning Man, a cultural arts festival that draws upwards of 70,000 people for a week on a desolate lake bed in the Black Rock Desert north of Reno, Nevada. Burners dress in outrageous costumes and nudity is commonplace. I was amazed at how many beautiful women, when given an opportunity, were more than willing to bare their beauty. However, I was not witnessing liberated people in a natural setting, but rather the bizarre response of human beings to 2,000 years of sexual repression. As sexually liberated as we imagine ourselves to be, there is still plenty of repression to go around. And what goes around comes around in the form of distorted aberrations. Pornography use appears to be more prevalent in fundamentalist, repressive religious cultures than in secular groups. That includes evangelicals, Mormons, Muslims, and Buddhists. Studies indicate that the more religious, the more likely a person is to consider pornography sinful and the more likely they are to deny using it. Yet, searches for sexual content on Google are significantly higher in religiously conservative states.[9] As every addict knows, repression spawns a cycle of shame and guilt that leads to more acting out, and unless the source issues are faced, it is an endless process.

One could view Augustine's toxic and repressive theology as the mask he used to cover his shadow. Unfortunately, what he was unable to bear in himself, he projected onto others and onto women in particular. This conflict is revealed in his relationship with his mother. In his *Confessions*, he expresses a deep and abiding love for his mother. He shared with her the platonic spiritual love of the Blessed Virgin Mary, but in his bedroom, he lusted for a fleshy erotic embodiment of a Mary Magdalene, the good-girl whore. As we will later discuss, this sort of ambivalence is not uncommon and is typical of men who have a disconnect between their pelvis and their head—the missing link being their heart.

Original Inadequacy

Original Sin moves in mysterious ways. Although few of us think about Original Sin in our daily lives, many of us experience a far more insidious form of it—an unspeakable emptiness called Original Inadequacy—the feeling that no matter what you do, how hard you try, no matter how much you have or achieve, it's never enough. In fact, you're not enough. You need more beauty, strength, intelligence, training, love; you need to lose weight, have bigger breasts, smaller breasts, and tighter abs; you must try harder, work harder, read more self-help books, earn more money; and above all, you need to "make something of yourself" and "become somebody." Why? Because you were born unworthy, and you must prove yourself.

A few years ago, I spent the day at Esalen with my middle daughter, Jhana. I wanted to show her where the New Age movement began. The Esalen Institute is perched on a rocky crag in Big Sur, along the northern California coast overlooking the Pacific. We drove up from Pismo Beach on Highway 1 in the early morning light through redwood forests and dense fog and arrived just in time for breakfast. People in loose-fitting garb and hand-woven caps and scarves huddled around worn, wooden tables. The air was thick with the smell of coffee, Constant Comment tea, eggs, and granola. It was a flashback to the Sixties, only everyone was forty years older. I felt immediately at home and smiled, murmuring to Jhana, "These are my people; this is my scene." I had come of age with the human potential movement, and we were standing at ground zero where Alan Watts and Fritz Perls held court with impromptu lectures, and cultural icons like Joan Baez, Henry Miller, Abraham Maslow, and Hunter S. Thompson hung out.

We spent the day walking the grounds, soaking in the hot tubs, and enjoying the recently renovated bath house with floor-to-ceiling glass walls overlooking the ocean. I stood outside the doorway of workshops in session to catch the drift and eavesdropped on conversations at the lodge over lunch as attendees discussed their issues (or "hang-ups" as we used to call them) and offered each other advice. And then it hit me like a bad acid trip: the whole self-help movement is based on the premise that we need improvement, that we are wounded, damaged, and in need of therapy, support, and psychological salvation. It was the same old Original Sin story dressed up in natural hemp and faded blue jeans, seeking redemption at the dawning of the Age of Aquarius. I was slightly nauseous. I had spent my entire life working through my own feelings of inadequacy and those of my patients. In that moment, I realized that we were like a congregation of penitent lemmings huddled on the edge of the continent—separated from the immense natural beauty surrounding us by a glass wall of our own self-absorbed feelings of inadequacy.

While we reward the industrious with material success, there is often an unspoken hidden dark side, a compulsive drivenness that stalks a person with certain uncomfortable feelings of inadequacy. The moment they pause to rest, the feelings are upon them, and they must move on. No grass grows under their feet. As long as they can stay one step ahead, they can keep the painful feelings of inadequacy at bay. After all, *there is no rest for the wicked.*

I've heard the same story from countless patients: ten or more years of incredible output, working longer and harder than most people could even imagine, let alone do. Finally, one of the wheels comes off and they end up a smoking wreck on the side of the road with a heart attack, stroke, cancer, autoimmune disorder, or some other dreadful disease. Feelings of inadequacy can literally drive a person to work themselves to death. It happens all the time.

When Original Sin is combined with an all-seeing, omniscient God who tracks your every thought, word, and deed, we have created an Orwellian "Big Father," with no place to hide. The burden of this inescapable guilt and shame of one's inadequacy can easily become overwhelming and turn into a ruthless, self-fulfilling prophecy, "proving" our human frailty and sinful "fallenness." Forgive me, Father, for I am a sinner and the image of a bloodied man nailed to a cross is the credo of a religion that glorifies self-hatred and suffering.

At the mythic, religious core of Western culture lies a toxic, fear-centric operating system: fear of God's wrath; fear of punishment; fear of inadequacy; and perhaps worst of all, fear of being unloved and banished. But fortunately, at the philosophical, rational core of our operating system, we find a much kinder approach, which we will turn to next.

▲▲▲▲▲▲▲

In brief:

Shortly after the founding of the Roman Catholic Church in the fourth century CE, Saint Augustine radically reinterpreted the Genesis story of Adam and Eve in an attempt to reconcile his inner sexual conflicts with the teachings of the Bible. The result was his theological invention of Original Sin, which has come down to us in a secular form as Original Inadequacy. Many of our feelings of inferiority—fear of being judged, shame, and guilt around pleasure, particularly sexual pleasure—can be traced to Original Sin. Knowing how this depraved concept entered the cultural matrix through a historical twist of one man's hang-ups can help us untwist it in our own lives.

Considerations:

- Growing up, what messages did you receive about being a good person?

- Do you believe in sin? If so, where does it exist?

- Notice the inner conflict and tension that arises when you experience temptation. How does it feel in your body?

- When you make a mistake, what do you say to yourself? How do you judge yourself?

- When you feel your life is lacking, breathe into the insufficiency and know you are already whole and worthy of love.

CHAPTER 4

The Ethics of Pleasure

My life is my message.
—Mahatma Gandhi

EIGHT HUNDRED MILES TO THE NORTHWEST OF JERUSALEM ON THE BROAD PLAINS of the Attica basin in ancient Athens a very different culture and approach to pleasure developed, one that emphasized the importance of reason as the touchstone of truth. Greek philosophers sought to understand the world in terms of natural phenomena without recourse to gods or superstition, giving birth to what would become the modern liberal arts education and the scientific enterprise.

While I vaguely recalled this from college, it wasn't until I met Frank Taylor, a retired University of Florida Classics professor, that I came to understand just how interesting and valuable studying the ancient Greeks could be. Frank, a charming British fellow, was of slight build by Yankee standards, but he made up for it with a keen intellect and a kind, knowing look in his eye. He was the aging father of a friend who brought him to Boulder to care for him in the last days of his life. As I had never studied Classics, I asked Frank if he would teach me.

Every few weeks, I'd stop by for an afternoon visit and bring a pastry to share. Frank would put on a pot of strong Earl Grey tea, and we'd sit across from each other at a small dining table. He carefully cut the dessert into two pieces, and as the steam rose from our cups, the stories began to swirl. He told me of his proudest hour as a centurion in the British army during WWII, leading a company of a hundred men, how he became a Classics professor after the war, and his love of the Finnish epic poem *The Kalevala* and Dante's *Divine Comedy* that inspired him to learn Finnish and Italian so he could read them in their native tongue. He often spoke affectionately of his wife, Carol, who had died of throat cancer the year before. She continued to communicate with him from the other side through odd occurrences like an inexplicable draft of cool air with the faint scent of her perfume suddenly wafting through the room. One day he found her favorite ashtray made of thick glass perfectly cracked in two. It was obvious how much he loved her and how strongly he believed (hoped) he would soon be reunited with her. He was a man who had come to the end of his life and relished in its retelling.

Frank deeply admired the Greeks for their noble ideas. "It's useful to study them because they were so much like us and yet lived in very different circumstances," he told me. "Seeing the world through their eyes can give us another perspective from which to see our own in the present day." In the brief time we spent together, Frank did teach me the essence of Classics. "In the end," he said, "all we have is our stories." Frank's true occupation—like the poem singers of *The Kalevala*, who travelled from village to village through the dense forests of northwest Russia reciting the 22,000 lines of the epic to keep their oral tradition alive—was a keeper-of-the-stories.

The Greeks

Before exploring what the ancient Greeks had to say about pleasure, it's important to understand the cultural context in which they lived and taught. These philosophers were nothing like today's tweedy, narrow-shouldered academics, contemplating lofty principles, cloistered within ivied walls. They were passionate, charismatic leaders and mystics who lived and breathed their philosophy in communities that gathered around them to study and practice the living spirit of their teachings.

For the ancient Greeks, the most important philosophical question was how to live a good life, which they defined as a question of ethics, one of the three branches of Greek philosophy. Unlike the theoretical study of epistemology (truth) and physics (nature), ethics was (and is) of urgent, practical import because it provides the foundation and overarching context that guides our daily actions and gives meaning and purpose to our life.

Today we think of ethics as being synonymous with morality, harking back to the Tree of Knowledge of Good and Evil. But, if you recall our discussion from Chapter 2, this turns out to be a perversion of its original meaning. For Aristotle, *ethos* (ethics) had to do with the development of one's character, which in turn was shaped by *arête* (virtue). Virtues were not codes of conduct like the Ten Commandments etched in stone. They were skills a person acquires to perfect their character, become an excellent human being, and fulfill their highest potential. Thus, the goal of ethics was not to be a "good" boy or girl, but to become a virtuoso of your life in the same way as you might master the violin. This ideal of self-mastery is beautifully expressed in Albin Polasek's sculpture, *Man Carving his Own Destiny*. In this extraordinary piece, a man wields a hammer in one hand and a chisel in the other as he hews his lower half free from the rock—literally shaping and revealing his character in an act of conscious self-creation.

In Aristotle's famous treatise, the *Nicomachean Ethics,* dedicated to his son Nicomachus, he lays out the virtues needed to secure a good life. The key, he argues, is to strike a balance between the extremes of excess and deficiency, which is the golden mean, similar to the "middle way" in the Buddhist tradition.

Balance is an extremely

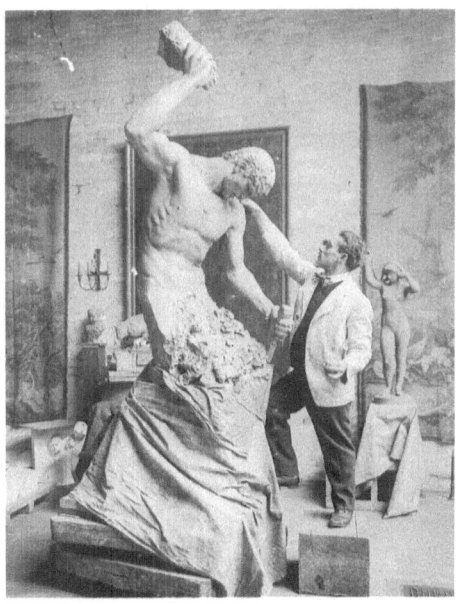

Figure 2: Albin Polasek posing with his sculpture, *Man Carving his Own Destiny* c 1918.

useful concept that applies to every aspect of life, from using just the right amount of salt when you cook to balancing your checkbook to standing on one leg in tree pose. When applied to the good life, it means finding the sweet spot where all the important aspects of your life—health, relationships, work, and connection to Source—are developed in equal measure. If you find yourself lacking in some areas, take heart; balance is not an easy thing to achieve and is, at best, a moving target. I once asked Peter Davidson, a professional juggler with Air Jazz, how he coped with the pressure of juggling on stage. "You'll always drop some balls," he answered. "I approach every performance as a work in progress."

Aristotle describes how to "juggle" various life skills. Take, for example, the virtue of courage. A person who fears nothing is foolhardy, while one who runs from danger is a coward. In between these two extremes is courage. Likewise, generosity is the mean between the excess of wastefulness and the deficiency of stinginess; truthfulness (about one's self) is the middle way between bragging and low self-esteem; temperance is the balance between indulgence and asceticism. The same sort of analysis can be carried out for gentleness, wittiness, prudence, friendliness, ambition, and so on.

Aristotle believed a person can be educated to make these distinctions to the point that they become second nature and part of one's character and disposition. "We are what we repeatedly do," he noted. "Excellence then, is not an act, but a habit."[1] He recognized that life is far too complex and nuanced to be governed by fixed moral precepts set in stone. Rather, his ethics were flexible and based upon his faith in humanity's original goodness. In other words, a person properly educated will have developed the necessary character to respond appropriately and skillfully to any situation. It's in this sense, Cicero claimed, "virtue is its own reward."[2]

The distinction between morality and virtue (*arête*) is crucial. With morality, you are motivated to do the right thing out of fear of punishment; failure means you are a "bad" person. With virtue, you do the right thing because it leads to a happier life, and failure simply means you need more training and must try harder next time. It's the difference between

The Ethics of Pleasure

a fear-centric life driven by the anxiety of punishment and a love-centric (or "*aah*-centric") life drawn forward by joy and delight.

As a young man, I received a valuable lesson in ethics during a walkabout on the back streets of Djakarta. I came across a small group of men huddled around a piece of cloth with a large red dot and blue dot painted on it. The dealer twirled a block of wood about the size of a stick of butter with each side painted in alternating red and blue, then slammed a wooden cover over it, at which point players placed their bets on the corresponding red or blue dot. The dealer then lifted the cover to reveal the winning color. It was a lively scene and money was changing hands fast.

I was intrigued because I thought I could see the color just as it was covered. I made my way into the inner circle and put a few *rupiahs* down on the red dot, sure I would win. But as he lifted the cover, the rectangular cutout fit loosely over the block, and he imperceptibly rolled it, changing its color from red to blue. I lost. Not quite believing my own eyes, I doubled down and bet again. But this time, as he was about to lift the cover, I grabbed his wrist to prevent any funny business. Suddenly, everyone fell silent and the men turned toward me with a menacing glare. The game was up; they were in cahoots, and I was the mark. I released the dealer's wrist and slowly backed away.

Returning to my hotel feeling victimized, I told the young desk clerk what had just happened. He shook his head and said in a serious voice, "Sir, you're an educated man. You should have known better." He was right. But until that moment, I had never connected education with ethical behavior. Imagine how civic life would be transformed if the best educated among us were also the most ethical.

Over and above the common virtues, Aristotle described two special *arête* that are a natural consequence and completion of the others. The first is magnanimity from the Latin *magnus* (great) and *animas* (spirit or soul), hence, "great-souled." To be a great-souled person is first and foremost to consider one's self worthy of great deeds and therefore to conduct one's self honorably. Again, notice the contrast between Aristotle's *aah*-centric motivating principle based on nobility and the rewards of a good life compared to Augustine's fear-centric motivating principle based on Original Sin and the fear of punishment.

According to Aristotle, great-souled people can be identified by their willingness to take major risks without regard for their lives and live independently, in accord with their own values; disinterest in mundane affairs, praise, and gossip; frankness in expressing opinions; lack of anxiety; interest in artistic and useless activities rather than merely productive ones; and a tendency to move slowly and speak in a deep steady voice.

The second overarching virtue is the pursuit of *kalon* (beauty), the willingness to act for the sake of beauty as an expression of one's own beautiful character. For the ancient Greeks, success or failure was not the ultimate goal. The goal was to live a noble, beautiful life and to be remembered well rather than to survive at any cost. There was no shame in failing if you failed beautifully. As my father used to say, "Better to die on your feet than to live on your knees." In the end, magnanimity and beauty are the essential ingredients for a good life and are what made Homer's heroes heroic. Can you imagine what the world would be like if, instead of choosing our political leaders for their Machiavellian cunning, we chose them for their Aristotelian magnanimity and beautiful character? Why is it that with such a brilliant start, our ethical development has progressed so little in the last 2,000 years? Is it because of a flaw in our human nature or a deficiency in our educational and religious institutions? Given the global nature of our predicament, I suspect the answer is a little of both, which is all the more reason to radically upgrade the ethical training of our cultural institutions beginning with ourselves and our families.

After Frank died, I learned from his daughter that he took his role as a major in the British army seriously, conducting himself nobly to uplift the spirit of his men. After the war, he brought the same magnanimity to his work as a professor and won numerous awards for his teaching excellence. He lived a good life, and as a keeper-of-the-stories, his life was truly his message.

In search of the good life

When we think of Greek philosophy, a lineage of three brilliant thinkers—Socrates, Plato, and Aristotle—comes to mind. Socrates taught that a good life is synonymous with a virtuous life, a life guided by the practical wisdom of *arête*. His student, Plato, defined the good life in more metaphysical terms. Plato believed there was a *summum bonum* (highest good), an ultimate goal toward which all human activity is directed and which is pursued for its own sake.

In Plato's famous Allegory of the Cave, people start out in chains and are forced to look straight ahead at a shadow puppet play projected on the cave wall (kind of like people today glued to their smartphones). Because they live their entire lives in the cave, they mistake the shadows for reality. Once a person manages to break free and climb to the surface, they behold reality as it is, illuminated by the sun—the *summum bonum*. If this sounds familiar, it's because the creators of *The Matrix,* the Wachowskis, were inspired by Plato's allegory. Do you take the blue pill and stay in the cave or do you take the red pill in search of illumination and liberating truth?

Aristotle, Plato's student, was more scientifically inclined and defined the highest good in practical terms. He claimed, "Happiness is the meaning and purpose of life, the whole aim and end of human existence."[3] Like Plato's *summum bonum,* this was a teleological argument based on the ultimate goal of things. We work to make money so we can buy things. We buy things to improve our life, and we improve our life so we will be happy. But unlike work, money, and buying things, happiness is something we pursue for its own sake. *Pleasure is its own reward!*

Happiness, however, is a poor translation of Aristotle's original Greek term *eudaimonia*. The prefix *eu* means "good," and *daemon* means "spirit," hence "good-spirited," which encompasses the notion of well-being and human flourishing.

The Greeks believed a person is born with a sacred, animating spirit, a *daemon,* that accompanies them throughout their life. Walt Disney films often portray the *daemon* as the hero's alter ego in the form of a small animal, chipmunk, bird, or cricket sidekick. The Romans referred to it as one's genius (from *jenn* or "genie" as in Arabian folklore). The ancients inhabited a polytheistic cosmos teaming with *daemons* to whom one would make humble offerings to secure good fortune in this world and the next.

When Aristotle says, "*Eudaimonia* is the meaning and purpose of life, the whole aim and end of human existence," he is saying *eudaimonia* is the final goal of the good life. Thus, it can only be assessed at the end of one's life, just as the accuracy of an arrow hitting a target can only be determined at the end of its flight. "To be happy," Aristotle wrote, "takes a complete lifetime; for one swallow does not a Spring make."[4] Only by looking back over the whole of your life can you assess if you fulfilled your potential and achieved your best and highest use.

In the late summer in Boulder, a magical light sometimes descends over the valley. It happens when the sun sets behind the foothills in the west and the last dying rays reflect off dark clouds to the east. In those fading moments of twilight, colors take on an extraordinary, otherworldly hue. It is in such reflective light that the full spectrum and meaning of one's life is revealed.

This Greek understanding of "happiness" reminded me of my chats with Frank, as he reflected on the highlights of his life and shared his *eudaimonia* with me over a cup of tea. And true to his word, peering through the ancient eyes of our Greek forebears provided me with the parallax to see my own life more clearly.

German philosopher Friedrich Nietzsche also admired Greek culture for its nobility and beauty and developed an acid test for *eudaimonia* called the Principle of Eternal Recurrence: If you were given the opportunity to relive your life in every detail, would you choose to do it all over again? A life well lived, in other words, is a life worth repeating. You can also apply this principle looking forward: *Of the choices that lie before you, choose the one you would be willing to repeat again and again for eternity. Do this, and you are assured a life without regrets.*

Ethics, virtue, magnanimity, beauty, *summum bonum*, and *eudaimonia* are all about the higher mental and spiritual frequencies of the Pleasure Prism, which we will discuss in Chapter 8. However, it was Epicurus, a near contemporary of Aristotle, who most thoroughly contemplated and plumbed the depths of pleasure. Having prepared the groundwork, we are now ready to hear what this extraordinary man had to say about it.

▲▲▲▲▲▲▲

In brief:

A central concern for ancient Greek philosophers was how to live a good life—a goal they approached through the study of ethics. For Aristotle, this was a matter of training one's character in certain *arête*, virtuous skills, so as to appropriately respond to any and all situations, much like a well-trained martial artist. Virtue was understood to be a path of self-mastery to liberate oneself from illusion and achieve a good life described by Plato as the *summum bonum* (highest good) and by Aristotle as *eudaimonia* (good spirited). The degree to which one has succeeded can only be determined in retrospect at the end of one's life. Or, as Nietzsche suggested, by answering the question, "Would you be willing to do it all over again?"

Considerations:

- When you use the words "good" and "bad," are you making a statement about the quality of something or a moral judgment?

- How do you decide the right thing to do? Is it based on fear (punishment), love (reward), or habit (training)?

- Think of a role model, a personal hero you admire. What do you admire about them?

- To cultivate more magnanimity, beauty, and integrity in your life, what would you change?

CHAPTER 5

An Epicurean Conspiracy

▲ 1. The Law of Original Wholeness

> *Who controls the past controls the future.*
> *Who controls the present controls the past.*
> —George Orwell

For a philosopher, the only fate worse than being forgotten is to be misunderstood. Epicurus of Samos, whose name means ally or friend, lived in the fourth century BCE. His ideas inspired communities that flourished across the ancient Greek and Roman world for nearly 800 years. Yet curiously, unlike Socrates, Plato, and Aristotle, we know little about him, and the little we think we know is usually wrong.

According to the *Oxford Dictionary*, an epicurean is "a person devoted to sensual enjoyment, especially that derived from fine food and drink." There's only one problem. The "eat, drink and be merry for tomorrow we die" approach and its modern equivalent, "sex, drugs, and rock 'n' roll," is exactly 180 degrees opposite what Epicurus actually taught. If the definition were just 50 or 90 degrees off, we might attribute it to the vagaries of piecing together charred fragments of texts and the inevitable sands of time, but as we will see, this misinterpretation was deliberate and the result of a disinformation campaign that continues to this day. In fact, when you stumble across a word that is 180 degrees opposite its original meaning (e.g., *daemon*/demon), more often than not, it has been purposely manipulated, or more precisely, you are being manipulated. Hence, George Orwell's *1984* party slogan: "War is Peace; Freedom is Slavery; Ignorance is Strength." Some modern examples include the Department of War posing as the Department of Defense, disease care and disease insurance pretending to be health care and health insurance. These kinds of one-eighty inversions create knots in the mind that are surprisingly tricky to untangle because you must first negate the negation.

What was it about Epicurus's ideas that were so threatening, and who exactly was threatened? To answer these questions, we need to examine what Epicurus actually taught and the context in which he lived. Having been denied a fair hearing for over two thousand years, I will liberally quote him in his own words so that you can judge for yourself.

Although he authored over 300 works, only three letters and two groups of quotes remain. Above the gate to his garden school in Athens was a sign that read, "Stranger, here you do well to tarry; here our highest good is pleasure." Breaking with the elitism of his contemporaries Plato and Aristotle, Epicurus admitted women and slaves into his school, which puts him on record as the originator of egalitarianism.

Epicurus was a Doctor of Philosophy (Ph.D.) in the truest sense of the word. Like the Buddha, he approached his work as a form of *therapeia*: "A philosopher's words are empty if they do not heal the suffering of mankind. For just as a medicine is useless if it does not remove sickness from the body, so philosophy is useless if it does not remove suffering from the soul."[1] He diagnosed the cause of our existential suffering as the result of a profound confusion about pleasure and the fear of death and the gods. Accordingly, he developed philosophical antidotes to cure these afflictions.

He began by observing the inherent natural intelligence of a newborn who "seeks pleasure and rejoices in it as the highest good, and rejects pain as the greatest bad thing, driving it away from itself as effectively as it can."[2] Because the newborn is innocent and uncorrupted, Epicurus argued, "There is no need of reason or debate about why pleasure is to be pursued and pain to be avoided. These things are perceived, as we perceive that fire is hot, that snow is white, that honey is sweet. None of these things requires confirmation by sophisticated argumentation; it is enough just to have them pointed out."[3]

Having established the self-evident nature of pleasure and pain, Epicurus concludes the pursuit of pleasure provides the wisdom for living an ethical life:

> Practical wisdom is the foundation of all these things and is the greatest good. Thus, practical wisdom is more valuable than philosophy and is the source of every other excellence, teaching us that is not possible to live joyously without also living wisely and beautifully and rightly, nor to live wisely and beautifully and rightly without living joyously, for the excellences grow up together with the pleasant life, and the pleasant life is inseparable from them … this is why we say that pleasure is the beginning and the end of a completely happy life.[4]

Epicurus, like Aristotle, believed the most important philosophical question was how to live a good life, but he differed in how to achieve it. While Aristotle claimed, "happiness is the meaning and purpose of life," Epicurus took the analysis a step further, asserting that pleasure is the cause of happiness. Virtue (*arête*), as you may recall, refers to a skill, and Epicurus argued that the ultimate skill is the practical wisdom to live pleasurably, which naturally leads to a good (wise, beautiful, and honorable) life.

Epicurus's emphasis on pleasure technically makes him a hedonist, but we need to be discerning here. The term "hedonism", like pleasure and happiness, is another casualty of the culture wars for control of the pleasure narrative. The term comes from the Greek *hedone* (the goddess of pleasure), which in turn derives from the Sanskrit *hedys* and *svadus*, both of which mean "sweet." *Svadus* is cognate with our word *suave*, as in "he's a suave fellow." The Spanish *suave* captures the meaning more fully and describes the soft, smooth, silky, gentle, and agreeable characteristics that distinguish pleasure.

But not all hedonism is the same.

Take, for example, the Cyrenaics, a competing school that advocated the unabashed pursuit of sensual pleasures as the ultimate goal of life. They were into the lowest frequencies of the Pleasure Prism, arguing that physical pleasure is more intense and therefore more desirable than the abstract pleasures of Plato's mystical *summon bonum* (highest good) or Aristotle's *eudaimonia* (good spiritedness). Today when we call someone a hedonist, we are usually referring to the Cyrenaic kind of self-indulgent, sensual pleasure seeking.

Epicurus adamantly opposed the crude hedonism of the Cyrenaics: "Thus when we say that pleasure is the goal, we do not mean the pleasure of debauchery or sensuality, despite whatever the ignorant, disagreeable or malignant people believe."[5] Epicurus defined pleasure as "freedom from pain in the body and turmoil in the soul. For it is not continuous drinking and revelry, the sexual enjoyment of women and boys, or feasting upon fish and fancy cuisine which results in a happy life." Instead he advocated, "Sober reasoning is what is needed, which decides every choice and avoidance and liberates us from the false beliefs which are the greatest source of anxiety."[6]

His approach to pleasure was so spare and reserved that to the modern reader it may appear to be a form of asceticism. "Everything we do is for the sake of freedom from pain and anxiety," he wrote. "Once this is achieved, the storms in the soul are stilled. Nothing else and nothing more are needed to perfect well-being of the body and soul. It is when we feel pain that we must seek relief, which is pleasure. And when we no longer feel pain, we no longer need pleasure."[7] His was technically a form of *negative-hedonism*, in that he argued pleasure arises from the absence of pain rather than the addition of pleasure. Such reasoning is based on the false assumption that the opposite of pain is pleasure, which, as we will see in Chapter 11, is erroneous because they exist on the same end of a continuum.

Nonetheless, his understanding was nuanced. Epicurus's philosophy of pleasure was constructed on the biology of need. For instance, hunger is a form of pain relieved by the pleasure of eating. Once hunger is relieved, eating more does not bring additional pleasure; we have had our fill; we have reached our pleasure limit. (Apparently, he was not one for dessert.) Epicurus was a proponent of the middle way, which he called *ataraxia*, from the Greek *a* (not) and *tarassein* (disturbed)—a subtle undisturbed state in which all desire has been sated and one is without need or want—what today we might call peace of mind or equanimity. He claimed *ataraxia* to be the supreme pleasure! On this point, he was quite correct. *Ataraxia* is indeed one of the three gateways to Paradise as we will see in Chapter 18. However, he left out the equally sublime gateways of ecstasy and bliss. Incidentally, Epicurus considered the second-greatest pleasure to be friendship, which helps explain why his communities thrived for centuries.

▲ The Law of Original Wholeness

There has long been a debate among thinkers, East and West alike, as to the true nature of humanity. Epicurus believed our natural condition is not one of Original Sin, as Augustine claimed, or Original Suffering, as the Buddha taught, nor is it entirely neutral. When you remove pain and want from the body and fear and greed from the mind, what remains is *ataraxia*, or Original Wholeness—the first of the Seven Immutable Laws of Pleasure—a delightful openness to life like the original joy of a young child: fresh, alert, and present.

When my youngest daughter, Satya, was about two years old, it was a pleasure to watch her awaken in the morning, beaming with curiosity and joy. A leaded-glass crystal hung in the window catching the light. As it twisted, she would chase the splashes of rainbow color on the bedcover. Her enthusiastic delight drew me into her magical world and re-awakened my wonder and mystery of life's ordinary miracles. Hers was a pristine, unconditioned nervous system, a mind free of judgments, fears, or opinions. Some years later, Satya became aware of the preciousness of her innocence and would say, "I hope I never grow up ... and become a teenager," as she had seen happen to her older sisters. Of course, all of us must eventually leave the Garden, as the demands of the outer world take hold, but fortunately, as an artist, Satya can revisit this enchanted world through the magic of the creative process.

When Epicurus said, "We hold the greatest pleasure to be that which is perceived when all pain is removed,"[8] he is talking about the removal of pain from both the body and the mind. In our state of Original Wholeness, we are free from anxiety, free from the worry of past or future, and filled with a profound feeling of peacefulness—*ataraxia*. The Taoist sage, Laozi, came to a similar conclusion: "Be content with what you have; rejoice in the way things are. When you realize there is nothing lacking, the whole world belongs to you."[9]

Conspiracy

Epicurus's modest approach to pleasure was hardly a threat to the social fabric of his day. But his day was a long one, and after 800 years, a brash new religion came to dominate the philosophical landscape. In the fourth century CE, the pagan Roman Emperor Constantine raised Christianity from an obscure offshoot of Judaism to become the new state religion of the Roman Empire, sanctified with his maxim: "One God, one religion. One Emperor, one empire." The only problem was that Christianity was not yet one religion. To solve this problem, he convened the Council of Nicea and gathered some 300 bishops from across the empire to hammer out theological disputes and formulate an orthodoxy that would become the future Catholic church—"catholic" meaning universal, as in "uni (one) version." Specifically, the one and only version of Christianity.

Constantine and the nascent Catholic church shared a common vision: world domination. As for his faith, perhaps Constantine underwent a miraculous spiritual conversion, or maybe he was just making a shrewd political calculation. It's hard to say. What we do know is that he remained unbaptized until his deathbed, presumably to secure entry into heaven with a clean slate, absolved of all his worldly sins, which included, among other things, ordering the suffocation of his wife, and the murder of his son.

An Epicurean Conspiracy

The Catholics immediately leveraged the might of the Roman army to ruthlessly stamp out all competitors: first and foremost, dissenting Christian Gnostic sects; and second, pagans who worshipped other gods. The theological cleansing was so thorough that had it not been for the 1945 discovery of a collection of Gnostic scrolls in a sealed earthen jar in Nag Hammadi, upper Egypt, we would never have known what the other early Christian sects taught.

During this brutal period of theological cleansing, I suspect Epicurus was singled out for special treatment, not because of his ideas about pleasure, nor his pagan beliefs, which were modest, but because of his revolutionary ideas. He was on a mission to liberate humanity from "the false beliefs which are the greatest source of anxiety," namely the fear of death and the fear of the gods, two anxieties vital to the success of the Catholic Church.

Driving to work the other day, I saw these words written in bold capital letters on the marquee of a local church: "IN THE FEAR OF THE LORD ONE HAS STRONG CONFIDENCE. PROV. 14:26." Epicurus was 180 degrees opposed to this sort of fearmongering. He wanted people to be confident in their natural intelligence and trust prudent pleasure to guide them to the good life. To accomplish this, he needed to liberate the human mind from the fear of death and superstition.

The fear of death

Epicurus subdivided the fear of death into three types and developed effective antidotes for each:

The fear of a painful death, he argued, is of no concern because in any event, it does not last long and so can be endured. As fate would have it, Epicurus would take a strong dose of his own medicine. He died from the complications of a kidney stone, one of the most painful afflictions, known as "laboring under the stone." By all accounts, he bore it well.

The fear of dying, he argued, is baseless because logically, no one can experience their own non-existence: "Death is nothing to us, since while we exist our death is not, and when death occurs, we do not exist."[10]

The fear of being punished after death he dismissed with a more thorough argument based on his atomic theory of physics. The human soul, he asserted, is composed of atoms like the rest of the material world, only much finer. At the time of death, the atoms of the body and soul disperse. This remarkably modern scientific description negates the possibility of a post-mortem existence. Without an afterlife, there is no need to fear retribution. *No eternal soul, no problema.* For those who were still fearful, he offered my favorite remedy: "You don't fret about the eons of non-existence before you were born, so why dread an eternity of non-existence after you die?"[11]

Although his logic is compelling, our fear of death has a strong emotional hold because it is rooted in our biological imperative to survive. This is precisely where religion and superstition have their greatest attraction and where Epicurus's ideas posed a clear and present danger.

The fear of gods

Epicurus (like the Buddha) was an empiricist. He taught that it is better to claim ignorance than to accept something on the basis of authority or blind faith that cannot be verified by direct observation with one's own senses and that conforms to logical reason.

As for the gods, Epicurus was technically a deist. He did not deny the existence of gods, as they frequently visited people in their dreams, but he argued that they enjoy a sublime existence beyond our world and are unconcerned with human affairs. Therefore, people should not indulge in false opinions about them, beseech their help, or fear their punishment.

To sharpen his point, he offered the following quadrilemma and in so doing was one of the first to raise "The Problem of Evil," which has dogged monotheistic religions ever since:

> If God is willing to prevent evil, but not able,
>   then he is not omnipotent.
> If he is able but not willing,
>   then he is malevolent.

> If he is both able and willing,
>   then whence cometh evil?
> If he is neither willing nor able,
>   then why call him God?[12]

With surgical precision, Epicurus excised the malignant dread of the unseen world, not by denying its existence, but by denying its relevance to our daily lives. Rather than seek salvation and heavenly bliss in some future postmortem existence, he preached liberation now without fear in this life. It was this sort of down-to-earth thinking that prompted the twentieth century scholar Cyril Bailey to hail Epicurus "The apostle of common sense."

Imagine if, instead of speculating about life after death, we embraced a simple belief that after we die, we will either vanish as we do each night in deep sleep, or we are on to our next adventure. As Epicurus observed: "There is nothing terrifying in life to someone who truly understands that there is nothing terrifying in the absence of life."[13] When I ponder this simple aphorism, a subtle heaviness falls away and I feel lighter and freer.

But for those whose influence and legitimacy rests upon the existence of a menacing unseen, and therefore unverifiable netherworld, Epicurus's common-sense approach was a threat that had to be neutralized. For this reason, I believe, he became the target of a disinformation campaign. However, a profound idea, once inserted into the cultural DNA, is not easily deleted.

Epicurus's legacy lives on

Epicurus is without doubt one of the great unsung heroes of Western civilization. His ideas on natural science and the atomic structure of matter inspired the likes of Bacon, Galileo, and Gassendi during the renaissance, and later Einstein. He anticipated Heisenberg's Uncertainty Principle, a fundamental concept in quantum mechanics,[14] and his emphasis on self-reliance and simple living influenced Emerson, Thoreau, and Nietzsche.

The British social reformer Jeremy Bentham extended Epicurus's ideal of the individual to the body-politic and called it Utilitarianism based on the axiom: "It is the greatest happiness of the greatest number that is the measure of right and wrong."[15] Bentham, inspired by Epicurean ideals, vigorously advocated equal rights for women, freedom of individual expression, decriminalization of homosexuality, abolition of slavery and the death penalty, separation of church and state, and humane treatment of animals. He is known as the first patron saint of animal rights.

The crowning jewel of Epicurus's legacy was to be fulfilled by Thomas Jefferson, a self-avowed Epicurean: "As you say of yourself, I too am an Epicurean. I consider the genuine (not the imputed) doctrines of Epicurus as containing everything rational in moral philosophy which Greece and Rome have left us."[16] Jefferson was also a Christian and highly valued the teachings of Jesus the man, but like Epicurus was a foe of organized religion. In a letter to William Baldwin in 1810, Jefferson claimed the church has been "perverted into an engine for enslaving mankind, a mere contrivance to filch wealth and power to themselves."[17] Well aware of the political role of religion, in a letter to Horatio Spafford, Jefferson wrote, "In every country and every age, the priest has been hostile to liberty. He is always in alliance with the despot, abetting his abuses in return for protection of his own."[18] Moreover, the church "themselves are the greatest obstacles to the advancement of the real doctrines of Jesus, and do in fact constitute the real Antichrist."[19] Hypocrisy is just disinformation by another name—the proverbial wolf in sheep's clothing.

But when the "good" shepherd sodomizes his innocent flock, it is a hypocrisy that stinks to high heaven and becomes a heinous criminal act. According to a 2004 report released by the John Jay College of Criminal Justice, 4 percent of the Catholic clergy have been accused of sexually abusing a minor.[20] Even more disturbing is the institutionalized cover-up that enabled the abuse to continue for who knows how many centuries. Mark Jordan, a professor at Harvard Divinity School, attributes the cause of the cover-up to the "cult of obedience" that he likens to a Marine Corps military chain of command in which "the first loyalty is to the church."[21] This is not surprising because the early Catholic church modeled itself after the Roman army with a pope (Greek: *papas*, "father," commander-in-chief) followed by cardinals, archbishops, bishops, priests, deacons, and laity. The very definition of the word "hierarchy" comes from the Greek: *hierós* (holy) and árkhon (ruler).

Jefferson's outspokenness against the church made him a target of disinformation. In the presidential election of 1800, he was labeled a "howling Atheist." Yet in the final years of his life, he painstakingly pored over six copies of the New Testament—in Greek, Latin, French, and King James English—and with a sharp knife, cut and pasted Jesus's teachings into an 84-page volume known as the *Jefferson Bible*. He was clearly a deeply spiritual man and an Epicurean anti-religionist.

It is in the Declaration of Independence, written from Jefferson's own pen, that we find Epicurus's ideas re-emerging most brilliantly: "We hold these truths to be self-evident, that all men are created equal and are endowed by their Creator with certain inalienable rights, that among these are Life, Liberty and the pursuit of Happiness."

Here at the birth of the great American experiment, we can hear Epicurus speaking to us across the millennia loud and clear: self-evident truth (what can be confirmed with your own senses); all men created equal with fundamental rights (egalitarianism); liberty (freedom); and the pursuit of happiness (pleasure).

And the rest, as they say, is history. Today more than half of the 192 member countries of the United Nations have a founding document that can be called a declaration of independence. Notable among these are Japan's constitution and Ho Chi Minh's 1945 Declaration of Independence for the Democratic Republic of Vietnam. Epicurus's ideas continue to inspire and reverberate in the hearts of freedom-loving people the world over. *Never underestimate the power of a clear thought!*

From the Tree of Knowledge of Good and Evil, Original Sin, and hedonism to ethics, virtue, and *eudaimonia*, we've come a long way, retracing the Judeo-Christian and Greek philosophical origins of our Western cultural matrix. We've seen how these two different traditions have intermingled and at times clashed to shape our collective ideas and conflicted feelings about pleasure.

Throughout history, down to the present day, this tension has played out as a power struggle, not only for control of the pleasure narrative, but for the control of human consciousness—a "war on consciousness" for the very the soul of humanity. Are we fallen angels born sinful in need of salvation or are we born whole with vast potential in need of enlightened, ethical training? The First Law of Pleasure, Original Wholeness, makes it clear where I stand. We come equipped with biological hardware honed through billions of years of evolutionary trial and error just like every other living creature. Our uniquely human confusion about pleasure is the result of malware inserted into our cultural operating system. But as Epicurus reminds us, you should not take my word for it or anyone else's. In Parts 2 and 3, we will explore the underlying neurobiology and natural history of pleasure so you can see for yourself how pleasure works and come to your own conclusions.

▲▲▲▲▲▲▲

In brief:

Epicurus advocated a modest, restrained approach to pleasure. He considered the greatest pleasure to be *ataraxia*, peace of mind or equanimity, and the second greatest pleasure, friendship. However, his "liberation theology" of egalitarianism, freedom from the fear of gods, death, heaven and hell, and his incisive critique of the problem of evil threatened the Roman Catholic Church. In an attempt to discredit him, the definition of an epicurean was twisted 180 degrees to describe a devotee of fine food and drink. Nonetheless, his enlightened ideas persisted and are now on permanent display in the rotunda of the National Archives in Washington, D. C., within the Declaration of Independence.

Considerations:

- When you hear the word "hedonist," what images or judgments spring to mind?

- Investigate your anxiety. What is the worst that could happen? Is it death, or something else?

- Do you believe in an afterlife where you will be judged for your actions? If so, where is it located?

- Are people basically good, bad, or both?

- Can people be trusted to govern themselves or must they be led, and if so, by whom?

- Can you be trusted? What are the ways you trust or distrust yourself?

- In the war on consciousness, where can peace be found if not in your own mind?

Part 2: **The Science**

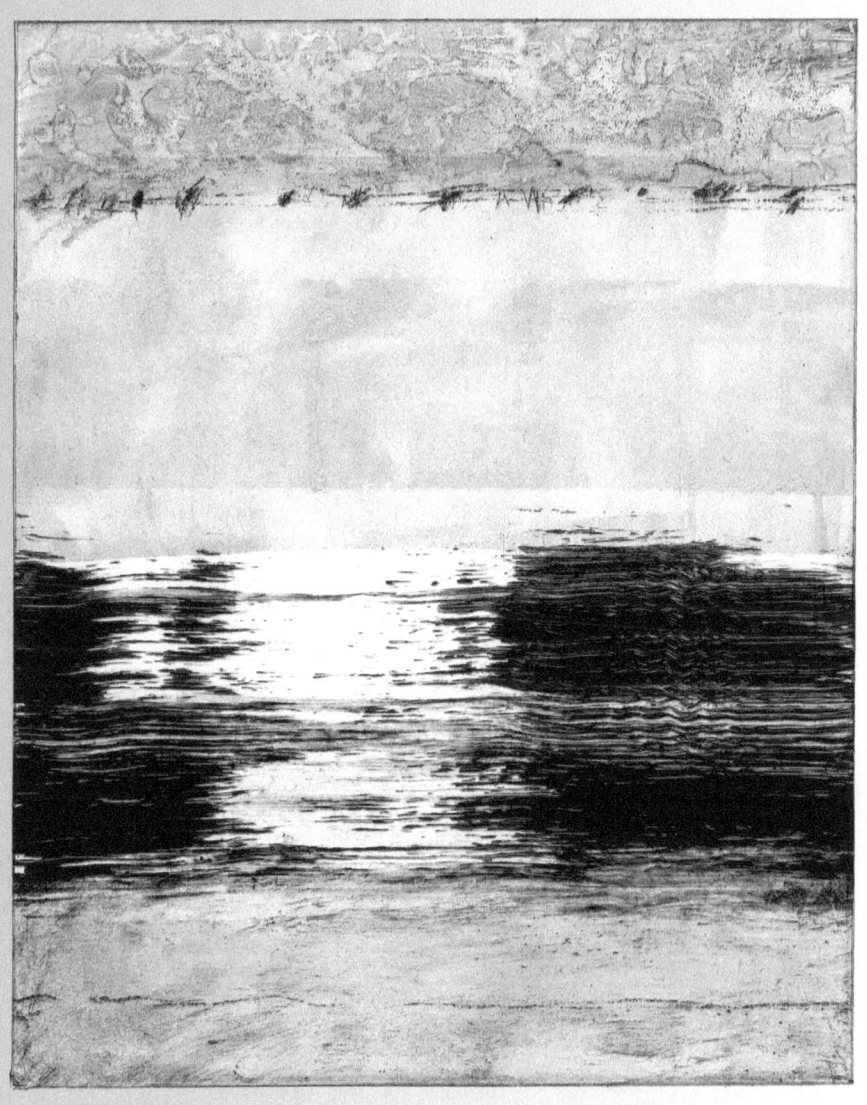

CHAPTER 6

The Anatomy of Pleasure

> *The human body is the best picture*
> *of the human soul.*
> —Ludwig Wittgenstein

As an undergraduate, I had a professor named David Hawkins, one of the smartest people I've ever known. He had a Ph.D. in physics and another one in philosophy. He encouraged me to attend the lectures of visiting professors even though the subject matter was way over my head. "You may not get all the words," he'd say, "but you can still hear the music." I recommend you do the same with this chapter. If you find this introduction to the neurobiology of pleasure a bit dense, don't sweat the details. They will change, in any event, as science learns more. Just sit back and enjoy the music.

Discovering the pleasure center

One day in the early 1950s, James Olds and Peter Milner reportedly stumbled upon the pleasure center when a thin electric probe went astray into a small cluster of neurons in a rat's forebrain known as the nucleus accumbens (located near the septum, which divides the two halves of the forebrain). While "nucleus accumbens" sounds impressive, most anatomical terms are simply Latin words that early anatomists used to describe what they saw, long before they understood their function. In the case of the N. accumbens, the cluster of nerves (called a nucleus) appeared to be leaning (think: recumbent bicycle) against the septum (a dividing partition), with one nucleus on either side. In older literature, this region was called the "rhinencephalon," or smell brain, harking back to our ancient past when we used to be on all fours with our snout close to the ground like a rhinoceros. The N. accumbens is thought to play an important role in reward, pleasure, and addiction.

By administering a small electrical impulse through the probe each time the rat approached a particular corner of its cage, it could be trained to spend more time in that corner, called conditioned place preference. At first, Olds and Milner thought they had provoked a curiosity response, but it seemed the rat "enjoyed" receiving the stimulation.

To test this hypothesis, they constructed a Skinner box, a device that allowed the rat to press a small bar that would send a tiny electric charge trickling down a wire electrode inserted into the pleasure center of its brain. They essentially created a high-tech, self-pleasuring machine, which they dubbed "intracranial electrical self-stimulation." Head-wired rats would endure scampering across an electric grid to tap the bar up to 1,700 times an hour, twenty days in a row, forgoing food and water to the point of exhaustion.

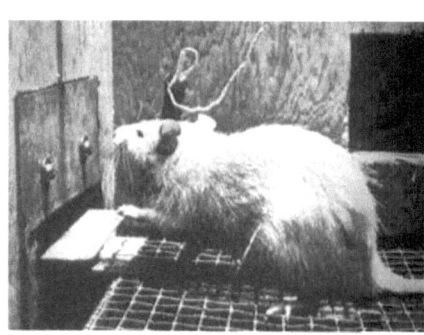

Figure 3: Head-wired rat.

Dr. John C. Lilly, of LSD and dolphin interspecies communication fame, found similar results in studies of head-wired monkeys, who would stimulate their pleasure centers up to 200,000 times before settling down to a daily routine of about 16 hours of bar-tapping and eight hours of sleep. It was both the intensity and the instantaneous reward that made tapping the bar so compelling. Sound familiar? Social media platforms such as Google, Twitter, and Facebook use similar Skinnerian marketing techniques to make their user interfaces "sticky." With every click, you get a small spark to your N. accumbens to keep you clicking for more.

These dramatic animal experiments set the stage for one of the darker chapters of medical research. In the 1960s, Dr. Robert Heath, chairman of the Department of Psychiatry and Neurology at Tulane University, took the next logical—but by today's standards horrifically unethical—step of head-wiring human beings. His subjects were mostly schizophrenics and severely depressed patients culled from the dank, dimly-lit back wards of Louisiana's state mental hospital. Using a dental drill and local anesthesia, he made holes in the subjects' skulls and then inserted electrodes deep within their brains in arrays of up to fifty at a time. Surprisingly, the procedure was relatively painless as the brain itself has no pain receptors.

Dr. Heath's brain experiments spanned nearly two decades and involved several thousand patients. One patient, identified as B-19, self-stimulated himself up to 1,500 times in a three-hour period. Dr. Heath observed: "During these sessions, B-19 stimulated himself to a point that he was experiencing an almost overwhelming euphoria and elation, and had to be disconnected, despite his vigorous protests."[1]

Sadly, the effects of electrical stimulation were short-lived, and once the current was turned off, the subjects returned to their prior dismal state. Dr. Heath's early brain-mapping attempts have largely been replaced by non-invasive neuroimaging techniques such as fMRI (functional magnetic resonance imaging) and PET scans (positron emission tomography).

Brain evolution

While Olds and Milner were probing the pleasure center, a brilliant physician-researcher, Paul MacLean, was studying the evolutionary development of the brain as a way to understand human behavior. Using detailed electrical brain mapping, comparative anatomy, and animal behavior research, he traced how the human forebrain evolved through three distinct stages, from reptile to early mammal to primate. His groundbreaking research led to his becoming chief of the Laboratory of Brain Evolution and Behavior at the National Institute of Mental Health (1971-1985).

The way to understand anatomy is to start at the beginning with embryology. Studying the development of an anatomical structure is like seeing a movie rather than just a single photograph. The fetal brain begins to form during the fourth week as three swellings at the end of the spinal cord, which develop into the hindbrain, midbrain, and forebrain. The spinal cord together with the hindbrain and midbrain make up what Maclean calls the neural chassis: "By itself the neural chassis might be likened to a vehicle without a driver."[2] Just as the chassis of a car with its frame, engine, transmission, and steering wheel performs essential functions, the neural chassis performs vital bodily functions such as respiration, circulation, digestion, and elimination, as well as more complex functions like self-preservation, alertness, posture, locomotion, and reproduction. The chassis is more commonly known as the brainstem. When a person is in a coma, it is the brainstem that keeps the engine idling even though no one's at the wheel in the so-called vegetative state.

Sitting in the driver's seat on top of the chassis is the terminal swelling of the spinal cord, the forebrain, which steers the action. This is where things get rather interesting because, "In the more advanced vertebrates

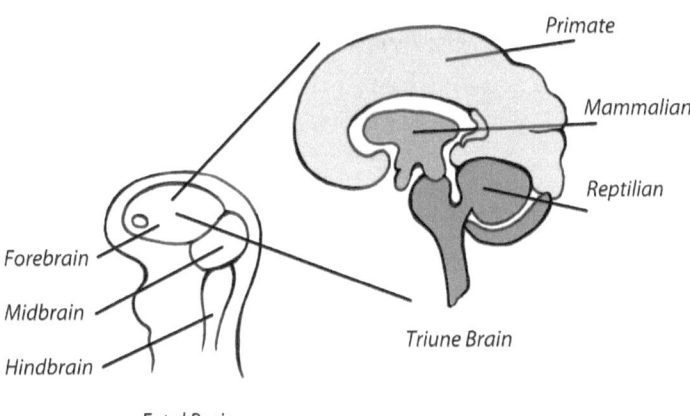

Figure 4: The developing fetal forebrain, midbrain, and hindbrain at four weeks gestation and the relationship of the fetal forebrain to the three divisions of the triune brain.

the evolutionary process has provided the neural chassis not with a single guiding operator, but rather a combination of three, each markedly different in its evolutionary age and development, and each radically different in structure, chemistry, and organization."[3]

Maclean called these three "drivers" the "triune brain," three brains in one. It represents the three evolutionary stages, reptilian, early mammalian, and primate, that take place primarily in the terminal swelling of the human forebrain. The preceding two swellings, the hindbrain and midbrain, which make up the brainstem chassis, have changed relatively little over time.

The reptilian brain is a simple affair that consists of a neural chassis with several knots of grey matter (clusters of nerves called ganglia). These few grey matter ganglia function as a primitive reptilian forebrain driver. A snake is essentially a long spinal cord with a small forebrain, which is why they have such flat heads.

Accordingly, reptiles can perform a limited range of behaviors beyond the vegetative functions, such as establishing pecking order, territoriality, aggression, defense, and mating rituals. I'm reminded of this when I pass a man in the street and we tip our heads in a gesture of recognition, which is what reptiles do when they cross paths.

It will take another 250 million years of evolution for the horny, leathery scales of the reptile to sprout soft mammalian fur. Along with hair came warm-blooded emotions and an enlarged brain case to accommodate a new expansion of brain tissue that wrapped around the ganglia of the reptilian brain. To early anatomists, it looked like a limiting (limbic) margin of tissue, hence the limbic brain. This limbic brain introduced a new emotional intelligence that enabled the nuanced social interactions necessary for herd living. And yes, we are herd animals!

A mere 50 million years ago, some mammals began to stand up on their hind legs and cast their gaze over the savannahs, freeing their front paws to manipulate the world in more creative ways than possible with a snout and mouth. That's when all the mischief started and we began to fashion tools and "think." The upright (and some might say, uptight) bipedal primate was born.

In primates, the thin layer of grey matter overlying the limbic and reptilian brains underwent a massive expansion folding in upon itself, greatly increasing its thickness and surface area to create a neocortex (*neo*, "new," and *cortex*, "bark"). In the modern human brain, the neocortical grey matter makes up 85 percent of its total volume and gives us our distinctive high brow.

Triune pleasure

My contribution is the simple observation that each of the three brains enjoys its own particular kind of pleasure: the reptilian brain seeks physical, sensual pleasures (sex and food); the mammalian, limbic brain seeks emotional pleasures (love and happiness); and the primate, cortical brain seeks symbolic, mental pleasures (status and meaning). These are the three evolutionary stages of the human forebrain that refract the three primary colors of the Pleasure Prism. The various shades and combinations of these primary colors create the diverse palette of pleasures we enjoy, from the drenching sweat of a hard workout to cozying up by a fire with a good book. Let's zoom in more closely to see how the anatomy works.

The desire center is located in a small group of neurons in the roof of the midbrain portion of the brainstem known as the Ventral Tegmental Area (VTA), Latin for "the underside of the roof." Desire is therefore a function of the reptilian brain, which explains why our habits, once established, seem to run on autopilot and are so hard to change. The VTA registers what is salient. Like a flashing warning light on a dashboard, it tells the forebrain, "Pay attention! A potential reward is coming!" which motivates us to move toward the reward.

The neurons of the Ventral Tegmental Area produce dopamine, the primary neurotransmitter of the reward system (i.e., the chemical messenger in your brain that gets you high). The midbrain VTA has two-way connections that project forward to the limbic brain and cortical brain known as the mesolimbic and mesocortical pathways, "meso" meaning middle for midbrain. Consequently, the VTA plays an important role in regulating emotions, love, and fear in the limbic brain and cognition, planning, and motivation in the cortical brain.

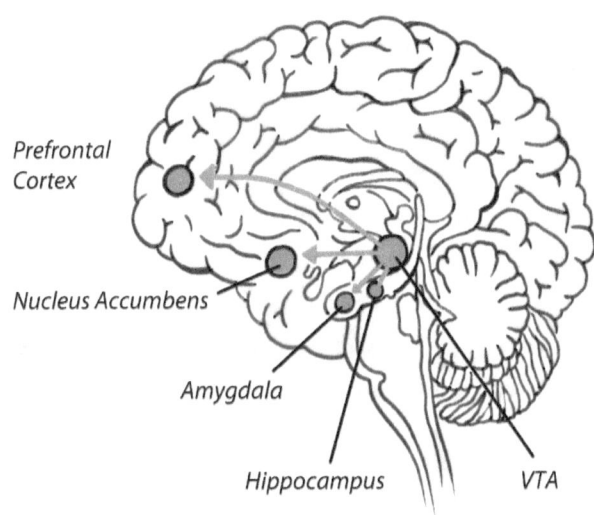

Figure 5: The Dopamine Reward Circuit: VTA-limbic-cortical pathways.

The mesolimbic pathway of the VTA connects to three key centers in the limbic brain: the N. accumbens (the pleasure center); the hippocampus (where long-term memories are stored); and the amygdala (which governs fear and aggression). "Hippocampus" is Latin for seahorse, and "amygdala" means almond. In other words, the underside of the roof in the midbrain connects to the recumbent nucleus, the seahorse, and the almond in the limbic brain.

Usually, desire and pleasure are closely coupled, one following the other, and we think of them as being practically the same thing: I want what I like, and I like what I want. However, they can become uncoupled at times. Have you ever really wanted something like a new electronic gadget or a cool jacket, and after buying it, it sat on the shelf or hung in your closet gathering dust? The uncoupling of desire and pleasure is particularly dramatic in addictions, where we have a strong desire for something but surprisingly little enjoyment of it. As many cigarette smokers will confess, smoking is just a bad habit, but one that is really hard to quit.

All pleasures, whether food, sex, drugs, rock n' roll, positive affirmations, acts of generosity, or spiritual communion, funnel into the same pleasure-reward circuits of the N. accumbens/VTA. Some artificially induced pleasures like cocaine and heroin are so intense, however, that they hijack the reward system and blot out more natural pleasures (as in, "blotto" drunk).

Neurobiologists are at the very beginning stages of unraveling an immensely complex human reward system, so be wary of oversimplified explanations. Dopamine is just one of over a hundred neurotransmitters in the brain. At the base of the limbic brain is a structure known as the hypothalamus (below the chamber) that secretes oxytocin, a neuropeptide that acts as both a hormone to initiate uterine contractions during childbirth as well as milk letdown for breast feeding, and simultaneously stimulates the VTA and N. accumbens to reward pair bonding, maternal behavior, and other prosocial behaviors. Much like head-wired rats, lactating female rats that have been trained to press a bar in order to retrieve their pups will press the bar continuously hundreds of times over multiple hours to see their pups or foster pups. In some contexts, oxytocin promotes social bonding while in others it distances. Monogamous prairie voles under the influence of oxytocin are attracted to their mates but exhibit aggression toward female strangers.

Understanding the basic neurobiology of the reward system helps explain a number of common behaviors. The connection between the N. accumbens/VTA and the hippocampus (memory center) accounts for how we remember a pleasurable experience and are motivated to repeat it in the future. The relationship of pleasure to the amygdala (fear and aggression center) is a little less obvious. Anatomically, the N. accumbens lies very close to the amygdala for a good reason. Think of a tiger chasing a gazelle. The VTA is turned on in hot pursuit (desire). The tiger must first aggressively take down the gazelle before it can enjoy the pleasure of eating it. Then the tiger must fearfully protect its kill from jackals and other interlopers. That's why disturbing dogs when they are eating can be dangerous and why jealousy can be such a violent emotion.

The mesocortical pathway between the midbrain VTA and the prefrontal cortex is especially important. The prefrontal cortex is located immediately behind the forehead and orchestrates our higher executive functions of planning, decision making, and predicting outcomes. It's like a mental sketch pad where ideas can be evaluated before we act, enabling us to figure out the best way to fulfill our brainstem desires. Equally important, the prefrontal cortex has an inhibitory function that can tamp down our reptilian temptations. For instance, a man sees a beautiful woman and experiences an immediate reptilian urge to kiss her. The prefrontal cortex puts the brainstem on hold as it quickly sorts through the options. It hatches a plan to strike up a conversation, get her telephone number, ask her out to dinner, and then kiss her. The prefrontal inhibitory pathways are not fully myelinated until the early twenties, which may explain why adolescents have spotty impulse control, much like two-year-olds have spotty bowel and bladder control. They lack control because their neurons are not yet reliably connected.

As mentioned earlier, the mesolimbic and mesocortical pathways that connect the midbrain VTA to the limbic and cortical brains are reciprocal; they go both ways. Just as brainstem desires can arouse strong emotions and whip the prefrontal cortex into thoughtful, premeditated action, thoughts and emotions can evoke strong desires. This sort of mental kindling is why advertising works. A drinker sees an attractive woman with a glass of bourbon reclining on a billboard sign and the thought of a drink coupled with sexual stimulation turns on his reward circuits to thirst for a drink.

This also explains why treating addiction is so difficult. If it were just a matter of quitting, we could lock addicts in jail for a month and turn them loose once they were drug free. The hard part is not stopping (an addict "stops" every night); the hard part is not starting again! As Mark Twain said about his tobacco habit, "Quitting is easy; I have done it many times." The mere thought of the drug, the sight of a liquor bottle, the smell of a cigarette, or walking by an old drug haunt can trigger the VTA to shower the N. accumbens with dopamine and arouse powerful cravings.

Normally, we aren't aware of having three different operators (brains) at the steering wheel because they work together seamlessly to give us a smooth ride. However, when we are under duress in a threatening situation or as the result of an addiction, the psyche can become dis-integrated as each brain attempts to drive in a different direction. At that point, we are internally conflicted and literally out of control.

What we typically refer to as the "unconscious" or "subconscious" is the functioning of our reptilian and limbic brains. Simply knowing this and paying attention to your reptilian habits and limbic emotions will allow you to feel more integrated and in control. For instance, have you ever found yourself late at night standing in front of your refrigerator, rummaging reptile-like through the shelves looking for something to eat and feeling emotionally conflicted about the extra calories, while a little primate voice tells you to shut the door and back away? It takes a healthy dose of humility to be honest with yourself and acknowledge your inner conflict. But the moment you do, *the moment you make the unconscious conscious, choice becomes possible and with choice comes freedom.* Interestingly, if you look just beyond the periphery of your vision, there is a mysterious fourth operator, the "witness," observing the whole process of your inner conflict. We will have more to say about this mysterious witness a little later in Chapter 8 as it holds an important key to your liberation and fulfillment.

It's as though the gods got bored one day and just for fun put a lizard, a rabbit, and a mischievous chimp in a small box to see what would happen. When the lizard's routine is undisturbed, the rabbit is feeling loved, and the chimp is absorbed in activity, then the three can get along rather smashingly. However, when a threatening predatory shadow flies overhead, the lizard darts under the nearest rock, the rabbit freezes with fear, and the chimp frets whether to run, keep still, or stand up and fight like an ape.

In a stunning example of art anticipating science, Maclean's triune brain model was familiar to the ancients in the form of a common mythological creature known as a sphinx. A sphinx is a chimera, a creature made from other animals, typically with a human or lion's head, an ophidian serpent's tail, and a furry mammalian body in between. That these unusual creatures are found throughout the world, often in pairs standing guard at temples, museums, and other auspicious portals, reflects the universality of our triune nature.

Now that you have some basic neurobiology under your belt, we will zoom out and examine the behavioral aspects of our sphinx nature, which will give you a much clearer picture of how the Pleasure Prism illuminates your daily life.

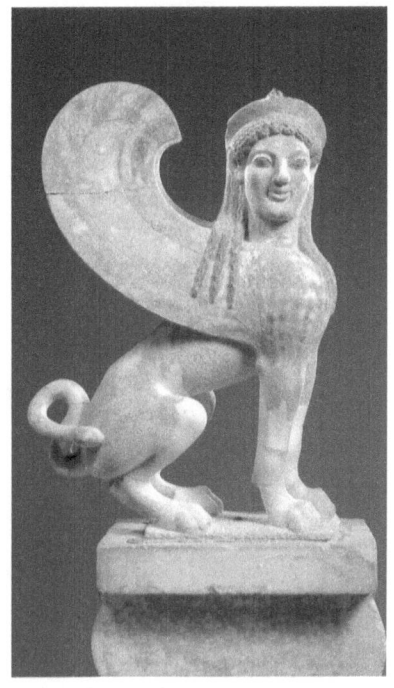

Figure 6: Marble sphinx capital ornament. Greek 530 BCE.

▲▲▲▲▲▲▲

In brief:

There are three basic *embryological* divisions of the human brain: the hindbrain, midbrain, and forebrain. The hindbrain and midbrain along with the spinal cord form the brainstem neural chassis. However (and this is where it can get a bit confusing), the forebrain "conductor" of the neural chassis also has three basic *evolutionary* divisions—reptilian, early mammalian, and primate—which form the triune brain (the reptilian, limbic, and cortical brains, respectively). Since the VTA desire center is located in the midbrain (part of the reptilian tail so to speak), *desire is a reptilian function*. The N. accumbens pleasure center resides in the limbic brain (along with the hippocampus memory center and amygdala emotional center) making *pleasure a mammalian function*. All three brains are interconnected in both directions by the pleasure-reward system, (i.e., the N. accumbens/VTA circuit). If this introduction to the triune brain is not crystal clear, not to worry, we will have occasion to return to these ideas a number of times and reinforce your synaptic connections.

Considerations:
- Check out your sphinx nature: the short tail you have tucked between your legs, the coccyx.

- Examine the lines and creases of the skin on the back of your hands—the remnants of reptilian scales.

- Notice your body hair was once thick mammalian fur.

- Brush your bangs aside and proudly display your primate highbrow. (You earned it, evolutionarily speaking.)

CHAPTER 7

Your Sphinx Brain

*The greatest language barrier
lies between man and his animal brains.*
—Paul Maclean

THE HALLMARK OF REPTILIAN BEHAVIOR IS EASY TO REMEMBER. JUST REPEAT AFTER me: *Reptiles like to repeat.* A reptile's day consists of a series of habits: crawling out of their hole, basking in the sun, defecating, feeding, an afternoon nap on their favorite rock, and a return to shelter, all carried out with monotonous regularity. They use the same defecatory post, and though there may be a shorter route to their favorite eating grounds, they take the familiar, long way around. Theirs is a life of repetitive, ritualized habit.

Enter the reptile

Consider for a moment your own reptilian habits. Do you take the same route to work each day? When you're out and about, do you have a favorite defecatory post, a favorite restaurant and table, a familiar watering hole where you gather with other local lounge lizards? From simple physical movements like brushing your teeth and walking, to more complicated tasks like lacing shoes, riding a bike, or making love, easily 70 percent or more of our lives are a function of our reptilian brain. Our inner reptile delights in the repetitive movements of gardening, jogging, fly fishing, washing dishes, knitting, beading, and other forms of handiwork. These "mindless" activities disengage the higher brain centers from the neural chassis like disengaging the clutch of a car, which allows our higher cortical functions to freewheel and provides a pleasant break from our mental machinations. Afterwards we feel calm and refreshed.

I received a valuable lesson in this one morning when I found myself sitting in a circle with five Korean women on a sweatshop floor in Denver. I was peripherally involved in a family start-up business manufacturing children's fleece clothing and was enlisted to help. The morning sun filtered through windows secured with wire grates and cast a diffuse, somber light on half a dozen vintage, industrial Singer sewing machines, each with a small metal gooseneck lamp, tired chair, and workbench. Cardboard cutout patterns were strung across the back wall like puzzle pieces. A kaleidoscope of fabric, spools of thread, and clothing in various stages of completion were strewn about. In the center of the concrete floor was a waist-deep pile of newly sewn children's fleece garments. One of the women handed me a pair of well-used scissors.

"Here, see," she said, holding up a tiny shirt with the seams turned inside-out, showing me the stray threads where the seamstress had paused in her sewing.

"Cut." She demonstrated, her fingers fluttering down the seams like butterfly wings, clipping off the threads and then, with a few deft movements, she pulled the shirt right-side out, exposing its pattern of brightly colored Ninja turtles.

"Then put, here." She tossed the shirt on the floor.

At first, I was annoyed that this was going to be a complete waste of a beautiful Saturday morning. But the women immediately dove in and I was swept along by their energy and focus. There was no talking just the sound of scissors snipping and the rustling of fabric. After about half an hour, I looked around at the women in the circle. They were absorbed in meditation, their faces Buddha-like in peaceful repose. It took us another hour to finish off the pile.

Completing our work, we stood up with a collective sigh and stretched our limbs. The women quickly cleared off a long work table and transformed it into a potluck spread of homemade Korean treats. As the women broke into animated conversation and laughter, the pungent smell of kimchi and soy sauce filled my nose, whetting my appetite.

"You want come fold clothes tomorrow?" my sew-master said with a crooked-toothed grin, plucking a chunk of pineapple from a bowl with her steel chopsticks as though catching a fly.

"Nah, back no good," I said, as I feigned a wince and motioned with my hand.

"Your work too hard!"

As we feasted, I realized my arrogance in thinking menial labor was beneath me. Repetitive work has its benefits. Looking at the pile of clothing, I felt a sense of accomplishment, a mental pleasure grounded in a calm, centered feeling that comes from working the body with repetitive motions. These women had given me a lesson in reptilian humility and how one can overcome difficulty with camaraderie and dignity.

Of course, institutions have long known the power of repetition. Religions are replete with reptilian rituals often performed together in groups—bowing, kneeling, fingering rosary beads, singing hymns, and chanting—that engage the body and mind in simple, direct ways. In certain lineages of Tibetan Buddhism, novices must perform prostrations, throwing themselves face down on a long, smooth board with hands placed on a folded towel to slide full length and then back to standing a hundred thousand times before they are deemed worthy to receive the secret teachings. Muslim clerics know that if you can get someone to kneel five times a day with specific hand gestures, vocalizations, and mental intention, you have one well-trained inner reptile. For the same reason, a great deal of military training is devoted to marching, saluting, singing, and other regimented group rituals. The Navy Seals borrow a saying from the Greek poet Archilochus. In a firefight, "We don't rise to the level of our expectations, we fall to the level of our training."[1] And it's no coincidence that men marching in military parades mimic the peculiar, staccato, high-step gait of aggressively posturing reptiles.

William James, the esteemed psychologist, called habits "the enormous flywheel of society."[2] He recommended putting as many of life's mundane activities as possible on automatic pilot to free the mind in order to ponder more interesting things. "Did you honor your inner reptile today?" might make a catchy bumper sticker.

If you've ever had a pet snake or turtle, you know how difficult it is to have a warm, fuzzy relationship with them. It's not just that they lack fur, it's because they lack emotions, which is another distinctive feature of reptiles. Don't take it personally. They don't bond with their offspring, either. After hatching, the baby reptile must flee into the underbrush, or in the case of the Komodo dragon, quickly climb a tree where it must live for the first year of life to avoid being eaten by its parents.

When my youngest daughter, Satya, was eight years old, we went to the pet store to buy some "pinkies"—helpless, hairless baby mice to feed her pet snake. The snake stalked the terrified mouse with rapt attention and devoured it without the least hint of enjoyment in its unblinking, cold, reptilian eyes. I suspect witnessing this violent sacrifice had something to do with her becoming a vegetarian not long afterwards.

Our emotional furry friends

The hallmark of mammalian behavior is also easy to remember, as easy as saying, "*mamma*," Latin for breast, as in mammary gland. Mammals are all about breast feeding and not surprisingly, "mama," or a close variant, was likely one of the first words you ever uttered (or should I say "uddered") as is true of newborn babes in many languages. Unlike reptiles that lay eggs, mammals are birthed naked and must be nourished at the breast. This in turn necessitated vocal communication to allow mother and baby to find each other for feeding, hence the beginning of language. And for the same reason, they must form a reliable emotional bond, hence the beginning of love. Since the breastfeeding-mother-infant unit is vulnerable to predation, there is an evolutionary pressure to select fathers who will stick around to protect and support them, hence the beginning of family. From the humble act of breastfeeding came the impetus for language, love, family, and civilization itself.

Evolutionary neurobiologists theorize the limbic brain developed in response to mammals living in herds, which necessitated more sophisticated behaviors called emotions. Emotions serve two important survival functions. First, they promote social cohesiveness through communication. The mother-infant bond serves as a template for love, loyalty, and altruism. For this reason, maternity leave is an extremely valuable societal investment and an enlightened society honors and protects the mother-child relationship. Second, emotions filter what is most critical to our survival from the deluge of incoming data and then amplify it, highlighting what must be remembered. For instance, many people remember exactly where they were (even what they were doing) during cataclysmic events like the collapse of the Twin Towers or the assassination of John F. Kennedy.

Because emotions are the key to remembering, they are also the key to learning. This has been demonstrated in experiments where young infants rapidly acquire language during face-to-face, human interaction but not when placed before a computer screen. The same is true of adults who learn more effectively in the classroom than online. Human relationships create an emotional need to please and fit in with the herd. This may explain why women, who are generally more emotionally attuned, are often better at learning languages and other social skills.[3]

As the word suggests, *e-motions* propel us into action. *E* is a common prefix which means "to move out" as in eject, exit, emerge, effluent, and emit. Emotions are the motive force that puts the wind in our sails.

And then there is play, a complex emotional behavior unique to mammals. Dogs chase each other and tumble in mock combat. We "horse around," play games, and throw parties. We play football, tennis, and other sports as forms of ritualized warfare. One of the most civilized human activities is to play music together. Through play we experience the pleasurable emotion of joy (This is fun!), which from a slightly different angle may be considered a form of love (I love this!).

Games, in addition to being fun, are an essential part of political craft. Roman emperors used "bread and circuses" to forge a collective political identity much like coliseum events today, which begin with standing, placing your right hand over your heart, and singing the national anthem (a salute to the nation and to our reptilian nature). Perhaps that's why China is now spending billions to develop soccer franchises as an emotional entrée onto the world stage—team China.

On the other side of the coin, tyrants routinely exploit the power of negative emotions, fear, anger, guilt, and shame to close ranks and turn the herd against a common enemy, often violently. Although we pride ourselves on our individuality, we have such a deep need to fit in that it can override our better selves. In the thrall of a mob, we can be moved to do things that we would never do on our own, from sporting a new fashion trend to groupthink to soccer stadium stampedes, riots, and ethnic cleansing rampages. Being a herd animal is a mixed blessing.

Paul Maclean in his textbook, *The Triune Brain in Evolution*, makes a startling observation: Truth-making (how we know, what we know) is a function of the emotional limbic brain, not the rational cortical brain. When it comes to controlling herd behavior, emotions always trump ideas, which is why political ads are long on feelings and short on reasons. If habit is the "enormous flywheel," then emotions are the "great glue."

With the evolution of the limbic brain, something else happens that is crucial to our story: pleasure and pain cease to be simply evolved instinctual drives. They are transformed into rewards and punishments and infused with powerful emotions, memories, meaning, and cultural associations. This transformation facilitates complex, nuanced social behaviors motivated by a vast palette of subtle shades of pleasure and pain.

A new brain called "me"

The hallmark of primate behavior is thinking. The neocortex, or cortical brain for short, is composed almost entirely of association neurons that interconnect various brain structures, enabling us to meld thoughts with images, memories, hopes, dreams, sensations, and actions—in short, the full spectrum of all that makes us human. Unlike early mammals that are primarily bound to the present moment, reacting to events as they occur, the cortical brain of primates brings past and future into vivid, imaginary existence. We can now learn from an experience long after the fact and re-interpret it, as well as anticipate what lies ahead. The cortex constructs a virtual map of reality and then hovers above it, outside of space and time. However, we can get so caught up in our virtual thoughts or two-dimensional images on a flat screen that we miss the far richer reality of the ever-present moment.

The cortex evolved to literally "think up" novel responses to the demands of our cultural and physical environment. Along with this newfound ability came a phenomenon called "me," the construction of an abstract agent, a self, who experiences the world. Earlier organisms possess only a rudimentary self-awareness limited to body sensations and instinctual self-preservation.

Beginning with our closest relatives, chimpanzees, bonobos, and a few other species such as dolphins and orcas, a fuller self-consciousness emerged. For the first time, matter became aware of itself! What we call the ego—me, myself and I—is an epiphenomenon of thinking, a pattern of discharges in the neocortex and associated body sensations. "I" only exists as an abstraction, a concept. It is not as real as say, your hand or leg, or a tree. As the Buddhists have long claimed, the self is an illusion, albeit a very convincing one imbued with emotions, memories, and body sensations.

Given that roughly 70 percent of our behavior is under habitual, reptilian control and that we are emotionally (limbic) driven herd animals, we can conclude that the majority of our behavior is subconscious, below or preceding cortical thought. In other words, the ego-self, that incessant, internal voice we call "me," is a relatively small part of who (or what) we actually are. For the same reason, the majority of interpersonal communications by some estimates is body language (55 percent) and tone of voice (38 percent), which leaves just 7 percent for the words spoken.[4]

Understanding the subtle ontological status of me, myself and I, as we will see in the following chapters, is an important step toward entering the three gateways to Paradise—ecstasy, bliss, and equanimity—and our collective survival.

▲▲▲▲▲▲▲

In brief:

Each of the three parts of our sphinx brain has its own unique experience of the world and associated pleasures. Reptiles are cold-blooded, unemotional, and seek repetitive, physical pleasures. Early mammals are warm and fuzzy and seek herd-oriented, emotional pleasures. Primates are thoughtful and rational and seek abstract, mental pleasures. Through the function of the limbic and cortical brains, pleasure and pain take on more complex social meaning and behaviors called reward and punishment. We experience these through an abstraction we call a "self," which ironically, is conscious of only a small portion of its true Self.

Considerations:

- Observe your habitual actions during the day: how you reach for a glass, scratch an itch, wash your face. Become conscious of your subconscious. Awaken.

- How do your emotions color your thinking?

- How do you know what is true?

- Who is in charge? Who should be in charge?

CHAPTER 8

The Pleasure Prism and The Light-Body

▲ 2. The Law of Colors

> *Spirit is our inner light made visible.*
> —JG

I FIRST MET PATTABHI JOIS, THE FOUNDER OF ASHTANGA YOGA, AT FEATHER Pipe Ranch in the Montana Rockies on the edge of Helena National Forest, in May 1987. My roommate, Richard Freeman, and I drove out to attend a seven-day workshop. Each day, fifteen of us lined up in two rows facing each other and went through the hour and a half primary yoga sequence while Guru-ji, as he was affectionately called, worked his way up and down the line adjusting people.

Pattabhi Jois was unremarkable in appearance with a round baby face, portly build, and a traditional Indian white *dhoti* neatly wrapped and folded about his waist. At first glance, you might mistake him for someone's father. But at seventy-two, his skin was smooth as milk chocolate, and he had the vigor and nimbleness of a man half his age. Quickly, with workman-like efficiency, he moved from student to student like a human blacksmith. His method was direct and forceful. He synchronized the student's breathing with a precise sequence of movements to heat the body like a bellows. Once the flesh glowed with sweat and became malleable, he applied pressure, using his whole body to bend and forge the struggling student into the prescribed position, or *asana*.

Each of us had our own particularly difficult *asanas*, and when one of us reached that point in the sequence, he would spend extra time, pressing us deeper into the pose whether we liked it or not. For me, it was *baddha konasana*, the bound angle. In this pose, you sit upright, hands clasping the soles of your feet with knees splayed open like butterfly wings. In the full pose, you turn the soles of your feet upward, as though opening a book, knees flat on the floor, and cantilever forward, placing your chin on the floor (in my case, a distant theory).

Each day when we got to *baddha konasana*, he would be on me, a foot on one thigh and a hand on the other, while his free hand pushed my head toward the floor. I fought back instinctively to keep my groins from being torn apart. "Aah...stiff-man," he mumbled, annoyed, as he let me up and moved on. His concept of the body and its anatomical limits was clearly different from mine. On the fourth day, I was, as usual, sweating, breathing hard, and struggling against him. This time, after pushing on me, he released his grip with his usual irritated grunt, but just as I inhaled with a sigh of relief, he thrust both my knees straight away to the floor with a whumph. It happened quickly and painlessly. I sat, stunned, bolt-upright with my hips completely open. He had been setting me up all week like a cat toying with a mouse, waiting to pounce at the precise moment when my defenses were down. I have never been that deep in *baddha konasana* before or since, but the lesson was unforgettable: what I believed to be my physical limits was nothing more than my mental resistance. What really got me, though, was that he knew my limits better than I did.

In many respects, our Western concept of the body is still stuck in a Newtonian model of ball and socket levers and pulleys operating on a machine-like platform of biochemical algorithms. While our detailed anatomical dissections and biochemical analysis have allowed us to peer into the tiniest dimensions of our physical existence down to a molecular level, they have largely ignored the energetic dimension of our being—the *élan vitale*, the vital impetus—that mysteriously animates and pushes life to evolve toward ever greater levels of self-organizing complexity. As William Wordsworth observed: "Our meddling intellect / Mis-shapes the beauteous forms of things: / We murder to dissect."[1] We destroy the very life force we wish to study in order to place it under the microscope. But the situation is far worse.

Western science does not even recognize the existence of a vital life force, let alone study it, as evidenced by the widespread dismissal and derision of vitalistic concepts. Such hubris is one of the consequences of having a *desert-ed*, dead cosmos for a cultural matrix. For other civilizations, the existence of a vital force is commonplace. It is referred to as *prana* in India and *qi* in China. The closest translation in English is "spirit" from the Latin *spirare* (to breathe). It is intimately related to consciousness, intelligence, and breathing which we will discuss further in Chapters 12 and 18.

▲ The Law of Colors

Let's now broaden our focus and incorporate the narrow, analytical method of taking things apart into a more intuitive, synthetic approach of putting things together. For this purpose, we will employ the optics of the Pleasure Prism to look beyond the purely physical, mechanistic view of the body into its subtle metaphysical nature and explore the relationship of the triune brain to our energy "Light-body." (See Figure 7.)

With the Pleasure Prism, we can break down a pleasurable experience into a spectrum of four colors or levels, the Law of Colors:

Level 1 Physical pleasure (red) Physical pleasures inhabit the realm of the reptile. They are sensual, immediate, and uncomplicated. You don't need to think about the pleasure of receiving a massage or relishing a tasty treat. In fact, thinking, "This really feels or tastes good," is a distraction from the present moment and diminishes the experience.

As we saw earlier, reptilian pleasures have a habitual, repetitive nature. The quirky, personal rituals athletes use to prepare for a game are good examples of this. Michael Jordan, who led the Chicago Bulls to six NBA championships, always wore a slightly longer uniform to cover his lucky North Carolina shorts underneath. (As the alpha male, the long-shorts style caught on and became the new "herd" standard.) Tennis great Serena Williams wears the same pair of socks throughout a tournament, ties her shoelaces in a specific way, and bounces the ball five times before a first serve and twice before a second. She has blamed major losses on not sticking to her routine.

Such rituals are based on the reptilian belief that by repeating a past behavior that once led to a successful (pleasurable) outcome, you can increase your chances for future success. We dismiss such rituals as superstitious or magical thinking, and from the perspective of the cortical brain, they are, but from the perspective of the reptilian brain, it's not about thinking. It's simply a matter of repeating what works. Recall that reptiles always take the same route to the feeding grounds even though shorter routes exist. After all, athletic skills like shooting baskets and hitting tennis balls are honed through countless hours of repetition and depend on a well-trained reptile.

Another telltale sign of reptilian pleasure is rhythm. Whether it's waking up at the same time each day and making your cup of coffee or tapping your foot to a primal drum beat, rhythm is a reptile thing. The gyrations of Elvis "the pelvis" and Jim Morrison "the Lizard King" are legendary. Or consider the rhythmic undulations of a temptress, pole dancer re-enacting the Fall of Man in some smoky strip joint. And there's nothing quite like swarming body-to-body in a mosh pit to get your inner "rep-tail" on.

Physical pleasure is red—the color of passion, power, lust, aggression, vitality, blood, and survival. It is the lowest frequency and the longest wavelength of visible light. Like the bass note in music and the foundation of a building, it represents the source of core strength in the body.

The physical center is located in the pelvis. In the yogic system, there are seven main *chakras* (whirling vortices of *pranic* energy) that correspond to the major ganglionic plexuses (key centers) in the peripheral nervous system. We will focus on just three. The first is the *muladhara chakra*. *Mula* in Sanskrit means "root, source, foundation." It is said the *kundalini*,

The Pleasure Prism and The Light-Body

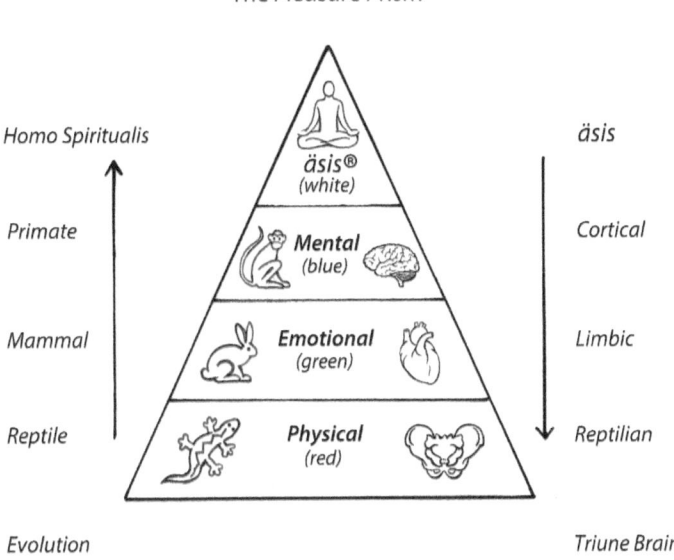

Figure 7: The four levels (colors) of the Pleasure Prism in relationship to the stages of evolution, the triune brain, and the human body.

or serpent energy, lies sleeping at the base of the spine coiled three and a half times. The *muladhara chakra* is depicted by a square, signifying stability. In Chinese medicine, the pelvis represents earth and *yin* essence. Accordingly, the strongest and most interior *yin* acupuncture point on the body is located at the perineum precisely halfway between the base of the genitals and the anus. Its name is *Huiyin*, the gathering point of all the *yin* channels of the body.

Level 2 Emotional pleasure (green) Emotional pleasures inhabit the realm of the mammal. As noted previously, love, happiness, joy, excitement, and fun are simply pleasures experienced at an emotional level, but what does that mean? What is an emotion? The answer is suggested by the anatomical location of the limbic brain, which is sandwiched between the reptilian and cortical brains. An emotion combines elements of both: sensations and thoughts.

When I say, "I feel excited," it means I feel alert and energized in the body. My eyes are wide open and thoughts of anticipation race through my mind. When I feel depressed, my limbs are heavy and my thoughts run dull and dark. I experience fear as a feeling of tightness and nausea in the pit of my stomach, my shoulders are drawn, and I have negative, worrisome thoughts. Anger rises up my back like a flame and curls my lips with self-righteous indignation.

We have difficulty talking about our emotions in part because our language is imprecise. We use the same word "feel" to describe a sensation (it feels soft) and to indicate an emotional state (I feel excited)—a body sensation *and* a thought. Such ambiguity presents serious methodological problems, especially for happiness researchers.

For instance, suppose someone asks, "Are you happy?" If I take that to mean, "Do I feel happy at this moment, brimming with warm, light sensations in my chest and a smile on my lips?" then, "No, I'm not particularly happy right now." But, if I interpret the question as, "Am I happy with my life in general?" then I would need to think it over for a moment, after which I might conclude, "Yes, I'm fairly happy with my life these days." The first interpretation of the question emphasizes the momentary physical aspect of happiness and the second its longer-term mental assessment. The potential for misunderstanding is even worse with cross-cultural studies that introduce a confounding layer of culture-specific expectations and perceptions. That's why it's difficult to compare the happiness of a Bushman living in a mud hut to the happiness of a Silicon Valley executive living in a mansion.

Emotional pleasures exist at the fluid boundary between physical and mental pleasures and contain differing proportions of each, which accounts for the many shades of emotional pleasure we experience. For clarity, I will refer to body sensations as the "body-stream" and mental thoughts as the "mind-stream." Take for example, the difference between happiness and satisfaction. Happiness is more body-stream—sensual and in the moment—and feels relatively hotter toward the red end of the spectrum. Satisfaction is more mind-stream—cerebral and independent of time—and runs a bit cooler toward the blue end of the spectrum. That's why it's possible to feel happy without being satisfied, satisfied without being happy, or "purplish," both at the same time.

Emotional pleasure is green—the color of spring, growth, and renewal when everything comes to life. Hence, it is associated with the environment, ecology, and sustainability. It is midway in the frequency and wavelength spectrum of visible light and conveys a feeling of calm harmony as when looking out over a field of grass or a forest canopy.

The emotional center is located in the heart region. In the yogic system, it is known as the *anahata chakra* (*anahata* refers to the *nada*, the unstruck, primordial sound that fills the cosmos). It is the fourth *chakra* midway among the primary seven and is depicted by superimposed upward and downward facing triangles, symbolizing the union of male and female and the balancing of opposites. In Chinese acupuncture, *Shanzhong* point, located at the center of the chest, is the controlling, gathering point of *qi* energy in the body.

Level 3 Mental pleasure (blue) Mental pleasures inhabit the realm of the primate. We delight in learning new ideas, solving puzzles, or reading a good book. The nostalgia of a fond memory steeped in sepia tones has its own delicate sweetness, as does the anticipation of a budding romance or the satisfaction of knowing you've done a great job. Then there are the acquired intellectual tastes for an elegant scientific theory, the spare beauty of a mathematical equation, the intricate composition of a piece of music, or the catchy lyrics of a popular song. Collectors enjoy the abstract pleasure of owning a signed original or other rare items. I experience a special pleasure when I wear the herringbone sweater my mother knitted for me.

A unique feature of mental pleasure is its ability to be self-propagating. The Chinese have a traditional blessing for newlyweds called "double happiness." I like to think of it as being happy about being happy. Like the power of positive thinking, simply telling ourselves we are happy, beautiful, and smart makes us feel better about ourselves. Indeed, positive thinking can spark initiative and increase the chances of fulfilling our desires. This effect has been popularized and shamelessly marketed as the "Law of Attraction." But, as we'll discuss in Chapter 18, desire is only half the equation.

One of the most important areas of mental pleasure is existential:

thinking that my life matters and has meaning and purpose. Such ideas comfort us. They give us an identity, a *raison d'être* (reason to be), and sense of belonging that immunizes us against feelings of insignificance and the terror of emptiness. According to Austrian psychiatrist and Holocaust survivor Viktor Frankl, "striving to find meaning in one's life" is an essential human drive.[2] For this reason, *work is more than just a way of earning a living; it's a way of earning a life.* When we are actively engaged, we feel inspired and know who we are and where we're headed. When disengaged, we dither, lose our bearings, and may even become suicidal.

Mental pleasure is blue—the color of the sky and ocean, vast and formless. It suggests dynamic change, lightness, and space. Its higher frequency and shorter wavelength are consistent with the more refined energy of the thinking process, which is abstract, insubstantial, and dream-like.

The mental center (as I'm referring to it here) is located in the region of the soft palate at the back of the throat. In the yogic system, it is called *talu chakra* (*talu* meaning "palate"), one of the lesser-known esoteric chakras, which has a profound effect on thinking. In Chinese medicine, it corresponds to *Renzhong* point, which is located where the upper lip meets the nose. This is an extremely sensitive and powerful point that is used for its stimulatory effect in emergency conditions such as loss of consciousness and also for profound calming in conditions of acute anxiety or mania.

Level 4 Spiritual pleasure (white) We now come to the highest level of the Pleasure Prism: the realm of *Homo spiritualis*, where we experience ecstasy, bliss, equanimity, and the rapture of deep connection. Unlike the previous three pleasures, it has no corresponding anatomical brain structure. Rather it arises when the physical, emotional, and mental brains have been well cultivated and integrated in a balanced way. What to call this ultimate level of pleasure is problematic. The word "spiritual," like happiness, has been so hackneyed as to be rendered almost meaningless. When speaking loosely I will sometimes refer to this fourth level as spiritual, and to be more precise, I will use the term *"äsis."*

The meaning of *äsis* is in its sound; it's an onomatopoeia. To get a feel for it, simply take a deep breath and exhale with a satisfying *aah* sound.

Now try it again with feeling *aah* ... Now once more with your lips closed. *Mmm* ... that feels good! (In Chapter 18 I will describe how *äsis* can be used as a mantra for a powerful pleasure meditation.)

Contrary to conventional assumptions, we reach the top of the prism not by transcending, but by descending. That is, we reach the highest pleasures not by denying our human biology, as though it were some unclean, mortal husk to be discarded, but by embracing it and descending into the murky depths of our mental, emotional, and physical levels of existence to bring them into enlightened harmony and balance. From the perspective of *äsis*, higher and lower lose their meaning. *The only difference between the sacred and the profane is in how we approach them.* In reality, you have to crouch before you jump; you have to dig a foundation before you raise a building; and you have to go down before you go up. To spurn the lowly for the high is to misunderstand the nature of reality and the nature of pleasure.

The color of *äsis* pleasure is white—a color that emerges when red, green, and blue light are combined in balanced proportion. White contains all the colors of the rainbow in much the same way as zero contains all the numbers of the number line. You can think of white light as an infinity of colors.

The *äsis* center is located a hand-breadth above the head. In the classical yogic tradition, the crown, or seventh *chakra*, is depicted as a thousand-petaled lotus blossom called *sahasrara,* meaning a thousand. In Chinese medicine, the highest, most *yang* point on the surface of the body is at the vertex of the head and known as *Baihui,* the gathering point of a hundred *yang* channels. It is the mirror image of *Huiyin,* the gathering point of *yin* channels at the perineum. In both the yogic and Chinese systems, the crown and root define the plus and minus poles of the Light-body that connect us to heaven and earth. Interestingly, we find a similar association in a king's crown whose earthly authority derives from receiving "divine goodness" from the heavens above.

The witness

At the *äsis* level, we encounter something supremely subtle and sublime called the "witness," the fourth operator—pure consciousness—that can dispassionately observe the other three brains. The term "pure consciousness" emphasizes the fact that consciousness is not something that we own or possess, any more than we own or possess the air that we breathe. (Recent research suggests that the brain may not actually generate the mind, but receives it, as a television receives a signal.) The mind is something that moves through us, animates, and enlightens us. At the same time, it underlies all that we experience and, like the breath, is so close to us that we hardly notice it. But there are even more subtle reasons we overlook it.

To begin with, just as a flashlight can't illuminate itself and no one can see their own eye, awareness can't be aware of itself. The moment you look for your awareness, it vanishes. I once had a vivid dream in which a second body had been seamlessly affixed to the backside of my body. Everything I saw, heard, smelled, tasted, touched, or thought was also being experienced by this second body. It felt wonderful and deeply satisfying to share my every experience intimately with another. Overjoyed, I looked back to see who it was, but because it was affixed to my back, I couldn't see anyone. A moment later, I awoke with a profoundly peaceful feeling and this thought: *Could it be that the soulmate we seek is our very own consciousness?* Ever since that expansive dream, the loneliness that had often stalked me was transformed into an intimate companionship with a consciousness far beyond myself, both vast and profound, yet closer than my own breath.

What made this dream so extraordinary is that, technically speaking, when immersed in pure consciousness, there is no "I" to objectify it; there is no "self" and therefore no self-awareness. There is only pure awareness. But in the dream, I could "feel" my consciousness.

The word "consciousness" is slippery; it's hard to wrap our mind around because it's so huge. Awareness is much more manageable. I can focus my awareness on my computer screen or the bird outside my window at will. I can narrow it to a fine point for laser detail or broaden it to take in a large view like a search light. Yet, consciousness and awareness are one and the same thing. Awareness is just a particular, personal experience of universal consciousness. The Hindus describe this as the relationship between *Brahman* and *Atman*, where *Brahman* is a river of consciousness (the signal) and *Atman* is like a pipe placed in the river (the receiver) around which the water flows.

If all this seems a bit confusing, don't worry. We will approach this paradox of the particular and the universal from a number of different directions and by the end of the book, you will have an intuitive grasp of it. Ultimately, *äsis* pleasure is not something to be understood intellectually; it is something to be experienced. I describe how in Chapter 18.

A classic image of pure consciousness from ancient Egypt and Asia is that of a lotus blossom, which humbly takes root in dark, muddied waters that others shun yet each morning spreads open its petals, pure and unstained, to receive the illumination of the sun, the clear white light of the *summum bonum*, the highest good.

Rethinking the body

The body is much more than we think. Our conventional Western view reminds me of old anatomy textbooks, which had transparent overlays so that as you turned the page, you first see the muscles, then the organs, nerves, blood vessels, and lastly the skeletal bones. In medical school, we added a few more layers and looked at the tissues and cells, first under a light microscope and then under an electron microscope. Finally, we looked biochemically, down to the level of molecules in the DNA within the cell nucleus. Such is the incredible penetrating power of analysis.

The Eastern view takes a different approach. Asians didn't do dissections, which in the days before refrigeration must have required some serious fortitude. Instead, they stepped back and looked at the body from a phenomenological perspective and tried to understand how it works by analogy to nature: the flow of water and wind, sun and moon, heat and dampness. Both the ancient Indian yogis and the Chinese Taoists perceived channels—*nadis* and *meridians*—through which the vital energy of the body flows. The yogis added a few more overlays, subtle bodies called *koshas*, sheaths. Each of these sheaths was envisioned to be composed of increasingly finer grades of energy. The innermost sheath is known as *anandamaya kosha*, the bliss body, or what I am describing here as the Light-body.

The Triune Brain and Light-body

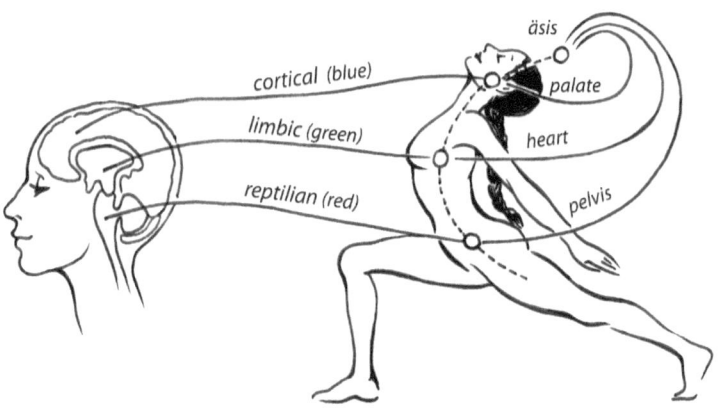

Figure 8: The triune brain and the four vital pleasure centers of the Light-body.

Consciousness is often compared to light because both illuminate. The Pleasure Prism describes how a pleasurable experience is refracted through the "optical" properties of the triune brain to illuminate the Light-body. Like a rainbow, there are no sharp edges that separate the different colors. Rather, we experience different frequencies and wavelengths of pleasure dynamically shifting and blending one into the other like the colors of oil on water. Thus, a pleasure encountered at one level quickly swirls into the others. Hearing a familiar song on the radio can trigger strong emotions that mentally transport us back to our college days. Knowing we've helped someone with an act of kindness can generate warm emotional feelings. Indeed, we often find meaning and purpose in our lives through service to others, which can make giving more gratifying than receiving.

Physical pleasure is at the base of the prism for a very important

The Pleasure Prism and The Light-Body

reason. All pleasures, regardless of where they originate, whether at an emotional, mental, or *äsis* level, quickly soak through to the physical plane and generate pleasant body sensations. *It is ultimately these pleasant body sensations that define not only what feels good, but the very meaning (the experiential referent) for words such as good, beautiful, meaningful, and other positive attributions, which are simply different refractions of pleasure.* You can observe this for yourself. The next time you lay your eyes on a beautiful object, such as a mountain peak, a work of art, or an attractive person, notice that as your eye moves over the object, subtle pleasant sensations begin to stir and stream through your body. The same thing occurs when we are in the company of good friends, receive praise for a job well done, or get goosebumps walking through a redwood forest. *Every pleasure is ultimately experienced in and through the Light-body.*

The Pleasure Prism is a luminous map whose secrets, if you know how to interpret them, can lead you back to the Garden of Eden from whence we came. Within each of the three *chakras* noted above, there resides a vital pleasure center which we will locate anatomically in Chapter 18. When these three vital centers are fully activated and aligned, we spontaneously experience *äsis*, the clear white light of pure consciousness, which is nothing other than ecstasy, bliss, and equanimity. The instant Pattabhi Jois slammed my knees to the floor into *baddha konasana* and I was sitting bolt upright, it was like a light switch had been turned on. For a few moments, the gates had opened and everything, within my body and without, was extraordinarily vibrant and clear.

▲▲▲▲▲▲▲

In brief:

In Part 2, we traced the evolution of pleasure from reptiles to mammals to primates and described how we are heir to all three. In the process, our thinking evolved from the analytic to the synthetic and from the physical anatomy of the triune brain to the metaphysical anatomy of the Light-body. We have seen through the lens of the Pleasure Prism that words, such as "good," "beautiful," "meaningful," and other positive attributions are merely different refractions (frequencies) of pleasure. At the *äsis* level we encounter the witness—pure consciousness—the clear white light that illuminates all that we experience and mysteriously animates our physical body and is the medium through which the *élan vitale*, *prana*, and *qi* propagate. We will have more to say about these subtle aspects as we delve deeper into the phenomenology of pleasure in preparation for our approach to the three gateways to Paradise: ecstasy, bliss, and equanimity. For now, here is a summary of the terrain we've covered:

Level	Triune brain	Pleasure	Color	Characteristic	Light-body (chakra)
1	Reptile	Physical	Red	Habit, ritual	Pelvis (*muladhara*)
2	Limbic	Emotional	Green	Love, happiness	Heart (*anahata*)
3	Cortical	Mental	Blue	Abstract, meaning	Palate (*talu*)
4	Integration	*äsis*/Spiritual	White	Ecstasy, bliss, peace	Crown (*sahasrara*)

Considerations:

- Practice focusing on body sensations (the body-stream) rather than thinking (the mind-stream). Thinking is an abstraction which distracts us from the reality of sensations.

- Pause at moments in the day to behold the mystery of your body and existance. Be *aah*struck.

- Notice the different colors and shades of the pleasures you enjoy (physical, emotional, mental, and *äsis*).

- Notice that you are noticing!

Part 3: **The Natural History**

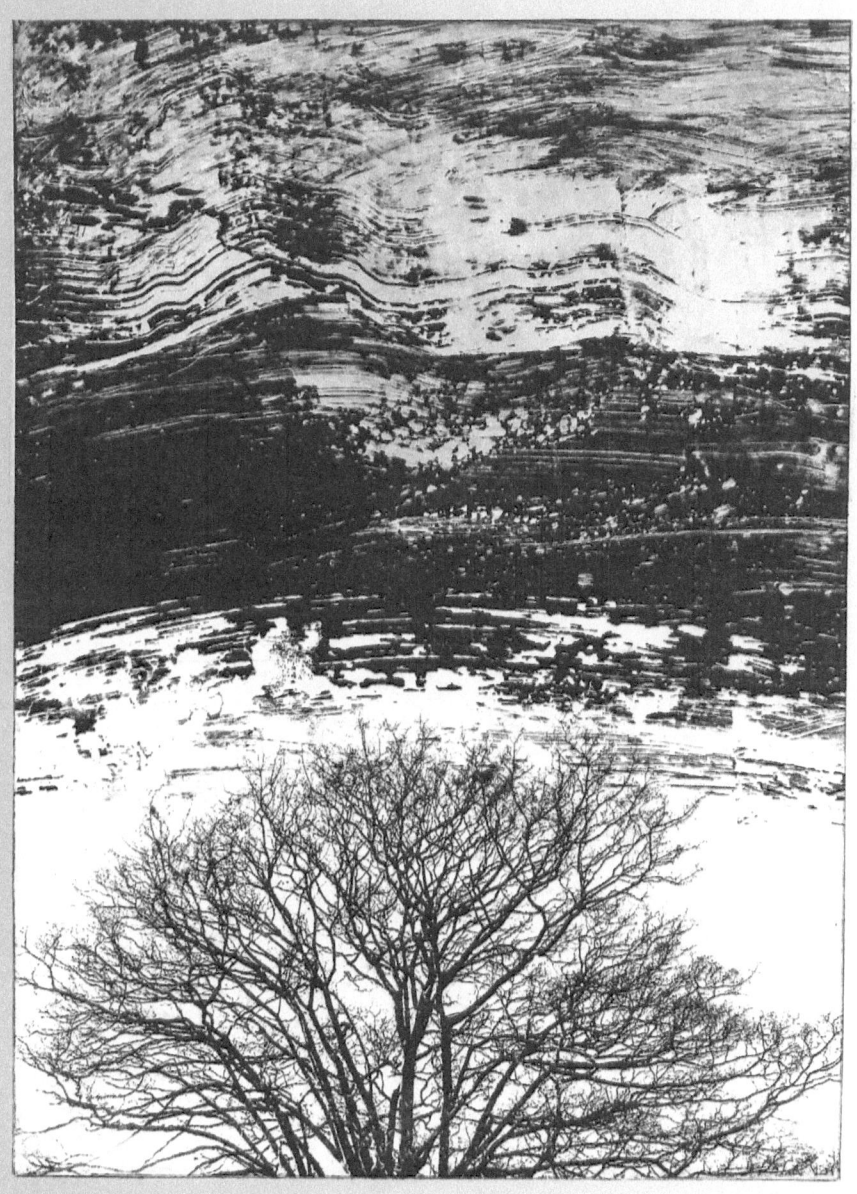

CHAPTER 9

Real Compared to What

▲ 3. The Law of Contrast and Comparison

> *If one only wished to be happy,*
> *this could be easily accomplished;*
> *but we wish to be happier*
> *than other people,*
> *and this is always difficult, for we believe*
> *others to be happier than they are.*
> —Baron de Montesquieu

OUR EXPERIENCE OF PLEASURE ULTIMATELY DEPENDS ON OUR PERCEPTION, but perception is a funny thing. It is much less objective than we imagine. We assume that we all inhabit the same world. While this may be objectively true in terms of what can be measured, each of us experience a different world. A dog sees a world of muted shades of yellow and blue four to eight times less distinctly than we do, but smells a world fifty times more richly scented. A bee sees flowers in ultraviolet colors, and a bat hears ultrasonic sounds in 3-D. Consider the silent and sightless world of a tick. It climbs to the tip of a blade of grass guided by its skin's sensitivity to light, and when it smells butyric acid, an odor emitted from the sebaceous glands of mammals, it detaches into free fall. Talk about blind faith. If it's lucky enough to land on its prey, it uses a special organ tuned to 37 degrees Celsius (the temperature of mammalian blood) to find a suitable spot to bury its eyeless, earless head and feed.

Each organism perceives and experiences its own world according to its biological needs. In the early 1900s, biologist Jakob von Uexküll dubbed this relationship of an organism with its environment *umwelt* (German for "environment"). He understood this to be a dynamic relationship through which an organism both shapes and is shaped by its surroundings.

The same is true at an *intra*-species level. Each of us experiences our own world, our own *umwelt,* known only to ourselves. There is no way to know if my enjoyment of a peach is the same as yours. What we do know is that each of us is born with a unique composition of neurotransmitters and receptor sensitivities. The differences in our biochemistry are far greater than the differences in how we look. These individual variations incline us in a particular direction and then become amplified or diminished by our environment and personal history that ultimately shapes who we become. An artist, for example, sees beauty and is sensitive to color just as a musician is to sounds and a writer is to words. A scientist sees how things work and an entrepreneur spots business opportunities. As writer Anaïs Nin observed, "We don't see things as they are, we see them as we are,"[1] and what we are is a living process in an endless dance with our environment.

It's all relative

Our senses are not like a mirror passively reflecting the outer world. They continually adjust to the ambient light, sound, smell, taste, and touch and actively shape the world we experience. When we walk into a florist shop, we are immediately struck by a thick, humid fragrance hanging in the air, yet within moments, this refreshing experience fades imperceptibly into the background. We feel the initial thrust of an elevator, but then, feel that we are standing still. Even the most experienced pilots, within moments of initiating a banked turn, feel that they are flying straight and must rely on their instruments for a true orientation.

Have you ever had the jarring experience of looking out the window of a train and suddenly feel yourself lurch backwards, only to discover that the adjacent train was pulling forward? Our perception of something as basic as stillness and motion, as Einstein keenly observed, is entirely relative. For example, at this very moment, you are spinning around the earth's axis at nearly 1,000 mph suspended by your feet and wheeling about the sun at 67,000 mph. And if you're not feeling queasy yet, that's just for starters. Our sun, along with the rest of the stars in our Milky Way Galaxy, is spiraling around a massive black hole at the galactic center at 490,000 mph, and our local group of galaxies is barreling through space at nearly 600 miles per second—that's over 2 million mph![2] If you like to travel, consider this: a year from now, you will have traversed some 19 billion miles of space! So, the quaint image of the earth circling the sun like a merry-go-round is only true relative to the sun. From an astronomical frame of reference, the earth and other planets are corkscrewing through space, following the sun as it circumnavigates the galactic center—a journey of about 230 million years, known as a galactic year.

▲ The Law of Contrast and Comparison

The relative nature of perception—the ceaseless contrasting, comparing, and adjusting to our environment—is literally hardwired into our nervous system. Each neuron has a resting voltage across its cell membrane that is raised or lowered by tiny increments as electrical charges are received from other neurons in its network. Moment by moment, the individual neuron contrasts and compares its current voltage to its resting voltage. When the voltage falls below a certain threshold, the neuron depolarizes, firing a spark of information down the line. Thus, each neuron functions as a tiny digital switch that is either "on" or "off," like the billions of transistor switches embedded in the silicon chip of your computer. Ultimately, it is the synchronous discharging of millions of neurons blinking on and off in ever-changing patterns in your brain that creates sensations, thoughts, emotions, and muscular movements—your entire conscious experience—much like digital bits and pixels create simulations on your computer screen.

Zooming out to the next level of organization, we come to the five senses—eyes, ears, nose, tongue, and touch—which also work in terms of contrast and comparison. We are as blind in a blizzard whiteout as on a pitch-black, moonless night. It is the alternating light and shadow that allows us to see. Similarly, the white noise of a waterfall is as deafening as the silence of a forest blanketed in freshly fallen snow. When you hold your partner's hand at the movies, you need to squeeze it from time to time to let them know you're still there. Without contrast, we are senseless, blind, deaf, tasteless, and numb.

Asians believe there are six doorways to consciousness—the usual five, plus thinking. This makes "sense" because what we think powerfully affects our perception. Thinking also works by contrast and comparison. To think, we must first break reality into conceptual pieces, symbols, words, numbers, and images. Then, applying the rules of grammar and logic, we contrast and compare one fragment to another to develop a unit of meaning. These chunks of meaning are then assembled in an orderly way to form an idea which, when woven together with other ideas, creates something called understanding. That's what I'm doing now as I write these words and what you're doing as you read them.

Confusion, on the other hand, is a form of mental white noise where jumbled thoughts cascade through the mind like a cataract. In contrast—and by comparison—when you experience a profound state of calm, the broken pieces of reality are restored to their Original Wholeness and the mind-stream meanders smoothly like a gentle brook. Notice that in both extremes of profound confusion or profound calm, contrast and comparison ceases and thinking is momentarily suspended as with the other senses. As we will see, the ability to suspend thought is an important skill to master, especially if you wish to enjoy the higher frequencies of pleasure.

It cuts both ways

Like many things, our greatest strength can be our greatest weakness. It all depends on how we use it. On the plus side, we have an ability to habituate and continuously re-calibrate our awareness, relegating what is unchanging and constant to the background so what is novel stands out. This adaptability allows us to walk through a forest with chirping birds and dappled light, yet remain alert to the snapping of a twig or a shadow moving through the underbrush, which could make the difference between getting dinner or being dinner. This same ability has allowed us to adapt to the sweltering, equatorial jungles of Africa and the frigid tundra of the Arctic, making the entire globe habitable.

On the minus side, the dulling effect of habituation makes us a restless lot, forever in search of greener pastures. Habituation is the mother of appetite, ambition, aggression, and a fondness for conquest, often violent. It stamps every pleasure with a limited shelf life. As a result, no matter how plentiful your food or lovely the scenery, no matter how big your house or beautiful your partner, no matter how much money you have in the bank or stellar your success, you eventually get used to it, take it for granted, and become bored. Stale pleasure is no pleasure at all, and we soon begin to look for new, more exciting experiences—a change of scenery, a new restaurant, a new lover, a Cyrenaic indulgence, perhaps. If, as William James said, habit is the enormous flywheel of society, it is also the great leveler, reducing what was once fresh and stimulating to humdrum routine.

For better or worse, our nervous system is hardwired for novelty. Habituation constantly resets the baseline expectations in our VTA brainstem, ratcheting our desires ever higher, insuring our perpetual discontent. In an economy that depends on selling next year's model and measures success in terms of one's net worth and an expanding GDP, our discontent and insatiable appetite are actively cultivated (and exploited) with multimillion-dollar marketing campaigns.

Are we destined then to be consumer-slaves to an endless product cycle in pursuit of more and more … of everything? Are we fated to be like mealworms in a sack of flour that consume themselves into oblivion, poisoned on their own waste? Avoiding this mealy outcome requires a radical change in many areas of life, especially how we go about teaching our children about pleasure.

Growing up with contrast

I was shocked the first time I heard my three-year-old daughter say, "I'm bored." She must have picked up the word at daycare like a communicable disease, and I had to think fast to come up with an antidote. "There's no such thing as boring," I said. "There are only boring people … you don't want to be a b-o-r-i-n-g person, do you?"

I taught my daughters instinctively as my father had taught me. He believed that education was 80 percent exposure, so I exposed my girls to a wide range of experiences, particularly high-contrast ones like skiing in Beaver Creek, Colorado, with our friends, the Landis's, through a raging blizzard. The snow was coming down horizontally and sandblasting our faces with stinging cold, which got worse the faster we skied. My girls were suffering, but the only thing we could do was keep going to get to Beano's Cabin, a posh restaurant on the mountainside. It was heavenly to come in from the biting cold, step out of our ski boots into cozy slippers, and sit down to a fabulous meal while the tempest raged outside.

On another occasion, I took my girls from Denver to Las Vegas on a Greyhound Bus, naively thinking it would be like travelling by bus in the Third World with a cross section of people. I was wrong. In America, only poor people ride "the Dog." At one point, Satya couldn't sleep because the guy in front of her smelled so bad. At three in the morning, we arrived at the bus-cleaning stop and everyone had to get off and sit under the glaring light of the station canteen. When we finally made it to Las Vegas, we stayed at the kid-friendly Circus Circus hotel and the next night had front-row, balcony seats at the Bellagio to see Cirque du Soleil's enchanting performance of "O." It was the high contrast that made these experiences memorable. The blackest nights have the brightest stars. It's just the way the nervous system works.

It was no small feat to raise my girls with a sense of value and appreciation in a wealthy town like Boulder, where entitlement is a way of life. It's crucial because if a person lacks gratitude, they will never know true wealth.

Another important area of childhood development is adolescent rites of passage, which serve to contrast and demarcate one's entry into adulthood. Unfortunately, aside from the occasional religious confirmation, *bar mitzvah,* or debutant party, coming of age is often given short shrift in the West. In many indigenous cultures, a child is not recognized as a full member of the tribe until she or he has undergone a ritualized death and rebirth, which can be extremely strenuous and entail real mortal risks.

Among the Tikuna people of the Amazon, a girl is separated from the tribe for up to a year and lives in isolation in a small thatched shelter in the jungle after her first menstruation.[3] Her only human contact is her grandmother, who instructs her in many skills, from weaving, plant cultivation, and medicine to caring for a baby and being a wife. It is a deep, cross-generational experience that honors both the adolescent and the elder. At the end of her seclusion, the young woman is adorned in elaborate dress and feathers and brought wrapped in blankets to the *maloka,* a communal gathering house where a huge feast awaits. Like a butterfly emerging from its chrysalis, the blankets are removed to reveal the beautiful metamorphosis that has taken place, and the entire village celebrates with food, dancing, and song for three or four days.

One of the most intense rites of passage is that of the Pentecost Islanders of Vanuatu. Young boys must "land dive" headfirst off platforms as high as sixty feet with vines tied about their ankles. The vines are carefully prepared by their family to have the precise length and tensile strength (stretch). The ritual demands tremendous courage and a true leap of faith, as the ideal dive allows the boy's crown to just graze the earth to ensure a bountiful harvest.

Adolescents know at a cellular level that they must "die" in order to be reborn. Because we lack meaningful rituals to empower our youth, millions of adolescents are lost, clinically depressed, muddling through, half-dead, half-born. This is reflected in the morbid aesthetics of goth and heavy metal subculture. Drug taking is in part an attempt to assert one's independence through an act of defiance (recapitulating the parent-child dynamics of the "terrible twos"). How many senseless "accidental" deaths, homicides, and suicides—which account for nearly three quarters of all teenage deaths—could be prevented by providing a real initiation into adulthood?

In my case, I had two self-styled initiations. Both revolved around speed. At age fifteen, my friend Mark and I would wait until his father fell asleep and then push his black 327 Chevy down the long driveway onto the road to go for a joy ride. We'd stop under a street light, pop the hood, and remove the air cleaner to make the engine sound throatier. After a night of cruising, we'd sometimes end up on County Line Road, a long, straight stretch of highway over rolling hills through dense forest. Because it bordered two counties, it was unpatrolled by the local police. Mark would floor it, and I'd watch the speedometer needle disappear past 120 mph (called "burying it"). And then, just for kicks, he'd turn off the headlights for a few long seconds as we hurtled through space, suspended between life and death. I seriously doubt we would have felt a need to do such a crazy stunt if we knew that someday, we'd be land diving in front of the whole village with our ancestors bearing witness from the other side.

My second initiation happened when I turned twenty. I had just read Nikos Kazantzakis's novel *Zorba the Greek* and was hungry to taste life and follow Zorba's example of living passionately to the full. At one point, Zorba tells the boss, "While experiencing happiness, we have difficulty in being conscious of it. Only when the happiness is past and we look back on it we suddenly realize—sometimes with astonishment—how happy we had been."[4] I reasoned the key to living a good life must be to create beautiful memories, which meant engaging the moment boldly, taking risks, and trusting the unexpected. That summer I found a cheap flight to Europe, bought a Triumph 650 Bonneville motorcycle in London, and drove 4,000 miles as far north as Sweden and as far south as Greece. (I am indebted to my father, who clearly understood what was at stake and sent me off with his blessings.) I knew from the moment I got my motorcycle that someday I'd have to open it up to see how fast she could go.

That day happened on the Autostrada superhighway, which winds down the spine of Italy. Like the Autobahn, it had no speed limit. My motorcycle and I were well broken in and there was not a car in sight. It was a calm, slightly overcast day with a smooth, straight road ahead, when I decided to go for it. I put my feet on the rear pegs, laid my chest on the gas tank and wound the throttle wide open. At 100 mph, the bike began to vibrate, but there was more to go. At just over 120 mph, she topped out. I have never had a more exhilarating and terrifying forty-five seconds.

But the risk of speed wasn't enough for me to become a man. I had to face my own death. At the end of my trip, I met up with a college girlfriend in Athens and rode up to an overlook of the city that had a military installation at the top. On the way down, I was showing off, driving faster than I should down the winding, potholed road. The last thing I remember was leaning hard into a tight turn when all of a sudden, a thick steel bumper was coming right at my shoulder. A military truck was barreling up around the blind bend and failed to honk its warning horn. Reflexively, I straightened up the bike and began downshifting. The next thing I knew, I was on the side of the road with the bike on top of me. Julie, who was wearing my helmet, slid free. Neither of us was hurt (besides my leg getting banged up a bit), and the bike was amazingly undamaged. Later, I came across the truck at a restaurant stop and matched up my bike with the bumper to find out what happened. A half-inch round steel flag post jutting out from the bumper at a forty-five-degree angle had struck my handle bar, knocking us out of the path of the truck. "Two equally steep and bold paths may lead to the same peak," Zorba told the boss. "To act as if death did not exist, or to act thinking every minute of death, is perhaps the same thing."[5] I had tempted the fates and luckily survived my appointment with death. That summer I became a man. I had learned how to live on my own and create beautiful memories through high-contrast experiences, which set the course for the rest of my life.

When it comes to contrast and comparison, nothing is starker than life and death. But living on the perilous edge is not sustainable, as every adrenaline junkie knows. What if we could experience life and death more subtly without risking life and limb? There is a way, a very simple, elegant way of dying to our momentary experience that is the secret to ecstasy, bliss, and Epicurus's equanimity (*ataraxia*).

▲▲▲▲▲▲▲

In brief:

Perception is a highly personal, subjective experience. Every organism inhabits its own world (*umwelt*), which it perceives through the lens of its unique neural receptors and past experiences. At the same time, the mechanism of perception itself is continually modulated by the Law of Contrast and Comparison, which is occurring at every scale of our nervous system from the level of the neuron to our six senses. As a result, we rapidly habituate, making us eminently adaptable and at the same time, restless for novel experiences. The ultimate high-contrast experience is found at the edge of life and death, which, as we will see, can also be achieved more subtly in ordinary daily life.

Considerations:

- Walk through the world with humility. Realize that your perception is just one of many. The grass, trees, and birds—every living creature—experiences its own world. Look carefully at a flower blossom and imagine what a bee sees.

- Notice how all perceptions arise, peak, and fade.

- Although boredom is uncomfortable, it holds some important lessons. If you are willing to investigate, you'll discover boredom is actually quite interesting at which point, you'll never be bored again.

- Choose a beautiful landscape feature, perhaps a favorite tree or rock or overlook, as an emotional reference point. Notice how your experience of it changes with the time of day, season, and your mood.

- Take a chance on life and try something new!

CHAPTER 10

Increasing Your Pleasure Capacity

> *I do not understand what the man*
> *who is happy wants*
> *in order to be happier.*
> —Marcus Tullius Cicero

My father used to say, "A hunk of bread, a piece of salami, and a beer—what more could a man want?!" Somewhere in my twenties, I followed his example and took up the habit of drinking a beer with dinner. I relished my nightly beer, and as my medical practice grew, I drank better beer.

One day, my roommate Richard, while glancing at a pile of empty beer bottles gathering dust in the corner of the kitchen like spent cartridge shells, said in his gentle, understated way, "I see you're collecting quite a few bottles." A hint of advice, as subtle as the faint odor emanating from the bottles, was in his voice. He wasn't commenting about my lack of domestic tidiness but was suggesting I clean up something much closer to home.

"Yeah, maybe it's time to take a little of my own medicine," I sighed, "and give the beer a rest."

I stopped the next day. I was surprised how much I missed my nightly brew. At first, I thought it was the dry, sparkling taste that I craved, but then around dinner time I noticed I was getting a little edgy. "Hmmm … just one beer, and I'm really missing it," I thought. "It's irritating not getting what I want." But what did I want? What was the beer giving me?

Some things are most clearly seen in the rearview mirror. Beer had been a comfort, a reward for a hard day's work, my nightly treat for being a "good boy." After a few weeks of abstinence, I decided to drink a bottle and observe its effect: the anticipation of reaching for a cold one; the satisfaction of prying off the cap with a pop and smudge of vapor; pouring the golden liquid along the side of the glass to release its spirit slowly; the familiar tang on my palate; and a strange, stale, bitter aftertaste that I hadn't noticed before.

A half hour later, a soft dullness spread over me like a fuzzy, warm blanket, easing the stress from my body. I felt more relaxed, safe, and content. The next morning, during my daily meditation and yoga practice, I was surprised to detect a slight, yet distinct decrease in clarity and focus. Could this be the dregs of a subtle hangover? Numerous follow-up experiments confirmed that indeed it was. But there was more.

After going weeks without a beer, I could spot exactly when my desire for one arose. Usually, it followed a hard day at the office. This made sense because alcohol is a central nervous system depressant, a "tranquilizer." The reason people become animated and gregarious after a few drinks is because alcohol initially depresses the prefrontal cortex, the good boy part of the brain that inhibits inappropriate behavior. When the good boy is sedated, we feel less inhibited, less self-conscious, and more charming, at least in our own mind. Keep drinking, however, and the depressant effect spreads to other brain regions and becomes more obvious as the system begins to shut down, leading to slurred speech, decreased coordination, stupor, loss of consciousness, and ultimately, death.

I started to notice something odd. After a great day hiking in the mountains or a vigorous workout, when I felt really good basking in the warm afterglow of an endorphin high, that same old hankering for a beer would reappear, seemingly out of nowhere. Why would I want to take a dulling depressant when I was feeling so great? For that matter, why do

Increasing Your Pleasure Capacity

people travel a thousand miles to go skiing in the Rockies and, in the midst of all that immense beauty, feel the urge to drink heavily? In the early days when skiing was a small European sport, it was not uncommon to see someone skiing with a wineskin *bota* or taking a nip out of a silvered flask on the chair lift. After the lifts closed, the drinking continued with *après ski* socializing.

Once on a river trip, a group of friends and I floated for days down a glorious canyon. I was shocked at how much drinking went on. Margaritas before breakfast and a large, orange watercooler lashed to the raft for refills throughout the day. Why does such magnificent beauty whet the appetite for drink?

This paradox crystallized for me in 1994, when I put together an eight-week, stress-reduction program to teach my patients how to transform their lives through breathing, yoga, and meditation. At the end of the program, we sat in a circle to discuss how our lives had changed and fill out a questionnaire. The results were astounding. Out of 194 participants, 92 percent reported improved ability to cope with stress; 91 percent said they had an increased sense of well-being; 74 percent described a marked improvement in severe pain; and 62 percent stated they had reduced medications or eliminated them. I thought I had found the Holy Grail. But, twelve months later, only about a third of the participants had made these practices a regular part of their lives. What was most puzzling were the two-thirds of participants who had reported benefits and then slowly slid back into their former misery.

I had led the proverbial horse to water; it drank from the stream, tasted its sweetness, and then wandered away complaining of thirst. If we are pleasure-seeking organisms, then why would we not do the very thing that makes us feel good? That old haunting question reared its curious head once again.

After examining this phenomenon from every conceivable angle (including my own backsliding), I came to a startling conclusion: *Just as we have a limited capacity for pain*—at a certain point in the dentist's chair we beg for the Novocain—*we have a limited capacity for pleasure!*

I know, it sounds counterintuitive. We think, "Pleasure, I can handle it, just bring it on." Like a beer commercial, we imagine ourselves reaching for all the gusto surrounded by a bar full of cheerful people with frothy mugs in hand. But that's simply not the case. The truth is, we can only take so much pleasure; our capacity is limited.

In more extreme cases, there is a condition known as pleasure anxiety. This is particularly problematic in men who become so sexually excited that they ejaculate shortly after entry or perhaps, even worse, can't muster an erection at all. When the pressure is on and the outcome of a basketball game comes down to a single penalty shot, it's easy to clutch at the free throw line of life. It happens all the time. I had a patient who was one term paper away from graduating college, and she never turned it in.

Most of us are unaware of our limited Pleasure Capacity, as was the case with Victor (not his real name), a Brit I met at the Writer's Bar in Chiang Mai, a local watering hole for expats and would-be-writers. Victor was an amicable bloke in his early fifties with a portly heft and ruddy cheeks. An old Asia hand, he was heading up an NGO refugee program in neighboring Myanmar. When we got around to the subject of my book, he listened with keen interest.

Part way through my rap on St. Augustine and Original Sin, which I was writing about at the time, he interrupted me and said, "My friend, you just put into words something I have been feeling my whole life but didn't know quite how to express." Thoughtfully working his mug of beer, he continued, "It had always been there in the background, a certain awkwardness with my body. Yes, you might even call it shame, but I never really noticed it till I got over here and started having oil massages. I know what you're thinking, but it wasn't about sex. It was about allowing myself to be touched and letting myself enjoy it. I found it difficult to relax. I'd get tense inside and couldn't let go and get into it." Then leaning forward, in a low voice, he said, "You know it took me over a year and quite a few massages, sometimes twice a week, before I started to loosen up. Those kind women with their hands, in the most intimate way, taught me how to relax and enjoy myself." I was happy for him, and at the same time sad

Increasing Your Pleasure Capacity

that it had taken him the better part of his life to learn such a basic thing.

I now understood the experience of my patients who relapsed after the stress-reduction program. As they began to make healthier lifestyle choices, they changed. They began feeling so good that they were no longer sure of who they were. Once a patient who suffered migraines, after her headaches went away, confessed, "I don't know what to do without my migraines."

The reason a chronic illness can be so difficult to treat is because it requires not only getting rid of the illness, but getting rid of the sick identity and narrative that goes along with it. Faced with this choice, some patients would rather return to their less happy, albeit familiar, state of suffering. Such is the power of identity. Patients have become furious with me for daring to take away their illness story. The participants who relapsed had simply exceeded their Pleasure Capacity and couldn't sustain their higher level of well-being. They found excuses to avoid their daily practice and allowed old habits to creep back in the kitchen door like a chastened dog. I realized that, like my patients, I, too, was backing away from pleasure. It was this realization that eventually led me to discover the crucial role of the Pleasure-Pain Threshold.

▲▲▲▲▲▲▲

In brief:

Just as we have a limited capacity for pain, we have a limited capacity for pleasure. It is often this limited Pleasure Capacity that prevents us from making the life-affirming changes we seek. We can see this when we find ourselves avoiding activities that make us feel good—perhaps reaching for a central nervous system depressant like alcohol in the midst of a beautiful experience. Once we realize that we have a limited Pleasure Capacity, we can learn how to increase it, which incidentally, can be a lot of fun (if you can handle it)!

Considerations:
- When things are going well, identify what is working.

- Cultivate what works while allowing for the natural ebb and flow of life.

- When you get off track, start over again with humility, patience, and persistence.

- In the midst of a pleasurable experience, notice if tension arises in your body. How does it change your experience of pleasure?

- Soften, relax, breathe, and allow yourself to feel good. Observe what happens.

- Can you imagine yourself being a happy person who enjoys life? What would you have to let go of to be that person?

CHAPTER 11

The Sensual Continuum

▲ 4. The Law of Thresholds

> *Life and death*
> *exist on a continuum*
> *of awareness.*
> —JG

WE TYPICALLY THINK IN BINARY TERMS, SUCH AS HOT AND COLD, TALL AND short, light and dark, but these merely define the extremes of a continuum with many gradations in between, which is why we have thermometers, light meters, and tape measures. Pleasure and pain are also on a continuum, but not in the way most people think.

While we can objectively measure the intensity of say, temperature or height, there is no way to objectively measure pleasure. As we discussed in Chapter 9, each of us dwells in our own *umwelt* and enjoys our own personal sunset, ice cream cone, love, joy, meaning, purpose, and God. It is this subjectivity that makes the social sciences "soft" in contrast to the measurable "hard sciences" like physics and chemistry.

To see how this works, let's perform a thought experiment with the question we originally began with: What is the opposite of pain? You'll need to use your intuitive, artistic eye rather than the objective eye of a scientist. Imagine a continuum, a Sensual Continuum, based on your perceived intensity of sensation. Perception is a function of both the objective, measurable intensity of a stimulus and your subjective sensitivity to the stimulus and therefore is intimately related to your level of consciousness, or awareness. For instance, to rouse someone who is drunk, whose nervous system is depressed with alcohol, you may have to yell and shake him, while to wake a young child may take only a gentle whisper or light touch on the cheek.

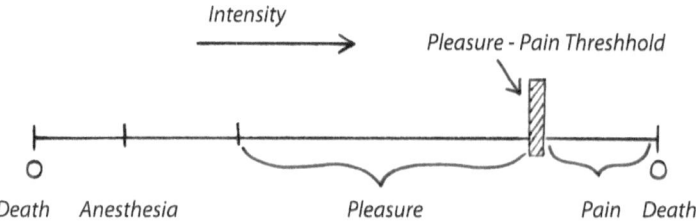

Figure 9: The Sensual Continuum of perceived intensity.

We can construct a Sensual Continuum that begins at zero, at the left end, indicating death, the complete absence of sensation. As we move to the right, the sensual intensity increases. Now, if you were to undergo a surgical operation, the most important doctor you need, after a competent surgeon, is a good anesthesiologist to keep you from feeling any pain and squirming under the knife. They accomplish this by administering drugs in the form of IV sedatives and anesthetic gasses to depress (desensitize) your central nervous system and level of consciousness. The realm of anesthesia hovers in a twilight zone somewhere just short of death. This reminds me of an old joke:

A mother gets the bill for her son's tonsillectomy. She's shocked at the cost and complains to the anesthesiologist, "I can't believe you charged me $1,500 to put my son to sleep. It only took twenty minutes to take out his tonsils."

Anesthesiologist: "I only charged you $500, ma'am. It cost a thousand to wake him up again."

We've come a long way since anesthesia was induced by drinking half a bottle of whiskey or placing a thick leather cap on the patient's head and rapping it sharply with a wooden mallet. Back then, a surgeon's skill was gauged by how quickly a limb could be amputated with a knife and saw, about sixty seconds.

▲ The Law of Thresholds

Let's follow your perceptual changes on the continuum as you awaken from surgery. Once the surgery is completed, the anesthesiologist weans you from the anesthetic. The first signs of consciousness appear with a return of primitive reflexes such as pupils constricting to light, the gag reflex, and increasing blood pressure and pulse in response to pain. These are the objective signs an anesthesiologist uses to gauge your depth of anesthesia. You then enter a stuporous state and gradually become more aware of your surroundings as your cortex regains control of the neural chassis. You are kept in the recovery room until you return to a normal baseline neurological function.

Each morning we make a similar, though less extreme journey, from unconscious sleep to wakefulness, some of us more stuporously than others. There are degrees of waking up, from hitting the snooze button to rising from bed and stumbling into the bathroom to making breakfast. On the weekends, I like to linger in the sweet, twilight half-sleep, drifting between worlds. In many spiritual traditions, the day begins with formal practice in the early morning hours before dawn when the veils between the worlds thin. If I awaken in the middle of the night, I often take the opportunity to meditate and might use a candle or the red light on my headlamp to avoid jarring my consciousness as I set up my meditation cushion.

As we move toward higher levels of sensation along the continuum, let's imagine that you go to a spa to get a massage. The mere anticipation as you lie down on the table can arouse a whisper of pleasurable relief as you are enveloped by the sound of relaxing music and the scent of warm oil. The first touch of the masseuse piques your attention, moving you further along the continuum, and each nurturing stroke sends ripples of delight through your body like smooth stones slipping into a pond. As the masseuse presses more deeply, your awareness increases, and so does your pleasure. But at a certain point, as she leans in deeper, probing muscle and sinew with thumbs and elbows, releasing unconscious knots of tension, things start to get edgy. You are approaching a no man's land where pleasure rubs up against pain, and you encounter the strange paradox of "it hurts so good," an exquisite, unbearable sensation that you want to give into and at the same time resist.

You have arrived at the Pleasure-Pain Threshold, a limiting wall beyond which further increases in intensity lead to frank pain. In a nightmarish scenario, if the masseuse were to keep increasing the pressure, the pain would turn into bruising tissue damage, and at a certain point you would pass out from the intensity, lose consciousness, and then die, returning to zero from whence you came. All our pleasure and pain, the entire spectrum of our lives, exists within this limited bandwidth of intensity bounded on either end by death. Welcome to the fourth law of pleasure: The Law of Thresholds.

Where pleasure meets pain

There are several important lessons to be gleaned from our thought experiment. To begin with, we can now answer the question posed at the beginning of the book: *The opposite of pleasure and the opposite of pain are the same thing—anesthesia, no feeling at all.* Pleasure and pain are on the same end of the continuum. They are neighbors, sharing a common wall—the Pleasure-Pain Threshold. Increase the intensity beyond this point, and what was pleasurable a moment earlier turns to pain.

Take an itch, a peculiar sensation that straddles both sides of the threshold. The first few scratches of a mosquito bite feel heavenly, but keep digging at the pale mound of flesh and it turns into excoriating pain. If you have the presence of mind to scratch lightly around the base, you can play at the edge of the threshold, have your relief and enjoy it too.

We can state this as a general principle: *Maximum pleasure is found at the threshold just before it turns into pain.* This is where excitement meets danger, where positive meets negative, and we come up against our perceived limitations. It is within this extreme borderland that the risk-taker and the sadomasochist seek their "kicks." Like the end of a bone, it's also a place where we grow.

Each level of the Pleasure Prism—physical, emotional, mental, and spiritual—has its own perceptual continuum of intensity and Pleasure-Pain Threshold. Here are some warning signs that you are nearing the edge:

> **Physically**, it's the point at which the breath becomes unsteady, the jaw tightens, nostrils flare, shoulders rise, and we stiffen and begin to tremble.
>
> **Emotionally**, it's where our patience grows thin and we become irritable, angry, depressed, or anxious. We may tremble from sheer emotional intensity and cry.
>
> **Mentally**, it's where our thinking becomes hyper-critical, obsessive, vague, and confused.
>
> **Spiritually**, it's where we become dogmatic, intolerant, self-righteous, and lose touch with our humility, humanity, and higher knowing.

It can be fun to challenge yourself, push your limits and play at the edge of the threshold, but it's not a place you can inhabit. It's too extreme and unstable. But step back a few paces, and you can drop into the sweet spot where you can breathe easy and ride the currents of high-quality pleasure without the edginess and at the same time develop your Pleasure Capacity. (In exercise physiology, it's the difference between aerobic and anaerobic training.)

What makes things tricky is that the threshold is not a fixed wall but continually shifts, moving in closer or further away, depending on how well you've slept, the time of day or month, what you had for dinner the night before, your mood, expectations, level of training, age, and countless other factors.

Still, at any given moment, *the Pleasure-Pain Threshold determines your Pleasure Capacity.* To increase your capacity for pleasure is to increase your capacity for pain, which is nothing other than to increase your capacity for life! This is easier to do than you might think. All it takes is a willingness to open yourself to the "life-stream," which we will discuss next.

▲▲▲▲▲▲▲

In brief:

Our physical, emotional, mental, and spiritual lives are experienced along perceptual continuums of intensity. Pleasure and pain are on one end of the continuum and anesthesia (the absence of experience) is on the other. Each continuum is bounded by a Pleasure-Pain Threshold that defines the point at which pleasure turns into pain. An important skill is to learn when to lean into and when to lean back from the threshold, which continually shifts throughout the day and throughout our lives. Think of it as a form of training that increases your capacity for pleasure and your capacity for an *aah*some life.

Considerations:

- Notice how the intensity of your body sensations (the body-stream) continually fluctuates through the space-time continuum of your body.

- When eating, track the intensity of pleasure from the first bite to the last. How does your stomach feel if you stop eating before you're full? How about your mouth?

- Patiently refine how you work with your Pleasure-Pain Threshold.

- When exercising, explore the limits of your Pleasure-Pain Threshold with honesty, kindness, and sensitivity.

- Try doing the same thing emotionally with your intimate relationships.

CHAPTER 12

Go with the Flow

The river is everywhere.
—Herman Hesse

ONE OF THE HARDEST THINGS TO LEARN IN MARTIAL ARTS IS TO STAY FLUID in the face of a physical threat and not contract in fear. The Japanese have a training method called *misogi,* which uses cold water immersion to simulate fear. The initial shock literally takes your breath away, followed by panic and gasping for air. This reflexive response often results in cold water drownings where a person plunges into freezing water and gasps, filling his or her lungs with water, and then sinks straight away. *Misogi* is traditionally performed on New Year's Day in a body of water or beneath a waterfall for spiritual purification.

So, when I saw an announcement for the annual Polar Bear Club swim at the Boulder Reservoir on New Year's Day, I seized the opportunity. The desolate, snow-swept prairie was an unlikely setting for a New Year's celebration. Food vendors set up concessions in the parking lot and loud music blared from speakers bolted to aluminum scaffolding. A large portable hot tub truck was nearby to warm intrepid bathers. Spectators milled about a large blue hole cut through the ice about thirty yards across and nearly as wide. On the far side was a low fence of mylar banners, as you might see at a ski race. It was a nearly perfect day with a cloudless, deep cobalt-blue sky and a hint of alpine breeze.

I stripped down to my trunks and made my way awkwardly over the glazed, granulated snow to the edge of the hole. The Polar Bear swimmers had already come and gone, and two small groups of enthusiasts were now standing waist deep in the water. On one side, half-a-dozen bathers in sunglasses were eating frozen yogurt and drinking cans of soda and beer as though it were a typical hot summer day at the rez. They were in the "mind-over-matter" denial camp. On the other side, people were hollering, jumping, and splashing wildly to dispel the intensity of the freezing cold. They were in the "emotional-expressive" reactive camp.

Standing at the edge of the ice, I centered myself with slow, deep breaths down to my lower belly, a place the Japanese call the *hara*. Fear is a contraction, but it's not possible to contract if you're breathing deeply. I waded into the icy water midway between the two groups up to my waist and stopped. Then, turning back to face the mountains, I pressed my trembling hands together in front of my heart to gather the two opposing feelings welling up within me, which ironically were being acted out by the bathers on either side. I tried to find the middle way, as half of me was trying to be calm and brave, while the other half wanted to scream and run away.

My skin tingled as though pricked by a swarm of tiny needles. As the cold penetrated deeper, I began to quiver and then started to vibrate like a tuning fork from the base of my spine to the top of my head. Then suddenly, everything became crystal clear, elemental and immediate—the sky, the mountains, the breeze, the water. I was fully alive, straddling the exhilarating edge of the Pleasure-Pain Threshold somewhere between life and death.[1] After a few minutes, I made my way back to land and eased into the maternal warmth of the hot tub. The contrast of going from an icy windswept prairie into a steaming hot pool is a rare Epicurean delight, one the early Native Americans surely relished in their winter lodges alongside hot springs.

The Lakota Sioux have a saying, *hoka hey*, "Today is a good day to die." It was this spirit that made the Native Americans such formidable warriors. The samurai were also known to be fearless, throwing themselves so completely into battle as to transcend the fear of death, which is essentially no different from the absorption of a Zen master in deep meditation or an artist fully engaged in their work. Cold water training has given me a way to connect with my spiritual-warrior self, purifying the fear from my mind and body. The same purification can also be achieved with heat. Every Japanese home has a dedicated hot bath known as the *o furo* ("o" meaning "honorable" bath). It is customary to first sit on a small stool by a water spigot, and with a small bucket and washcloth, thoroughly scrub your body with soap and water. After cleansing your body, you immerse yourself in the tub to cleanse your soul. In this way, the whole family can use the same water. In Zen temples, the bath water afterwards is used to scrub the floors. If you ever visit a traditional Japanese temple, the shiny luster of the wooden walkways is from the accumulated years of human oil in the bath water.

The lesson of cold water training is to surrender to the cold. This is both counterintuitive and paradoxical because the moment we surrender and breathe into the cold: we feel it more; it becomes more intense; yet we suffer less. This is something you have to experience for yourself to comprehend. Going with the flow is also a reliable way to expand your Pleasure-Pain Threshold.

The life-stream and the body-tube

Going with the flow has more to do with what's flowing through you than the flow of events around you. The body is essentially a tube. Food goes in one end and out the other. The other thing that flows through this tube is your life, experienced as sensations (the body-stream) and thoughts (the mind-stream.) These two streams combine to form the "life-stream." Whatever challenges we might face, no matter how difficult or complex, they occur within these two streams of sensation and thought. (To be complete, there is a third phenomenon of conscious awareness: the witness. If the life-stream is a wave, consciousness is the medium through which the wave propagates.)

The life-stream is a universal phenomenon. In Hebrew, it is called *ruach*; in Greek, *pneuma;* and in Latin, *spiritus.* Why then, does Western science reject the concept of an animating vital-force? This mind-body split can be traced to the Catholic church, which claimed exclusive branding rights to the *Sanctus Spiritus*, the Holy Spirit. No one else was allowed to speak of "spirit" for fear of being burned at the stake for witchcraft and other heresies.

In the seventeenth century, French Catholic mathematician René Descartes cut a shrewd theological deal with the church that made possible the unfettered study of science. All things (*res* in Latin) that possess spirit, soul, and therefore mind, he called *res cogitans*. Everything else, *res extensa* (things extended in space) is without spirit, soulless—matter that God set in motion according to the rules of mathematics. Descartes argued that these two realms were mutually exclusive and independent. Henceforth, *res cogitans* was to be under the dominion of the church and *res extensa* the domain of science.

This simply formalized the ontological hierarchy we encountered in Genesis where God is superior to the universe, mind is superior to matter, the soul is superior to body, and the flesh is merely a necessary evil. Only the spirit is pure. At the same time, it reinforced the notion of a dead, clockwork universe, which we'll discuss in Chapter 20. The scientific ignorance (ignoring) of the vital force in all creatures and things (*res extensa*) is the result of monotheism.

The Asians took a more open-source approach. The life-stream—*prana* in Sanskrit, *qi* in Chinese, and *ki* in Japanese—is a familiar, everyday concept. In Chinese, strength is *li qi,* and climate is *qi hou*. In Japanese, electricity is called *denki*. In yoga and Chinese medicine, the life-stream is understood to circulate through the body along certain channels or meridians referred to as the *nadis* in Sanskrit or *jing-luo* in Chinese. I've practiced yoga and acupuncture for over thirty years, and it still amazes me that the existence of a phenomenon as obvious as vital force is hard for the Western mind to acknowledge, let alone grasp.

Existentially, we are standing in a river of sensations and thoughts. Life is so challenging that few of us can stand in this rushing river entirely naked. Instinctively, we brace ourselves against the torrents to prevent being overwhelmed and washed away. To visualize how this works, recall that the Sensual Continuum is bounded at either end by zero. We can join these two ends together to form a belt around the body-tube with the Pleasure-Pain Threshold acting as a cinch or buckle. As with a well-fitting belt, there is an optimal tension. When the life-stream becomes too intense, we feel uncomfortable, sense danger, and contract. The belt is drawn tight, crimping the tube. Crimping the tube causes resistance, and like a garden hose, pressure builds up behind the constriction. Each of us has our own habitual ways of getting "gripped" or "bent out of shape." These emotional-muscular constrictions become the chronic gut, back, shoulder, neck, TMJ, headache pains, and banes of our existence. They may also appear as mood disturbances, irritation, anxiety, depression, and malaise. Consequently, any definitive solution to these problems requires opening the tube, which is precisely what yoga and acupuncture are designed to do.

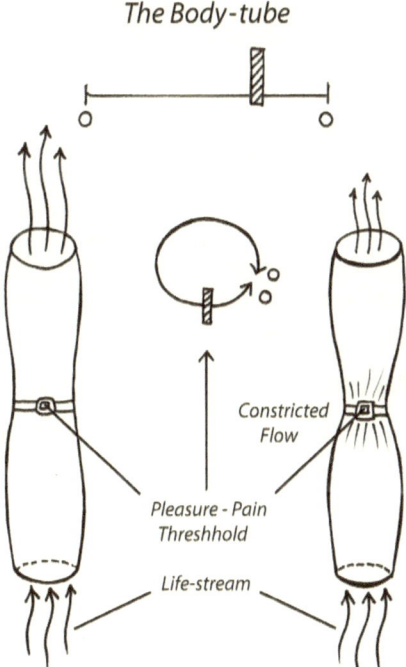

Figure 10: The body-tube with the Sensual Continuum as a belt and the Pleasure-Pain Threshold as the buckle.

Working with pain

There are, of course, times when contracting is necessary to protect ourselves, like pulling back from a hot stove or cringing from a blow. And sometimes pain is unavoidable, as in childbirth or a toothache. At these times, I try to make good use of the pain.

Although pain may be unavoidable, suffering is optional. It depends on how we stand in relationship to our pain. The life-stream flows through the body much like the flow of electrical current through a wire as described by Ohm's Law:

$$V = I \times R$$

where V is volts, I is current, and R is resistance. In our case, the voltage corresponds to the back pressure that builds up behind the resistance (constriction) in the body-tube. We experience this pressure as suffering:

$$\text{Suffering} = \text{Pain} \times \text{Resistance}$$

For any given intensity of pain, the more we resist, the greater the pressure and the more we suffer. Conversely, the less we resist, the more life flows through us and the less we suffer. It's all about opening the tube.

Pain can teach us a great deal, if we approach it intelligently. As a young girl, Satya had a more intense emotional life than her sisters, which would cause her to burst into tears at the dinner table or to lie on her bed crying into her pillow. When she was about five years old, I tried to help.

"Sat, you know when you get those strong feelings, they start like little green vines growing up around your ankles. What can you do?"

"Breathe?" she answered.

"Yes ... and then what happens?"

"They go away?"

"No Sat, when you breathe into your feelings, the vines grow even bigger and take over your whole body. It can feel really scary and then ... poof, they go away!"

To tell a child not to cry—to not feel what they feel—is a violation of their spirit. It creates an unholy (unwholesome) double bind that cripples and deadens a person. Emotions are a natural phenomenon that come and go like internal weather. And just as no one controls the weather, no one controls their emotions. We can't change the way we feel. We can, however, change the way we stand in relationship to our feelings. When it's hot, we can wear shorts and when it rains, use an umbrella. By embracing the truth of our experience with radical acceptance, we move with the flow of our *internal* nature. How we choose to express ourselves in the *outer* world is a separate matter.

I tell my patients there are two kinds of suffering: the usual kind that leads to interminable suffering and creative suffering that leads to the end of suffering. The creative kind requires a willingness to feel the pain. Not gratuitously as some form of penance, but as a way to study the mechanics of suffering to free ourselves of it. Like a leaf floating down a creek, if we contract in fear when we get into white water, we become dense, sink to the bottom, and get stuck in the mud. It feels like the world is passing us by and it's depressing. But if we stay open and keep afloat, we get around the next bend where the water runs calm and new adventures await.

This is more than a metaphor. A woman once told me how she fell out of a white-water raft and got sucked under into a swirling pit. She balled up in fear, and tumbled like in a washing machine, completely disoriented. Running out of air, she remembered the words of the river guide: "If you get caught in white water, relax and stretch out your limbs." She did and was instantly swept downstream and back to the surface.

Resisting pleasure

The thing is, we not only tighten up around pain and fear; we also tighten up around pleasure and joy. The Buddhists refer to this as grasping, clinging, and attachment. It is an emotional, muscular contraction, only around pleasure. It's a contraction caused by trying to hold onto the object of our desire, the wanting of more pleasure. As with any contraction, *grasping is a form of resistance that decreases the life-stream and diminishes enjoyment.*

The difference between a connoisseur (Epicurean) and a glutton (Cyrenaic) is that the connoisseur savors pleasure rather than devours it. William Blake wrote:

> He who binds to himself a joy
> Does the winged life destroy;
> But he who kisses the joy as it flies
> Lives in eternity's sunrise.[2]

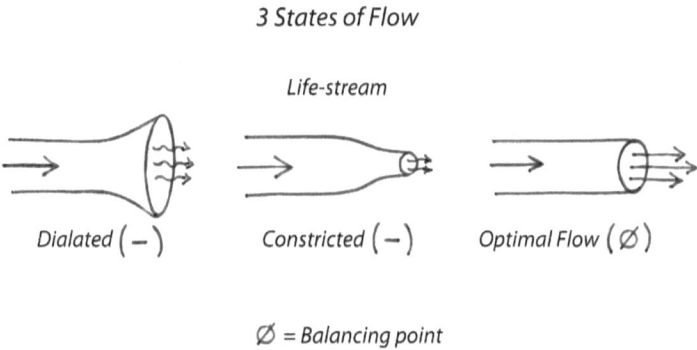

Figure 11: Optimal flow of the life-stream requires the balancing of desire and surrender. Note, dilation occurs from excessive surrender.

The key to enjoying life is to be fully present in the moment, neither grasping nor pushing away. We can express this as:

$$\text{Joy} = \text{Pleasure} \times \text{Conductance}$$

Conductance equals the inverse of resistance: the ease with which the life-stream flows. (For a detailed discussion, please see the appendix: "The Amadeus Equation.") In other words, learning how to keep your body-tube open in the face of pain carries over directly to the experience of pleasure.[3] When delightful sensations are streaming through your body, loosening the buckle of the Pleasure-Pain Threshold increases your capacity to enjoy them.

Go with the Flow

Simply put, if you wish to experience contentment, you must be able to hold content. If you wish to experience fulfillment, you must be able to fill up. Pleasure, contentment, and fulfillment require optimizing the life-stream, which in turn requires developing a specific skill set—the balancing of desire and surrender—the sixth law of pleasure. We will begin with desire.

▲▲▲▲▲▲▲

In brief:

Your body is a tube through which your life-stream flows in the form of thoughts (mind-stream) and sensations (body-stream). The Sensual Continuum acts as a belt around the body-tube and controls the volume of the life-stream according to the limits of the Pleasure-Pain Threshold. Like a garden hose, there is an optimal nozzle setting that allows you to water the plants at the far edge of the garden. This maximal flow occurs when desire and surrender are balanced and we are neither grasping after pleasure nor cringing from pain. The next time you are confronted with a painful situation, notice that the more you resist, the more you suffer; and conversely, with pleasure, the less you grasp, the more you enjoy. In other words, as you near the Pleasure-Pain Threshold, remain open, breathe deeply, and allow the life-stream to flow through you.

Considerations:

- Finish your morning shower with a cold-water rinse. Breathe into the sensations and all will be revealed.

- Sensitize yourself to your vital energy—observe the myriad sensations streaming through your body.

- The quality of your life-stream is reflected in the quality of your voice, breathing, body movements, thinking, and mood.

- Wisdom begins with acknowledging the truth of your inner experience and then allowing this information to guide your actions.

CHAPTER 13

The Evolution of Desire

*Remember that sometimes
not getting what you want
is a wonderful stroke of luck.*
—Dalai Lama XIV

Before pleasure came desire. Recall that in the evolution of the human forebrain (Chapter 6), desire is located in the reptilian brainstem and came online long before the mammalian pleasure center. Dopamine, the primary chemical messenger produced in the desire center, first appeared 500 million years ago in the sea pansy, a cousin of the jellyfish (phylum, *cnidaria*) where it served to initiate muscular contractions and to perform the unique function of bioluminescence, a visual form of desire. Think of lightning bugs blinking like a flashing neon sign on a warm summer night, attracting mates and potential food sources, as well as young kids with butterfly nets and glass jars. The distinction between desire and pleasure is an important one.

Wanting

Desire is about "wanting" in all of its forms. We experience it most directly through primal urges such as appetite, lust, and craving, which in turn fuel the more complex animal spirits of passion, greed, ambition, competition, jealousy, and envy. Scientists shy away from such emotionally charged words, preferring more neutral, sterilized terms such as stimulus, incentive, salience, and motivation.

By whatever name you call it, desire is essential to life and propels us forward into the future, for without wanting there would be no movement, and without movement there can be no life. That's why attempts to eliminate the human appetite—through religious proscriptions, Prohibition, the War on Drugs, and self-discipline—is like trying to suck air out of a flask, doomed to fail. Sure, you can coerce someone to curb their desires through social pressure and the threat of punishment, but as we saw with Original Sin, turning a person against their own nature leaves them internally fractured and weakened. This is the very definition of perversion: to turn about, or in this case, to turn against.

Most of the time, we are only dimly aware of our desires because they originate in the deep recesses of our reptilian brain, below cortical consciousness. Like a butterfly, we flutter through the day following a daisy chain of desires from one to the next—rising from bed, reaching for a glass of water, going to the store, meeting friends, and so forth—as we move along the Sensual Continuum. It is only when we need to make a "conscious" decision to purchase an item, pursue a love interest, or some other important activity that our desires come into sharper focus. Still, what we really want at the deepest level of our being can be a deceptively difficult question to answer, a subject we will examine later.

On the other hand, if we attempt to deny the truth of our desires, it only drives them deeper into the subconscious where they can fester and turn into perversions. It is this unconsciousness that makes desire, particularly perverse desires, so powerful, and why politicians, priests, gurus, coaches, celebrities, and other pillars of society are so susceptible to corruption. In their attempt to be a "good" role model, they often suppress their dark side. As a result, the more righteous and dogmatic, the deeper the denial and the more potent the perversion. As the saying goes, *the bigger the front, the bigger the back*.

Ted Haggard, founder and superstar pastor of the Colorado Springs New Life mega-church and past president of the National Association of

Evangelicals, frequently railed against homosexuality from the pulpit. In 2006, a gay prostitute discovered Haggard's true identity and outed him. Haggard had been paying the young body builder for methamphetamines and sex during a three-year liaison. Lord Acton's dictum, "power tends to corrupt, and absolute power corrupts absolutely,"[1] holds true because power attracts the ambitious and then inflates their ego, exposing the underlying fault lines in their character. The ancient Greeks described it more poetically: "Those whom the gods would destroy, they first drive mad with power."[2] Power provides the means of abuse and denial provides the unconscious perversion.

The converse is also true. When we have the humility and honesty to bring our urges and temptations into the light of day and consciously acknowledge them, they lose their power, at which point choice becomes possible. For this reason, awareness in and of itself is a potent agent of change. This is why virtually every imaginable weight-loss diet works (temporarily) because it makes us pay attention to what we put in our mouths. *The path to freedom begins with awareness.*

According to the Gnostic Gospel of Thomas, Jesus said, "If you bring forth what is within you, what you bring forth will save you. If you do not bring forth what is within you, what you do not bring forth will destroy you."[3] This is the most concise statement of health and disease I have ever heard. The truth exists, and because it exists, it exerts a force in the world and therefore will always come out, but in one of two ways: straightforward—which may be awkward, even painful, but is essentially healthy and in service to life—or in a *sinister* way (from the Latin "left-handed") which leads to disease.

Ultimately, what makes a desire perverse is its denial. That doesn't mean we should give free rein to our every desire, which would be foolish, as some desires are harmful. What I am saying is that to make a wise choice about what desires to pursue, we first must become conscious of them. Obviously, we cannot control what we are not aware of, just as we cannot have a conscience without being conscious. This is where the Greek idea of *arête* (virtue) comes in and why learning how to skillfully work with our desires is an important virtue to master. It begins with bringing forth our true nature, our Original Wholeness, which includes our alienation, brokenness, and depravity. There is no light without darkness, and true compassion for ourselves and others becomes possible only through seeing our own human nature in all its glory and wretchedness.

The Zen teacher, Thich Nhat Hahn, at a conference with over a hundred psychotherapists in Granby, Colorado, told a story about pirates off the coast of Vietnam who would plunder, murder, and rape local fishermen and their families and then throw them into the sea. He described their brutality with such tender sadness that there was no room for blame. "Looking deeply in meditation," he said, "I realized that if I had grown up in poverty, neglected and abused, as these pirates had been, I could have been one of them." It was a stunning confession for a spiritual teacher. Can you imagine what might have happened if Ted Haggard, looking deeply in prayer, had the honesty to come clean about his drug problem and sexual appetite? He might have become a cultural hero in the eyes of many by practicing what he preached and willingly mounting the cross of his own human frailty.

If you patiently observe the contents of your own consciousness, you will discover that all of humanity dwells within you, what Carl Jung called the "collective unconscious." Some religious groups condemn the practice of meditation for that very reason, claiming that "an idle mind is the playground of the devil." From the perspective of Original Wholeness, there are no good people or evil people; there are only people. As Martin Luther King wrote in a letter from a Birmingham jail and later repeated in a speech in Memphis on the eve of his assassination, "We are caught in an inescapable network of mutuality, tied in a single garment of destiny."[4] Thich Nhat Hahn, who was nominated for a Nobel Peace Prize by Martin Luther King, referred to this mutuality as "interbeing."

The problem is not desire—which is essential to life—but the things we desire and how we go about seeking them. But to get this right, to use our practical wisdom, as Epicurus would say, we first need to understand what desire is.

Need versus want

A major source of confusion about desire is the difference between *need* and *want*. Both are a form of desire. Indeed, for most of human history they were the same thing. We lived hand to mouth and only desired what we needed and needed what we desired. We first had to expend calories to hunt and forage before we could enjoy the fruits of our efforts. The calories expended and the calories enjoyed were essentially equal.

About 12,000 years ago, at the end of the last ice age, desire and need began to uncouple due to the domestication of plants and animals. Farming allowed humankind to harness the sun's photosynthetic energy and store its radiant calories in granaries and herds of cattle, thereby leveraging an individual's energy reserves and productivity. The resulting caloric surplus freed large groups of people from working the land, making possible the specialization of labor and ultimately the flowering of civilization. (After producers came priests, followed by a warrior and political class. Surprisingly, little has changed. The church, military, and government continue to be the primary institutional power brokers whose existence depends on the support and productive work of others.)

The ability to harness energy freed us from our brutish toil and opened wide Pandora's box. Pleasure was no longer limited to one's personal labor, but to the resources one could command. *For the first time, we could dream of wants beyond our needs, and the more sophisticated our technology became, the more we dared to desire.*

Needs are rooted in biology and therefore have a built-in, self-regulating Pleasure-Pain Threshold, such as quenching our thirst, eating our fill, or keeping warm. At a purely mechanical level, hollow organs such as the stomach, bladder, rectum, and seminal vesicles have stretch receptors in their walls that signal when they are full. Similar feedback sensors regulate myriad physiological functions from temperature and thirst to blood pH and CO_2 levels. However, once desire is uncoupled from biological need, there is no natural limit. The only limitation is our imagination, which can easily run wild. How can you tell, for instance, when you have enough status, power, money, possessions, or grain in your granary? There are no stretch receptors. Like the saying goes, *you can never get enough of what you don't need.*

Machine technology further accelerated the uncoupling of need from want, first by harnessing steam energy in the Industrial Revolution and then electricity in the modern era, enabling us to manufacture goods with unprecedented efficiency. Technology has so vastly improved our material lives that "in progress we trust" might easily become our nation's motto. Today, we are assured that 5G, self-driving electric cars, genetic engineering, and artificial intelligence will make our lives so much better.

Unfortunately, all our brilliant technology has done little to advance the human heart. The gap between our *technical know-how* and our *ethical know-why* has widened into a yawning abyss that threatens to engulf us. If we are going to save ourselves from the potential destructive power of our technology, we must transform our human heart from fear to love, and we must do it quickly, which is the purpose of this book.

An Epicurean solution

Epicurus was well aware of the difference between need and want. He distinguished three kinds of desires:

- Natural and necessary (want and need are identical).

- Natural but unnecessary (want and need are uncoupled).

- Unnatural and unnecessary (want uncoupled from reality), which he called "empty desires."

Empty desires are based on culturally contrived "empty beliefs" (false assumptions) that lead to "empty pleasures." Chief among these is the belief that we can find happiness through money.

When my children were young, I taught them that you can't buy happiness. Turns out that wasn't quite correct. If you're poor, you can buy happiness, but only about seventy thousand dollars' worth, according to a 2010 Princeton study—roughly the amount of money required for an average American to cover their basic (natural and necessary) needs for food, shelter, warmth, transportation, and so on.[5] Beyond this level of income, money and happiness uncouple. In other words, *not having money can make you miserable, but having it doesn't make you happy.* As billionaire investor Warren Buffet observed, "If you have a $100,000 and you're an unhappy person and you think $1 million will make you happy, it's not going to happen."[6]

Just as need and want uncouple at a certain level of prosperity, so do desire and pleasure. The things we desire and the pleasure we derive from acquiring them no longer correlate. The connection between the brainstem VTA (desire center) and the limbic N. accumbens (pleasure center) weakens.

Multiple lines of research confirm the limited ability of wealth to buy happiness. Add to this the Law of Contrast and Comparison and the leveling effect of habituation and it's easy to understand why the wealthy are no happier than the rest of us. They may even be less so, given their high profile and the burden of maintaining their possessions. A manager of high end condominiums in Florida told me her clients are always complaining about finding good help to care for their multiple homes. There are millionaires who feel inadequate in the company of billionaires and billionaires who compete to have the largest yacht in the marina. (Apparently size matters: the Mirabella V's 292-foot mast is so tall it can't fit under the Golden Gate Bridge nor navigate the Panama Canal). A chauffeur for a billionaire described how his employer would occasionally buy several expensive sports cars in a month, drive them a few times, and then add them to his warehoused collection of over a hundred cars. Despite his massive wealth, on his seventy-fifth birthday, the only well-wishers in attendance were his six salaried, personal aides. Real wealth cannot be measured in dollars alone, and as Epicurus noted, "not what we have but what we enjoy constitutes our abundance."[7] No amount of money can satisfy empty desires because empty desires lead to empty pleasures.

Intellectually, it's easy to understand that money can't buy happiness, but to grasp it emotionally and allow this knowledge to change the way you live your life is another level of comprehension. We live under the collective spell of a cultural matrix that is difficult to break. But it is possible. I remember having a family dinner at an Asian restaurant when my kids were young. At the next table was an even younger family of four. As we were getting up to leave, the father struck up a conversation and told me how he and his wife had both been in corporate America. When their kids were born, they left their jobs and bought a trailer home so they could focus on raising their children and would return to their corporate jobs once their kids were older. This couple was clear about their values and had the courage to live them.

In our perverse world where the many suffer from too little and the few suffer from too much, millions of people go hungry while 40 percent of Americans are obese and another 30 percent are overweight. Companies spend billions of dollars to transform empty desires into perceived needs. In 2016, Coca Cola, arguably the most recognized brand in the world, spent nearly $3 billion, more than Microsoft and Apple combined, to convince consumers Coca Cola is superior to water.[8] In the same year, the tobacco industry spent over $10 billion, $25 million each day—to convince people smoking is more enjoyable than breathing fresh air.[9] That's more than $1 million every hour. Imagine what our world would be like if we applied such marketing resources toward more life-renewing goals.

As long as we define ourselves through our possessions and branded logos, we'll remain harnessed to the matrix, turning the wheel of *samsara*, endlessly comparing ourselves to others, trying to satisfy our empty desires. As long as we live in fear, the fear of not having enough, the fear of loneliness, the fear of inadequacy, the fear of each other, there is no way out; it is a self-fulfilling prophecy of our own making. Our collective myth of "success" isn't working for any of us—poor or wealthy. But again *what is created by the human mind can be changed by the human mind.*

To take your life in your own hands starts with freeing your mind and raising your head above the dust and toil of the herd to see the larger picture of who you are, what you value, and what you actually need to secure your well-being. Epicurus was perfectly clear on this score. He valued freedom as the highest virtue and saw living simply as a way to achieve it: "Training yourself to live simply and without luxury brings you complete health, gives you endless energy to face the necessities of life, better prepares you for the occasional luxury, and makes you fearless no matter your fortune in life."[10] Epicurus understood the futility of pursuing wealth beyond our needs. He understood that the stress and anxiety of pursuing empty pleasures undermines the very happiness we seek and distracts us from the love and connection to ourselves, each other, and the world that is the true source of fulfillment. He was not interested in individuals "who show off the culture that impresses the many, but rather men who are strong and self-sufficient, and who take pride in their own personal qualities not those that depend on external circumstances."[11] When I take the measure of a person, I look at their character, not their possessions; I look at the level of their personal freedom and the quality of their life, not their social status.

More than a theory

These ideas are not merely theoretical. I have personally field-tested them in my own life and correlated them with the experiences of my patients. As many a writer will confess, a book takes on a life of its own. In my case, it became my life. It's hard to explain, but as I worked on the book, the book worked on me. As my thoughts and words aligned on the page, so did my life. I became more coherent, more authentic, more real.

Outwardly, my life was nearly perfect. I was a respected member of the community, had a beautiful office in a hundred-year-old, red sandstone cottage overlooking Boulder Valley, and lived up Sunshine Canyon in a Japanese-style home on five acres of pine forest that backed up to open space. My daily commute was seven minutes down the mountain with one stop sign. Along with raising three young girls, at one point, we had two horses, two goats, three dogs, and a team of nannies, cooks, and house cleaners to help out. When we were in town, passing strangers would occasionally comment, "You're such a beautiful family," and we were in many respects.

Yet despite all the good fortune, despite twenty years of raising kids and building a life together, my wife and I never found the friendship and deep trust that is necessary for a lifelong commitment. By 2012, my business was on the rocks and so was my marriage. The arguments at the dinner table, emotional pain, and discord were destroying all the goodness we had created. Something had to be done. So, I sold my medical practice, fixed up the house, and embarked on a year-long writing sabbatical and trial separation. Since I had arranged for my seventeen-year-old daughter to do a volunteer stint at a children's hospital in Cambodia, I travelled with her to Southeast Asia and eventually settled in Chiang Mai, northern Thailand for my retreat.

I rented a fan-room on the fourth floor of a small guest house. My abode was 20 feet by 12 feet, roughly the size of Thoreau's shack on Walden Pond. I had a bed, small desk, chair, and a waist-high refrigerator. In one corner was a sink with a mirror, and in the other, a small bathroom with a detachable showerhead and water heater. Three large windows with levered transoms faced west. All this for 4,000 Baht ($150) a month, including fresh linens, two bath towels, and a weekly cleaning.

From my perch, I looked down on the grounds of Wat Mueng Mang, the oldest of Chiang Mai's 300 temples, and could see the gold-leaf tops of six other stupas and the head of a large Buddha. In the morning, when I sat on my bed to meditate, Doi Sutep, the main temple overlooking the Ping Valley, was shining in the distance directly opposite me. Thoreau withdrew to the woodlands of Connecticut to get in touch with nature. I withdrew to the ancient city of Chiang Mai to get in touch with my human nature.

Being functionally illiterate and only able to speak a few words had its advantages. It freed me from the usual cultural expectations. I spent most of my days alone in silence, except for an occasional meal with a few expat friends and a monthly meeting at Writer's Without Borders above a local Italian restaurant. I lived like a secular monk and at times like a desperado on the borderlands between cultures, being nobody and going nowhere.

One morning, about halfway through my sabbatical, I heard a fateful knock on my door. Unaccustomed to visitors, I opened the door cautiously. As I stood half-naked in my wrap-around sarong, a young American woman handed me a large official envelope while her friend filmed me with her smart phone. "What's this?" I asked.

"You're being served!" she answered.

Apparently, this was a way for them to earn some money while traveling. After they left, I closed the door with divorce papers in hand, shaking as though I had just been violated. It took some hours to calm down. The security of my sanctuary would never be the same.

Thus began the formal dismemberment of my marriage, my family, and my former life. In the process of my divorce, I lost my relationship with my daughters, my house, and most of my material wealth. Aside from several short trips back to America to settle my affairs, I lived in Thailand for three years as it was the only place I could afford to live—financially and emotionally—until a job brought me back to Boulder. The first time I walked down Pearl Street Mall with its high-end restaurants and fashionable shops, I was shocked to see how much it had changed and how much I had changed. The contrast was disturbing. Walking by beautiful people sipping wine and eating fabulous meals at sidewalk tables, I realized just how far I had fallen from my previous life and was overwhelmed with a sense of loss. I easily could have judged myself a failure, a victim of life's capricious cruelty. In Thailand, I had been a relatively wealthy foreigner; here in my hometown, for the first time, I felt poor.

As I began to contract into self-pity, a mantra spontaneously came to my lips: *I am not my clothes; I am not my car; I am not my job; I am not my bank account; I am not my judgments.* With each repetition, the false illusions that had kept me chained to the matrix began to fall away and my authentic self rose closer to the surface. It was all just a contrast-and-comparison mind game. As the author of my own narrative, I could cast myself as a victim, a scoundrel, or a hero. The choice was mine. Allowing my emotional pain to flow through me without resistance purified my suffering, and with it came liberating insight. By the time I reached the end of the mall, I realized it was enough just to be an ordinary human being, living a modest life, doing the best I can.

It's one thing to think something; it's another to speak it and still another to write it. Ultimately, the point is to live it. Despite all my personal shortcomings, my loss and emotional pain has made me a bigger and better version of myself. These days I find myself smiling for no reason and delighting in the simple pleasures life offers with refreshed *sense*-abilities. I am lighter in every sense of the word.

To live is to be humbled. I still get snared from time to time in the seductive machinations of the matrix, but I cycle through the illusions more quickly, buoyantly, and with less resistance. The more I free myself of empty desires, the happier and more satisfied I become for reasons I will explain in Chapter 19. I am grateful that I could kneel and drink deeply from the Pierian spring and for the quiet inner peace that has graced my life. Even the tragic estrangement from my daughters has made this book all the more urgent and meaningful, for in the end, it is written to them.

Next, we will examine the underlying biology of the shiny lures that keep us plugged into the matrix and that makes them so attractive.

▲▲▲▲▲▲▲

In brief:

Desire is fundamental to our existence, which is why attempting to eliminate it is a perversion. If, on the other hand, we are conscious of our desires and "bring forth what is within us," choice becomes possible. For this reason, honesty and self-awareness are essential to freedom. Technology uncouples needs from wants, which leads to empty desires for things we don't need based on empty beliefs. Understanding the distinction between need and want, desire and pleasure, and the limitations of money can help free us from the empty pleasures of the matrix and develop a truly meaningful and fulfilling life.

Considerations:

- At the moment of desire, pause ... Do you feel the spur to action?

- Before you buy something, stop and consider if it is actually a need or a want.

- In the gap between desire and pleasure: experience freedom.

- It is said in the Upanishads: "As is your desire, so is your will. As is your will, so is your deed. As is your deed, so is your destiny." So, choose your desires wisely.

CHAPTER 14

Supersize Me

*Freedom is found
in the gap
between stimulus
and response.*
—JG

W E LIKE TO THINK OF OURSELVES AS FREE AGENTS, AT LEAST AS FAR AS THE thoughts we think and the desires we pursue. And yet, as we have seen, our thoughts and desires are, to a great extent, shaped and defined by the cultural matrix in which we live. As American-Hungarian psychologist Mihaly Csikszentmihalyi points out, "The essence of socialization is to make people dependent on social controls to have them respond predictably to rewards and punishments."[1] One of the more powerful ways in which this is done is through socially engineered stimuli.

In 1955, when McDonald's opened their first fast food restaurant, it offered a seven-ounce cup—about the size of an original bottle of classic Coke. By 1994, the burger giant offered a 42-ounce Coke (six times larger) along with bigger burgers and French fries. The larger Coke was in response to a supersizing race that the convenience store 7-Eleven kicked off in1980 with the introduction of a 32-ounce Big Gulp, followed by a 44-ounce Super Big Gulp a few years later, and eventually a staggering 64-ounce Double Gulp, practically a six-pack in a cup, in 1989.[2]

This bigger-is-better trend is, in part, the result of the Law of Contrast and Comparison and competitive market forces. It turns out that we are also biologically programmed to respond to specific kinds of supersizing. To understand how, let's turn to the Nobel Prize winning work of Nikolaas Tinbergen.

In the 1930s, Tinbergen, along with Konrad Lorenz, created the field of ethology, the scientific study of animal behavior as an adaptive evolutionary process. We encountered this approach earlier with Paul MacLean, who studied the behavior of reptiles, mammals, and primates to gain insight into the function of the human forebrain. One of the most well-known discoveries was Lorenz's observation that baby geese imprint on the first mother-object they encounter within thirty-six hours of birth. He quite literally stumbled upon it one day as a gaggle of goslings followed him around wherever he went. He realized they were following not him but his rubber wading boots.

Meanwhile, Tinbergen identified "fixed action patterns" at the core of animal behavior. These instinctive behavioral sequences are hardwired into the nervous system and once triggered, run to completion—something like a neurological reflex where tapping your knee causes your leg to fly out, only more complex. While studying the nesting habits of the Graylag goose, he observed that the mother will immediately attempt to roll a displaced egg back to the nest with the underside of her beak. He discovered the goose would perform the same fixed action with a golf ball, door knob, or even a soccer ball, indicating that it was not the egg, per se, but a target stimulus of "roundness" that triggered the behavior.

The target stimulus could be artificially amplified to create what he called a "supernormal stimulus," the equivalent of a "supernormal desire." He made a bigger-than-life plaster egg painted in bright Day-Glo blue with large black polka dots. When presented with a choice, the mother Graylag preferentially selected the super-sized egg to roll back to its nest rather than its own small, pale, dappled eggs. An egg the size of a soccer ball worked even better, despite the brooding bird repeatedly sliding off and having to heroically remount it.

In another experiment, Tinbergen constructed a two-dimensional cardboard cutout of a female butterfly enhanced with exaggerated dark horizontal body markings across its abdomen. Male butterflies preferred to mate with the cardboard cutout rather than a real female butterfly. Wings were not even necessary; the enhanced body shaft was sufficient. He could transform an average male barn swallow into an irresistible super-stud by simply darkening the male's chest feathers with a black magic marker. Head-wired rats tapping on a bar to stimulate their pleasure center is just a more extreme example of a supernormal stimulus fixed action pattern.

Stimulating human desire

As you've probably guessed, we humans also respond to supernormal stimuli that can evoke an oversized desire for a Big Gulp or an impulse to mate. The difference is that unlike animals in a laboratory, we engineer our own stimuli and then subject ourselves to them. One of the earliest examples of a supernormal stimulus is Venus of Willendorf, a 25,000 BCE figurine of a woman with exaggerated breasts and buttocks. Her counterpart can be seen in prehistoric super-sized phallic art and stone representations.

Fast-forward to the sixteenth century, and European women are wedging themselves into whalebone corsets to accentuate their waist-to-hip ratio and their male counterparts, not to be outdone, are sporting decorative codpieces fashioned from thick layers of cloth and velvet sewn into the crotch of their britches to accentuate their virility. Curiously, it was taboo to speak of male genitalia but

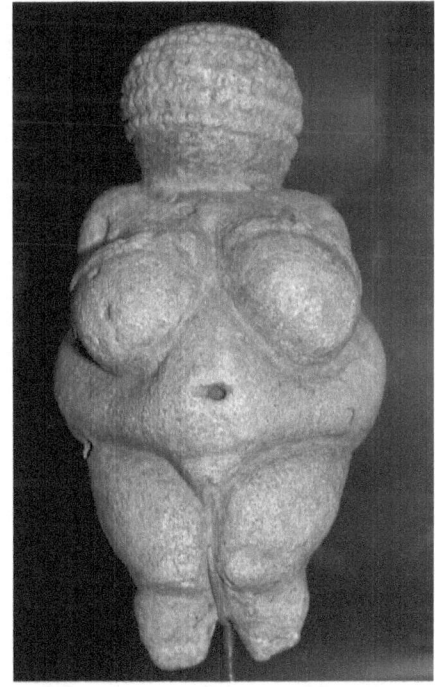

Figure 12: Venus of Willendorf. 25,000 BCE.

perfectly acceptable to strut about in public with a protruding codpiece.

I suspect the wedding gown with its peculiar train arouses some ancient ophidian preference for an elongated tail. Think of Angelina Jolie's captivating serpentine tail in *Beowulf* or the newly minted Her Royal Highness the Duchess of Sussex with her sixteen-foot-long bridal veil. According to Cambridge fashion historian Victoria Bartels, "We dress to construct an outward image of our perceived inner selves. The items we choose to adorn ourselves with are loaded with complex cultural messages."[3] Indeed, the aforementioned supernormal stimuli are examples of biological and cultural messages that are designed, among other things, to arouse the promise of pleasure. Despite our pride of place in the Great Chain of Being, it's an uncomfortably short step from a male butterfly copulating with a cardboard cutout to a man masturbating with a Photoshop-enhanced screen image. The most popular plastic surgery operation in the U.S. is breast augmentation, with some 300,000 procedures performed each year.[4] Interestingly, the fastest growing plastic surgery in men is confidence-inspiring chin implants, which surged 71 percent in 2011[5]. Such cosmetic surgeries demonstrate just how widespread and deep our feelings of original inadequacy run.

It's a con game to show someone attractive images of carefully prepped, idealized fashion models and then sell them "consumer" products to relieve the feelings of inadequacy these models arouse. A poignant example is the widespread use of skin lightening products among dark-skinned women. Forty percent of women in China, 61 percent in India, and 77 percent in Nigeria regularly use skin-lightening products, a $4.8 billion global industry in 2017.[6] And the obsession with fairer skin is not without cause. Studies demonstrate that lighter-skinned American black men and women receive more lenient prison sentences and are more likely to be employed compared to their darker counterparts.[7] The world has been sold the belief that "white" is better and millions of people purchase products to help them "fit in," despite the documented dangers these products entail.

Any of our senses can be the target of a supernormal stimulus. For our Paleolithic ancestors, salty, sweet, fatty tastes were a rarity that signaled a feast. Food manufacturers invest millions of dollars to develop artificial, supernormal taste enhancers and then promote them with supernormal advertising—full-screen shots of a bigger-than-life burrito steaming with melted cheese or an effervescent soda cascading over translucent ice in a perfectly lit, frosted glass. Deafening rock concerts, Las Vegas glitz, and a pampering spa massage are all sensual experiences that captivate us through supersized contrast and comparison.

Perfume can be a particularly potent stimulus. In college, I dated a French woman with glints of burnished gold woven in her brown hair. She was petite, slender, and shy like a delicate flower. Though forty years later I can't remember her name, I'll never forget how she smelled. I didn't notice anything unusual until I leaned in close to kiss her and entered her personal, perfumed space. It was earthy, sweaty, sexual, erotic, and primitive, like being in the den of a feral animal from which there would be no escape, nor any desire to escape.

The rituals we perform—folding hands in prayer, making the sign of the cross, genuflecting, saluting, and bowing—reverberate through our ancient subcortical reptilian and limbic brain circuits and powerfully motivate our behavior in unconscious ways. The same imprinting can be applied with a fearful intent. Think of the sound of beating drums and the blare of bagpipes as men rush headlong into battle and the oversized fear it arouses in those being attacked, or the image of the Twin Towers collapsing into a pile of rubble endlessly replayed in the weeks following 9/11. We have created our own digital screen equivalents of Tinbergen's oversized, Day-Glo eggs with flashing screen ads and other forms of click bait. Considering the huge amounts of resources governments and businesses invest to manipulate our collective consciousness, perhaps we are not all that different from lab rats in a grand social experiment.

Imprinting, as Lorenz demonstrated, occurs most profoundly early in life. With my girls, we felt pressured to introduce electronic media to give them a "head start" in the digital world. We also wanted to imprint them with healthy pleasures through music, sports, and playing in nature and didn't own a television. I often told them they were "mountain girls" with the hope that someday, when they found themselves in the big city, they would remember their roots and be less susceptible to its artificial, urbane pleasures.

We are entering a dystopia where digital screens and billboards flash commercials that know our desires before we do. Based on our internet searches, we are delivered prefiltered content that influences our behavior in everything from selecting a pair of shoes to selecting a political leader. The virtual reality of the matrix is becoming ever more compelling and pervasive. Its influence is reflected in a simple statistic: in 2018, one out of every five dollars in the economy was spent on advertising, and this number is projected to grow 3.3 percent annually.[8]

Still, desire is not something to be denied, but embraced, for only then can we understand how it works, avoid its pitfalls, and motivate ourselves toward healthy, life-promoting activities. We also need the countervailing balance of surrender to enjoy pleasure. We will explore surrender in a moment, but first we need to understand how pleasure cycles through time and through our lives.

▲▲▲▲▲▲▲

In brief:

Like other animals, we are biologically hardwired to respond to specific sensory cues that signal reproductive fitness and rewards such as food. These sensory stimuli can be artificially enhanced to create supernormal stimuli that trigger complex pleasure-seeking behavior akin to fixed action patterns in lower animals. Being aware of how we are being manipulated by these bigger-than-life stimuli with fast food ads, fake eyelashes, and Photoshopped celebrities can help immunize us against them.

Considerations:

- Notice when a specific sensory cue attracts your attention. Is it a supernormal stimulus?

- What physical characteristics are you attracted to in a sexual partner? Have they been artificially enhanced?

- Are you being manipulated by your favorite junk food? If so, how?

- What supernormal stimuli do you deploy to be more attractive?

Chapter 15

The Pleasure Cycle

▲ 5. The Law of Cycles

> *Artificial pleasures arrive stillborn;*
> *they have no life of their own.*
> —Mark Mitchell

Pleasure is not a state of being, but an activity, or more precisely, a fluctuation in the life-stream that spreads through the space-time continuum of the body as a wave. It can vary from a faint ripple of jasmine wafting in the night air to a thundering tidal wave of orgasmic ecstasy. We can characterize a wave in terms of its physical properties. Viewed through the Pleasure Prism (Chapter 8), we saw that pleasure comes in three fundamental colors (red, green, and blue), each with its own particular frequency and wavelength. These colors combine to create the full spectrum of physical, emotional, mental, and *äsis* pleasures that illuminate our lives. Next, we measured the intensity (amplitude) on the Sensual Continuum. Now let's go a step further and consider how pleasure varies through time (its temporal characteristics) and how this gives us a way to think about the quality of pleasure. Understanding the physical characteristics of pleasure will help us grasp the subtle metaphysical characteristics that lie ahead.

▲ **The Law of Cycles**

Imagine a pendulum swinging back and forth over the Sensual Continuum, seeking its balancing point. If we were to attach an inked stylus to the tip of the pendulum and run a piece of graph paper beneath it, it would inscribe a wave. Any phenomena, which rises and falls, cycles, pulses, oscillates, or vibrates about a balancing point can be described by a wave. The earth going around the sun, a cork bobbing on a lake, your heartbeat, breathing, light, sound, and molecular vibrations are all wave phenomena. Even at the tiniest dimension of reality—the quantum mechanical level of elementary particles—can be described by a wave, the Schrödinger Wave Equation. Thus, the whole cosmos is waving at every scale from quantum fluctuations to galaxies whirling through space, and all these waves interpenetrate to form the warp and woof of the very fabric of reality. Pleasure is also a wave. It's simply how nature works.

We can use our model of a pendulum to define three types of pleasure: when we push the pendulum to the right toward higher intensity (through an act of desire), we experience "active pleasure"; when we relax (surrender) and the pendulum swings back toward lower intensity, we experience "passive pleasure"; and when it zeros in on the balancing point, we experience "neutral pleasure," *ataraxia*, the equanimity that Epicurus so highly valued. Thus, the pendulum swinging back and forth over the continuum describes how we cycle through active, passive, and neutral pleasures—the Law of Cycles.

According to Occam's razor, the validity of a model is determined by its simplicity and explanatory power. Let's take it for a test drive and see how it works. Consider the pleasure of going for a run. From the moment you get up from the couch, put on your running gear, and stretch your legs, you are increasing your sensual intensity and moving into active pleasure. At first, you jog slowly to warm up and then as you pick up the pace, you encounter a little discomfort. You're approaching your Pleasure-Pain Threshold. In the case of running, this is known as the lactate or anaerobic threshold, the point at which energy production switches from aerobic to anaerobic metabolism. It occurs at approximately 85 percent of your maximum heart rate.

The Pleasure Cycle

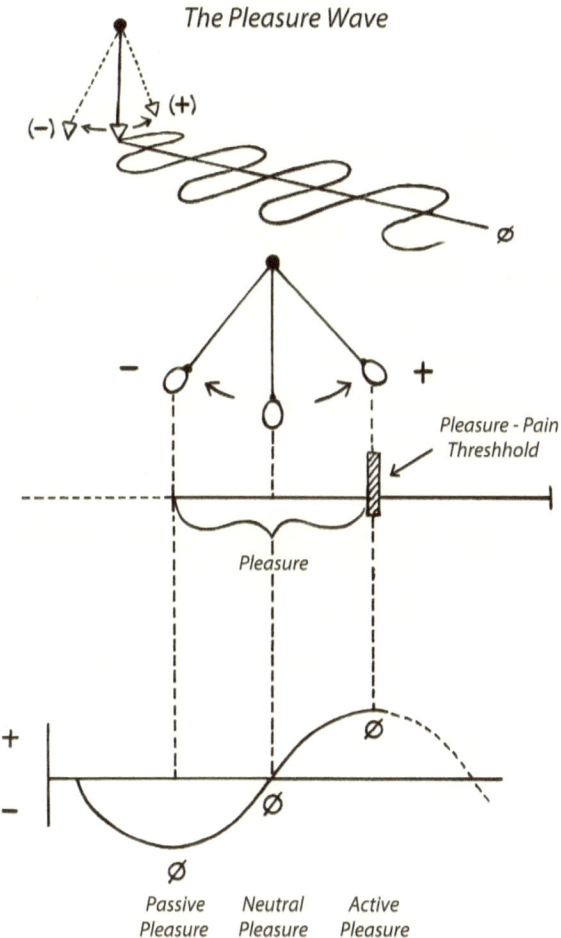

Figure 13: A pendulum seeking balance is a wave phenomenon. The Pleasure Cycle is a wave of active, neutral, and passive pleasures.

The purpose of the warm-up is to gently lean in to the threshold and nudge it to recede, which takes about five to ten minutes, depending on your level of conditioning. You know you're there when you break a sweat. Once this happens, you are firing at a higher metabolic rate, the discomfort fades, and you catch your second wind. Hitting your stride, you shift into high gear and glide over the road. You're deep into the run now and can comfortably handle the higher intensity. As you near the end, soaked with sweat, nostrils flaring, muscles flushed with blood, you push past your anaerobic threshold and sprint the last 100 yards at full power until your thighs burn and your lungs gasp for air.

You have reached your peak intensity, the crest of the wave, and from here it's all downhill. You begin to slow your pace, head home, and relax into passive pleasure. After the cooldown and shower, you bask in the sweet afterglow, which merges seamlessly into neutral pleasure as you return to baseline. The next day, you're ready to start all over again. Wash, rinse, repeat. This same basic Pleasure Cycle governs thirst, sex, and sleep, as well as emotional, mental, and spiritual pleasures.

Notice that you can enjoy moving in either direction along the continuum. Drug users refer to this as taking uppers (cocaine and methamphetamines that increase intensity) or downers (benzodiazepines and narcotics that decrease). Putting these data points together, we see that *pleasure is not so much a state of consciousness as it is a shift of consciousness.* The faster the shift and the greater the amplitude, the higher the contrast, the higher the high, the more intense the pleasure, and the stronger the desire to repeat it.

Pleasure is path-dependent. The enjoyment you experience depends on how you get there, specifically how fast and how intense. The thrill is in the acceleration: getting thrown back in your seat when you floor it, stepping off a plane in a foreign land, the infatuation of fresh love, or being blown away by the rush of a mind-altering drug.

The Pleasure Cycle also explains why we're such a restless lot, why after sitting we want to move and after moving we want to sit. As pleasure-seeking organisms, we need to shift our consciousness. The only question is how we go about it, and some ways work better than others.

Net pleasure

A useful heuristic device (conceptual tool) is a pleasure-time graph where the vertical Y-axis represents pleasure and the horizontal X-axis, time. Above the X-axis is euphoria (pleasure) and below, dysphoria (pain). Rather than focusing on how "high" you get (on the Y-axis), a more satisfying approach is to maximize the area under the curve, which measures the total amount of pleasure experienced over time. The net pleasure equals the area under the euphoric curve minus the area under the dysphoric curve.

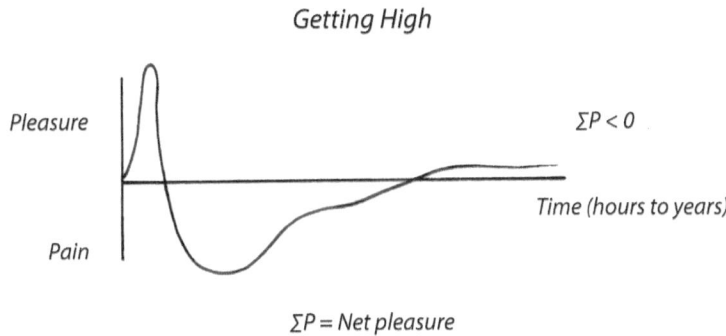

Figure 14: Getting high. The net pleasure is negative when you add up the area under the curves

For instance, drinking with friends late into the night can be fun, but the hangover and fatigue the following day may not be worth it. This is represented on the pleasure-time graph by a curve that peaks rapidly and then plunges below the baseline into prolonged dysphoria. Obviously, we need to strike a balance between momentary pleasures, their short-term consequences, and the fulfillment of achieving long-term goals. Epicurus was well aware of this calculus. In a letter to his friend Menoceus, he described it this way:

> Although pleasure is the greatest good, not every pleasure is worth choosing. We may instead avoid certain pleasures when, by doing so, we avoid greater pains. We may also choose to accept pain if, by doing so, it results in greater pleasure. So, while every pleasure is naturally good, not every pleasure should be chosen. Likewise, every pain is naturally evil, but not every pain is to be avoided. Only upon considering all consequences [the net pleasure] should we decide. Thus, sometimes we might regard the good as evil, and conversely: the evil as good.[1]

Think of it like making a financial investment with three possible outcomes: net positive return, break-even, or net loss. The best investment, according to Epicurus, is a safe, interest-bearing savings account: *ataraxia*. Although it starts as a low, humble curve on the pleasure-time graph, a daily modicum of equanimity powerfully compounds over time to create a resilient storehouse of well-being.

Delayed gratification

Another commonly confused idea is delayed gratification where the pleasure-time graph runs negative before turning positive. Barring certain dire circumstances, such as root canals, broken bones, and times of war, delayed gratification is overrated and an ineffective strategy to enjoy life. Many people front-load their lives with so much delayed gratification and get so good at it that by the time they reach their goal, they roll right past it and only glimpse the reward as it recedes in the rearview mirror. I witnessed this in my parents, who worked hard their entire lives, as immigrants often do, to give their children a better life. While my siblings and I benefited greatly from their sacrifice and efforts, I wish they would have taken more time to enjoy themselves along the way.

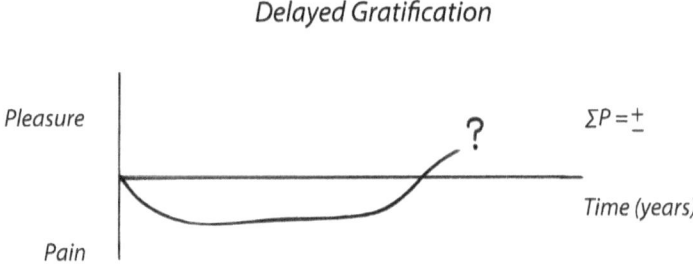

Figure 15: In delayed gratification, the net pleasure is uncertain because one's Pleasure Capacity often atrophies as a result of habitually denying rewards.

People often think of becoming a doctor as one long exercise in delayed gratification—slogging through four years of medical school and another three or more years of specialty training. When someone who is considering a medical career asks me about this, I tell them that time passes either way. The only question is: What do you want to be doing in the meantime? Time is elastic. When you look forward, it expands, and seven years sounds like an eternity. But when I look back on my medical training, it contracts into a tidy memory about the size of a diploma on my wall.

Intense training should not be confused with delayed gratification. Training by definition is designed to push the envelope of the Pleasure-Pain Threshold. I took satisfaction in the challenges of becoming a doctor—a kind of tough love. It was hard, but gratifying, which is not to say I didn't have moments when the intensity was way over the line. The difference is that with delayed gratification, we are stuck on the painful side of the threshold and stoically grit our teeth, counting the days until it's over. A life of delayed gratification is a life of denying our natural desire for pleasure. *Looking for satisfaction in the future is a fool's errand because pleasure can only be found in the present moment … or not. Pleasure is not a destination; it's the way.* If you focus on extracting the highest quality pleasure from each moment of each day, you will naturally be living life to the full.

Two caveats: don't be fooled by cheap imitations and look out for the Faustian bargain, otherwise known as a "loan." One of the main ways the matrix harnesses our energies is by offering the instant gratification of buying on credit in return for your soul. As writer Ambrose Bierce defined it, "Debt, n. An ingenious substitute for the chain and whip of the slave driver."[2] Or, as my father used to say, *A mortgage casts a shadow on the sunniest field.*

Authentic pleasure

Now let's see how the timing of pleasure can give us a straightforward way to think about the quality of pleasure. High-quality pleasure—authentic pleasure—is characterized by a healthy, intact Pleasure Cycle, whereas lower-quality, artificial pleasure has an unhealthy distorted Pleasure Cycle.

To get a feel for it, consider the quality of food, something familiar to all of us. We think about food in terms of taste, nutrients, and calories, whether it's organic and locally sourced, the care with which it is prepared, and how healthy it is.

I used to play a game with my girls where I would quiz them on what's healthier: an apple or applesauce? Applesauce or apple juice? Apple juice or apple pie? And then a tough one: an apple pie or caramel apple? Real food is natural and whole. It is grown in nutrient-rich soil with a minimum of chemicals and takes time and care to prepare from farm to table. Slow food is an apt description.

My parents raised me to be frugal, but not when it comes to food. The quality of food is particularly important for growing kids, so we invested the extra money to buy organic. We usually think of organic food as pesticide-free, but it has a deeper meaning. To be organic means to be derived from living matter. Living matter is biologically highly organized. In the language of physics, it is information rich. When you eat organic food, you are getting more than the list of nutrients, calories, sodium, and cholesterol on the label, you are eating life—the most vital nutrient of all. You are consuming high quality (intelligent) information. Life lives off of life. We are members of a "mutual eating society,"[3] as Alan Watts likes to point out.

Fresh vegetables are healthier because they have more life force than frozen or canned vegetables. If you take the same fresh vegetables, freeze dry and reduce them to a green powder drink, you have de-natured (removed the life from them) and severely diminished their informational value. Generally, the more processed a food is, the less wholesome, the less healthy, and the lower the quality. In short, the junkier. I grew up near Chicago, the home of Lay's potato chips, which had perhaps the greatest junk food jingle of all time: "You can't stop eating 'em." Why? Because junk food lacks nutrients and the empty calories leave us hungry for more. It's engineered to titillate the senses without delivering the goods (authentic pleasure).

The process of refining disrupts the organic balance and intelligence of real food. For example, you would have to chew twenty-seven feet of sugar cane stalk to get the nine teaspoons of sugar you can swallow in a few gulps of a twelve-ounce Coke.[4] Such convenience has made it easy for the average American to consume 100 pounds of refined sugar a year.[5] For the same reason, when natural products like coca leaves, coffee beans, and poppy flower resin (opium) are refined, they become abusable. In their denatured, concentrated form, a tiny amount packs a potent supernormal stimulus, but empty reward—the ultimate empty reward being death.

Using this sort of analysis, we can evaluate the quality of pleasure on a Continuum of Authenticity. At one end of the continuum are artificial (junk) pleasures and at the other are authentic (organic) pleasures. Artificial pleasures derive from empty desires—things we don't need—and, like junk food, leave us feeling unsatisfied. Authentic pleasures, in contrast, derive from and satisfy real needs. They are natural, whole, nourishing, and information-dense and take time to enjoy. Think "slow pleasure." We can state this formally in terms of the Law of Cycles: *High quality authentic pleasure is characterized by a healthy, robust Pleasure Cycle.*

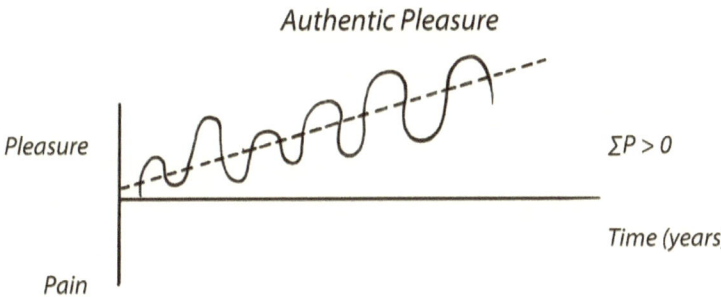

Figure 16: Authentic pleasure establishes a virtuous cycle of increasing net pleasure and vigor (amplitude) with a notable absence of pain and suffering.

With authentic pleasure, the enjoyment we receive is proportional to the effort we expend. Effort and reward (desire and pleasure) are closely coupled. The more you put out, the more you get back. Like surfing: the bigger the wave, the bigger the ride.

Growing up outside of Chicago, surfing wasn't an option, but there were a few small ski hills in neighboring Wisconsin. When I turned sixteen, my father took me to Austria on an American Youth Hostel ski club trip. I had my first formal lessons at the St. Anton Ski School, considered the best in the world at the time, and it was old school. Each morning we laboriously side-stepped up a bunny hill and then skied down, over and over again. The idea was to develop strength and make relationship with the snow on the snow's terms. It was humbling. But then in the afternoon, the instructor took us on the gondola to the top of the Valluga, a majestic mountain in the Lechtal Alps where the thin air and 360-degree view of the jagged mountains was literally breathtaking.

At the top, everyone was snapping pictures except an older Swiss woman. "Why aren't you taking any pictures?" I asked.

"My camera's up here," she said, pointing to her head. "I use my eyes; that way I will never forget." She was right. I can still see those mountains in my mind's eye like an old black-and-white photo. Not interposing a piece of technology between ourselves and reality allows us to engage the moment more fully and therefore more pleasurably and memorably.

Authentic pleasure has a natural barrier that weeds out the insincere. There are no shortcuts. They're not for sale. You can't buy the thrill of surfing a big wave, the ecstasy of skiing through deep powder, the satisfaction of playing a Bach cello suite, or the exhilaration of driving a golf ball 300 yards. The satisfaction of mastery must be earned the old-fashioned way, through effort (about ten years's worth, according to some estimates).

Artificial pleasures are artificial to the extent that they rely on technology. Technology uncouples reward and effort, short-circuiting the Pleasure Cycle, a cycle that has regulated human behavior since time immemorial. We can state this as a corollary: *A pleasure is artificial to the degree that it lacks a healthy Pleasure Cycle.*

For example, riding a chair lift is more artificial than side-stepping up a bunny hill; playing an electric guitar is more artificial than playing an acoustic guitar; Pilates is more artificial than yoga; pornography is more artificial than real sex; and driving a car is more artificial than riding a

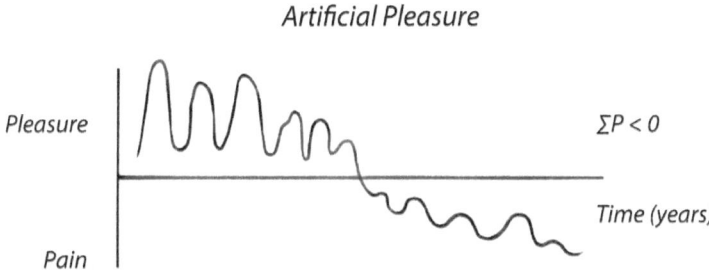

Figure 17: Artificial pleasure initially overdrives the Pleasure Cycle and over time, leads to decreasing net pleasure and vigor (amplitude).me).

motorcycle, than riding a bike, a skate board, and so on.

The point is that authentic pleasures, like organic food, are intrinsically healthy, satisfying, and self-regulating. They are less prone to abuse and most important of all, on the pleasure-time graph they are characterized by a notable *lack of dysphoria*.

While it is relatively easy to tell the difference between real food and junk food, the difference between authentic pleasure and junk pleasure is trickier in part because our lives are so bloated with artificial pleasures that we have a hard time imagining life without them. That's why it can be so refreshing to go camping or to take a trip to a Third World country and reboot our Pleasure Cycle.

Near the end of his life, the well-known Afrikaner, Sir Laurens van der Post, came to Boulder for a four-day retrospective. He wrote extensively about the Kalahari Bushmen, who are among the earth's oldest human inhabitants stretching back some 40,000 years. He showed a film clip of an encounter he had with a member of the *San* tribe. When their meeting concluded, the *San* fellow, barefoot, wearing only a loin cloth, and carrying a water stick, turned and walked off into the bush without looking back, which is their custom. Sir van der Post, decked out in expedition khaki and heavy boots, watched him for a while before returning to his well-provisioned canvas tent and attendants. In the film, he notes with admiration the bushman's connection to his environment and consummate self-reliance.

Despite the harsh conditions of desert living, the *San* highly value their leisure.[6] Children have no social duties aside from playing and much of their time is spent hanging out, conversing, making music, and ritual dance. Women enjoy high status and often head up the family, suggesting an ancient matriarchal lineage. When it comes to taking pleasure in life and family, who is more civilized and who is the primitive? Who is free and who is the slave? I suspect a *San* person would think the modern world strange, if not ridiculous. (Should our modern life collapse, I take solace in knowing that these hearty people will likely survive and like basal cells, regenerate the human race.)

I am not suggesting we return to a subsistent, hunter-gather existence. Technology has been a tremendous boon and improved our lives in countless ways. It's easy to forget that before the advent of modern medicine, existence was a tenuous affair where you could die from something as common as an infected cut or an abscessed tooth. Life was slow and arduous. In 1850, it took six weeks to sail across the Atlantic. By the 1950s, the world's fastest steam ship made the crossing in three and a half days. Today it takes just seven hours to fly from New York to London.

What I am suggesting is that we carefully consider the kinds of pleasures we seek and the impact they have on our lives. Generally speaking, authentic pleasures through thousands of invigorating wash-rinse cycles create a powerful rhythm, a vibrant pulsation that tones the body, tempers the mind, and makes us healthier, more integrated, and capable in the world. Authentic pleasures expand our Pleasure-Pain Threshold and increase our capacity for a robust life.

Intense, high-amplitude experiences (that do not derail us) stretch open our Light-body, enabling us to tune in to the higher frequencies of ecstasy and bliss. Unfortunately, our society avoids these higher feeling states as a matter of course. The usual bandwidth ranges on a spectrum of misery to fleeting moments of happiness with the midrange somewhere in the area of general drudgery. If you wish to increase your bandwidth, lean into your life and explore the limits of your comfort zone.

The Pleasure Cycle

The comfort trap

Countless people are lulled into a life of comfort based on the mistaken assumption that the opposite of pain is pleasure, and therefore as long as they are avoiding pain, they must be having a good time. They pad their lives with stuffed sofas, Lazy Boy chairs, and all manner of conveniences. Unfortunately, the "comfort-good/pain-bad" approach leads to a low-amplitude, shrink-wrapped life of inactivity, expanding waistlines, and chronic disease.

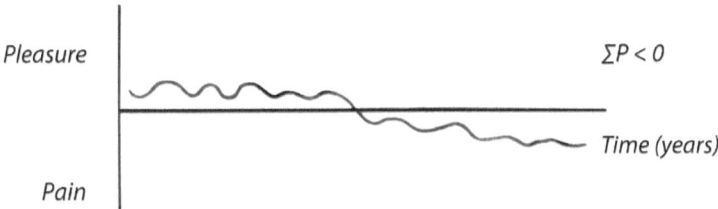

Figure 18: The comfortable life is a low flow state of diminished net pleasure and vigor.

The comfort trap often snares its victims early in life, something that can easily happen to the physically awkward child whose first experience of athletics is slamming into the Pleasure-Pain Threshold a few too many times. Or, the sensitive kid who dislikes competition, the overweight child who can't keep up, or the shy child who goes unnoticed and is never encouraged. Often it is not the pain of the physical threshold but the pain of the emotional threshold (bullying, ridicule, embarrassment, and shame) that discourages us from taking risks to expand our limits.

The walls of the comfort trap are lined with "slippery" artificial pleasures that tend to diminish us over time, making us weaker, less integrated, and less capable. That's why a pet dog is no match for a coyote and video gamers are pale shadows of the avatars they imagine themselves to be. The couch potato lives a tepid life of quiet desperation compared to the rich, multidimensional authentic life, which engages one across the full spectrum of their Light-body.[7]

We can enjoy the benefits of artificial pleasure as long as we engage in ample authentic pleasures as a counterbalance to maintain a healthy cycle. This requires a proactive approach. Modernity has made it possible to go for days without working up a sweat, and if we don't dial in regular exercise, it may not happen.

I performed a physical exam on a bright young man who had just graduated from MIT in physics and was on his way to Cal Tech to pursue a Ph.D. He was underdeveloped physically, so I suggested he work on his body.

"I like being thin," he protested.

"Really? What do you like about it?" I asked.

"I look good in a double-breasted suit," he quipped. He told me the dean of his college, when asked about physical activity, said, "I sometimes feel an urge to exercise come over me, but I lay down, and it soon passes."

Exercise is essential because it connects us to the real world and to ourselves in elemental, regenerating ways. That's why we call it *re-creation*. What's true on an individual scale is also true of the collective. Families, institutions, and empires go through their own kind of Pleasure Cycle. They start out lean and vigorous, but then go soft with privilege and hubris and eventually collapse from within. We may be witnessing this now with the general decline of our collective physical and ethical fitness and the creeping corruption rotting our institutions. Inevitably, the pendulum reverses its swing. As the ancients knew well, history is cyclical.

Think smooth

This brings us to the most important physical characteristic of all, which underlies every pleasure: smoothness. Like the touch of silk on soft skin, the taste of ice cream melting on the tongue, the sound of a Gregorian chant caressing the ear, the scent of lilac suffusing the nose, the ring of an eloquent thought illuminating the mind, and the oceanic bliss of dissolving into a spiritual epiphany, our nervous system is soothed by smoothness. Pleasure is mellifluous from the Latin *mel* meaning honey and *fluere* to flow. Pain, in contrast, is rough, jarring, jagged, erratic, torn, granular, and grating.

In fluid dynamics, it's the difference between "laminar flow" and turbulence. Whitewater river guides look for the smooth, glassy tongue of current, shaped like a downstream V where the water runs deep between the rocks. At the tip of the tongue the water breaks into turbulent ripples. We hear the same flow pattern in a singer's voice as a sustained note ends in an emotive vibrato. On the Sensual Continuum, the point at which the laminar flow of the life-stream breaks into turbulence marks the Pleasure-Pain Threshold.

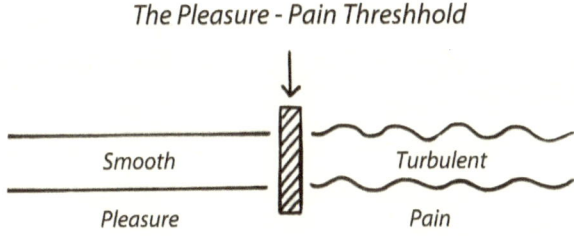

Figure 19: Pleasure is smooth; pain is turbulent.

We can sense the flow of another person's life-stream in the timbre, rhythm, and resonance of their voice because the voice is merely the breath made audible. I encountered a remarkable example of this while waiting for a flight at the Rio de Janeiro International Airport. Over the PA, announcing flight arrival and departure times, came the most sensual voice I have ever heard, as though heaven sent. My initial impulse was to go to her. It turns out I was not the only one. The announcer, Iris Lettieri, is famous for her sultry voice. According to a story on National Public Radio, an entire group of Japanese business men once missed their flight because her velvety voice had directed them to the duty-free shop, where they probably imagined they would meet her.[8]

Our mirror neurons, if well-tuned, vicariously reflect the inner flow of the life around us in people, animals, plants, rivers, and even the mountains and land beneath our feet. When the breath is smooth, the body is smooth, the mind is smooth, like a stream of oil poured from a cup or a speed skater gliding over ice.

▲▲▲▲▲▲▲

In brief:

Pleasure is a wave characterized by an amplitude (intensity), a crest (active pleasure), a trough (passive pleasure), a frequency (color), a rhythm (reptilian aspect), a time duration (net pleasure), and a quality (smoothness) that cycles through our life. To be a good surfer, you must learn to read the waves. It can be helpful to visualize pleasure as a pendulum swinging back and forth over the Sensual Continuum tracing a line on a pleasure-time graph. This analysis reveals that authentic pleasures have a robust Pleasure Cycle where effort and reward are coupled in a natural, organic way. Artificial pleasures, in contrast, rely on technology to leverage a relatively small effort into an outsized reward. As a result, authentic pleasures build character and increase our Pleasure Capacity, while artificial pleasures tend to fragment and weaken us.

Authentic Pleasure	Artificial Pleasure
Healthy Pleasure Cycle	Unhealthy Pleasure Cycle
Effort/Reward coupled	Effort/Reward uncoupled
Integrating	Disintegrating
Full spectrum	Narrow spectrum
Self-regulating	Dysregulating
Difficult to abuse	Easily abused
Slow	Fast
Strengthening	Weakening
Minimal equipment	Equipment intensive
Inexpensive	Expensive

The Pleasure Cycle

Considerations:

- What role does delayed gratification play in your life?
- If you are not enjoying your life now, what is it that you are missing?
- Take one of your favorite pleasures and assess its relative authenticity.
- Name a high-quality authentic pleasure that you engage in on a regular basis.
- Describe how you feel while doing it (active pleasure) and afterward (passive pleasure).
- When do you experience neutral pleasures and how would you describe them?

CHAPTER 16

Surrender: The Artless Art

*If you forget yourself,
You become the universe.*
—Hakuin Ekaku

SURRENDER IS A WORD THAT IS SELDOM USED IN THE MATRIX AND WHEN IT IS, IT is almost always in a negative context. It suggests defeat, weakness, giving up, all of which are anathema to our muscular, competitive, collective self-image. We aspire to be like the hero of Lord Tennyson's poem *Ulysses*: "To strive, to seek, to find, and not to yield."[1] This is the motto of a culture where getting what you want is called winning and synonymous with success.

But surrender is not wimpy and is as essential to life as desire. The Taoists likened it to the power of water whose yielding softness and humble willingness to seek the lowest level can overcome the strong and unyielding. If you have any doubt about this, check out the Grand Canyon, or consider the power of a tsunami. Laozi observed:

> Nothing is softer or more flexible than water, yet
> Nothing can resist it. That the weak overcomes the strong,
> that the hard gives way to the gentle—this everyone knows.
> Yet no one acts accordingly.[2]

Surrender is a state of relaxation, open receptivity, and non-attachment. It is essential because it brings us into the present moment.

We have seen how desire, from its brainstem cave, propels us toward a reward. Desire by its nature is future-oriented. It can deliver us to the gates of the Promised Land, but to enter within requires an act of surrender, for *whatever satisfaction we may seek can only be experienced NOW*. Indeed, the present moment is the only moment that exists, and if we are unable to give ourselves to it, if we are unable to surrender, we miss the very thing we are seeking.

But hold on … if the present moment is the only moment that exists, how could we be anywhere else? While we are always physically present in the "here and now," our attention may not be. We may be ruminating about the past or dreaming about the future, lost in our thoughts. We are so accustomed to our running, internal narrative that we mistake it for reality. "Life is what happens to you while you're busy making other plans," John Lennon quipped.[3]

It's not easy to be present in a culture obsessed with progress that looks to the future for satisfaction, driven by supernormal stimuli and hyperbolic ads. All of this makes surrender difficult to achieve—which is itself an oxymoron—for you can't try to surrender, just as you can't try to relax. Surrender occurs with the cessation of effort. It is a non-doing, a letting go, an allowing things to be as they are. You can't force your way into the present moment; you must abandon yourself to it.

In fact, no *one* can surrender because at the moment of complete surrender, there's no one there to surrender; we disappear like a rain drop in the ocean. All that remains is the mist upon the water, the witness, pure, *äsis* awareness, a condition of complete receptivity. At the instant of surrender, consciousness is an empty mirror that reflects what is before it. In the words of Zen master Dogen:

> Midnight. No waves
> No Wind. The empty boat
> Flooded with moonlight.[4]

Breaking it down

If all this seems a bit too mystical, here's a more analytical nuts-and-bolts approach.

When Niels Bohr was inducted into the Order of the Elephant at the Royal Danish Court for his groundbreaking work in quantum mechanics, he chose the ancient Chinese *Taiji* symbol (the *Yin-Yang*, black and white crescents interlocked in a circle) for his coat of arms. Inscribed beneath were the words *Contraria Sunt Complementa* (Opposites Are Complementary), a fitting salute to his famous Theory of Complementarity that asserts quantum objects possess opposing, complementary properties. The most well-known of these is wave-particle duality, where an elementary particle is simultaneously a discrete "billiard ball" that bounces off other billiard balls and a wave of energy that passes undisturbed through other waves. Which aspect is observed at any given moment—particle or wave—depends on the experimental setup used to measure it.[5]

We also possess two complementary modes of being: an ego-based discrete, separate self that desires things and an egoless, merged self that waves.

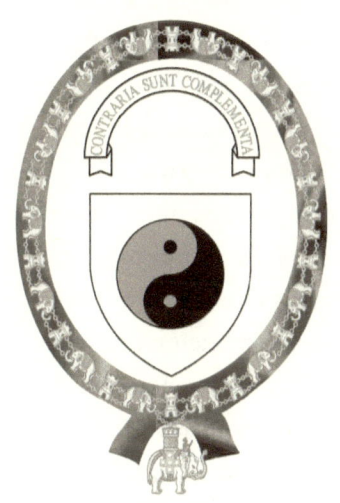

Figure 20: Niels David Henrik Bohr coat of arms. Awarded the Order of the Elephant, by the Royal Danish Court 1947. Nobel Prize in Physics 1922.

Which aspect we express depends on our moment-to-moment situation much like an electron remains indeterminate until a measurement is taken—in our case, the moment we act. When fearful, we contract and become a particle with hard boundaries, a "me-against-them" mode focused on self-preservation. When we are in love, we expand and join with others as a boundless wave. At times, we think only about our personal gain and benefit; at other times we want to save the rain forests and dolphins. Usually, we are in a vaguely self-conscious, indeterminate state, muddling through our day.

A stunning example of the fluid nature of self can be seen in stroke victims who might lose function of half their body and then neglect its care—not shaving half the face or treating a paralyzed limb as though it belonged to someone else. Neuroanatomist Jill Taylor, in her book *A Stroke of Insight,* gives a dramatic account of how she suffered a stroke one morning and experienced herself alternating between being in oceanic bliss merged with everything and being completely terrified and unable to dial the phone for help.

When we get stuck in the self-conscious ego-mode, the world breaks into two pieces—me and everything else—with "me" usually taking center stage. The ego serves an important function of self-preservation (don't leave home without it), but it's not the only game in town.

From the particle "I-perspective," it's easy to feel scared, alienated, and alone. Yet, upon closer inspection, the ego proves to be illusory. We can't point to it or touch this "me" because it doesn't exist in a material sense. Ontologically, "me, myself, and I" is merely a simulation, albeit a very convincing one, created by the life-stream of self-concepts and familiar body sensations. After all, how do we know we exist except for the sensations and thoughts that stream through us?

As far as I can tell, there is no unique, permanent me. In fact, most of our self-identity is not even our own. It's imposed upon us by the matrix and by the way people treat us, particularly when growing up. "I," to a great extent, is a social construction. Our current understanding of quantum mechanics has come to a similar conclusion: at the tiniest dimension of reality, there are no particles, only waves fluctuating in an endless quantum field.[6]

Letting go

Surrender is the art of letting go, principally letting go of fear, which is to let go of one's identification as a separate self. Because the ego is, in large part, a construction of thought, this is tantamount to a suspension of thinking, or more precisely, a letting go of our attachment to thinking.

And therein lies the problem: we are addicted to thinking because we are addicted to having a self and to suspend thinking is to lose our self. Humans in the remote past were less burdened by this problem because they engaged in less abstract thinking. In fact, the notion of a self as the basic social unit did not appear until the Axial Age. Previously, the fundamental existential unit was the family, clan, and tribe.

The cosmic irony is that the ecstasy and bliss we seek resides just beyond the ego's dread of non-existence. We are afraid to let go, and yet it is only when we surrender that we experience true fulfillment. This is the lesson of the *petite mort* (the little death) of orgasm that we will explore ahead.

As Westerners, we tend to be long on desire and short on surrender. Understanding how surrender works makes letting go easier, and like most things, we get better at it with practice. You can practice surrendering to a flower, the sound of cicadas droning on a summer night, washing dishes, or a traffic light. It takes but an instant to give yourself to the moment and disappear. I practice surrendering when I get into the swimming pool. I fold into a deep forward bend and then completely let go and tumble into the water. In the split-second it takes to reappear as me, the initial shock of entering the water (which I find uncomfortable) has passed.

Breakthrough at Mt. Baldy

Meditation is a formal way of practicing surrender. It's quite simple. My older brother taught me how to meditate sitting on the edge of his bed in about fifteen minutes. To deepen my practice, every few years I attended a week-long retreat called a *sesshin*, a Japanese term that means "to join heart and mind." When people asked me where I was going, I half-jokingly said, "I'm off to spend a week at 'Club Dead.'" The idea that one meditates to relax is a common misunderstanding. One meditates to be reborn; the only problem is, you first have to die.

To attend a *sesshin* is to step into a living Zen poem, the precise form of which was set down three hundred years ago. During the seven days of strict silence, a series of bells, gongs, and wooden clappers guide your every movement. Each day is divided into four practice sections, beginning with a sit at 3:30 in the morning and finishing with a small cookie and cup of tea at 9:00 in the evening. Wearing black monk's robes fastened about the waist with a cord of white rope, up to thirty-five people move through the day in single file according to the seating order in the *zendo* (meditation hall). You enter the *zendo* at the back door presided over by the *shoji* who performs the role of mother. If you have any personal needs, you ask the *shoji* for assistance. Sitting at the head of the *zendo*, presiding over the formal entry, is the *jikijitsu* who performs the role of father. No one speaks to him directly. His job is to keep time and maintain order by occasionally barking orders like "Quiet!" and "No sniffling!" If you have a runny nose, you let it run. At times the *jikijitsu* prowls the hall with a long flat stick and smartly strikes your shoulders with a loud "whack" if you dose off. The whack also breaks up body tension and can bring stunning relief.

Sitting periods are punctuated with walking meditation to revive the legs, performed quickly in chain gang, lock-step fashion. The strict regimentation is designed to deconstruct your individual self-identity with ritual dignity. Because each day is identical, it is like stewing in your own juices in a mirrored thermos bottle where all your projections are reflected back to you. After a few days, it becomes painfully obvious that any change in your experience is entirely a reflection of yourself.

The fourth day is typically the hardest and the most common breaking point of the week, where the long hours of sitting cross-legged build to a feverish pitch of deep bone and sinew pain. At this point, the existential situation becomes desperate, similar to climbing up a steep ridge line with a precipitous drop-off on either side. Slip off one side and you're lost in heaven; slip off the other and you're lost in hell. You might think, if it is simply a choice between heaven and hell, then why not leap into the chasm of heaven and disappear happily into bliss? But that would be a mistake. Heaven, you soon discover, can in an instant change into hell.

The only way to make it through is to stay balanced and continue climbing with calm equipoise, keeping your muscles soft and your mind open and accepting. But if you dare to resist the growing intensity, even for a moment, you tumble into a hellish grip of sharp, painful spasms. These can become knife-like stabs between the shoulder blades or twist up the low back in a dull ache of tightening knots or gnaw, with rodent-like teeth, at the tendons in your knees while you hang on by your fingernails, waiting for the bell to ring, signaling the end of the sitting period. The feedback is swift. Whether you experience peacefulness or excruciating pain depends entirely on the steadiness of your concentration and the depth of your surrender to the moment-to-moment unfolding of your experience. This is a paradox that you must experience to comprehend. Meditation is a way of learning how to balance desire and surrender at the most elemental level within your own body and mind. This is expressed in the posture of sitting perfectly erect and relaxed. Once the body is properly aligned, the mind pretty much takes care of itself.

In the Thai forest monk tradition, meditation master Ajahn Chah teaches, "If you let go a little, you will have a little happiness. If you let go a lot, you will have a lot of happiness. If you let go completely, you will be free."[7] But it can be difficult to let go if you don't know what you are holding on to, as I discovered when I was a fledgling doctor.

Modern medicine is a form of warfare; the goal is to ferret out the enemy called disease and destroy it by any means possible, whether with knife and cautery, drugs, radiation, or poisons. Medicine is serious business, and I was proud to be among the select few who could work 120 hours a week wading through the frontline trenches of human agony and suffering. By the time I finished seven years of formal training, I had become a lean fighting machine, humorless and deadened to my own pain. After all, in war, only the strong survive.

But denial comes at a high cost, as I would soon discover during a fateful encounter with an extraordinary Zen master, Sasaki Roshi. I was midway through the morning of the fourth day of a *sesshin* at the Mt. Baldy Zen Center outside Los Angeles when suddenly the immense difficulty of the situation boiled up inside me. A flood of raw emotions overflowed beyond my limits, and I began crying uncontrollably.

Breaking ranks, I bolted out of the *zendo* with tears streaming down my face and started running up the mountainside like a confused, wounded animal, stumbling over rocks and branches in the pine forest. Exhausted and unable to climb any further, I collapsed upon a large fallen tree trunk and struggled to catch my breath through sobbing tears. A few moments later, a vivid kaleidoscope of images tumbled through my mind, flashing the anguished faces and pained bodies of every patient I had ever hurt. Every flinch from a needle poke and every cringing scream as my fingers probed tender wounds had been recorded. Each image writhed through my flesh with convulsive spasms of tears like a knot being loosened from my body. At first, I was overwhelmed with pity for the suffering throngs of humanity that had passed through my hands. But then I fell into a bottomless pit of despair as their pain suddenly became more personal. My weeping turned into self-pity and fear that someday, I, too, might have to endure the torments that I had witnessed in my patients.

By that afternoon, I had regained my composure and was anxious to meet with Roshi. Every student is required to meet with him four times a day for *sanzen*, a brief, formal interview in which he asked, "Your *koan*?" and the student gives their answer. *Koan*, from the Chinese, *kung an*, is an ancient "question-answer" teaching method in Rinzai Zen. After gathering myself in meditation, I bowed out of the *zendo*, walked up the narrow path to the *sanzen* hut, and sat down on the bench to await my turn for the interview. After each encounter, Roshi rings a small bell and the next student in line, sitting before a table-top bell, picks up a wooden mallet, strikes it three times in response, and then runs down the path to the *sanzen* room. As one student leaves, the next enters quickly.

Entering the room with a standing bow, I approached Roshi, who was sitting on a low dais, and kneeled before him, bowing again. The moment of truth had arrived. We faced each other on the field of *dharma* to do battle, to manifest, no holds barred (this is the only time conversation is permitted during *sesshin*).

A stump of a man, Roshi fixed me in his unsettling, penetrating gaze. Across his lap he gripped a well-worn, menacing stick that was oddly twisted, as if it had been struck by lightning. "Your koan?" he asked.

Disregarding his question, my voice trembled, "Roshi, how can I, as a doctor, touch the suffering of my patients?"

He answered directly without hesitation, speaking from below his belly in broken English with a thick Japanese accent. "If you out in stormy sea and man falls overboard, do you jump in to save him? If you do, both you drown. Only if you are strong swimmer can you jump in to save him."

In a single blow, the piercing truth of his words fractured the enamel surface of my hard-earned, professional identity. Fine cracks now worked their way down into its very foundation, awakening a seed that had been lying dormant in the soil beneath. From that moment, a profound feeling began to stir within me. I was missing something terribly important, something I needed to find before I could jump into the roiling sea of human sickness and suffering. I needed to find a philosophical basis for the practice of medicine. Thus, began a four-year journeymanship that took me from working in emergency rooms up and down the central valley of California to martial arts training in Japan and studying acupuncture in China. During the *sesshin,* I had surrendered to the truth of the immense pain that I had unknowingly been carrying in my body, and the truth had freed me.

Surrender need not be difficult. When I lived in Sebastopol, I would drive on Coleman Valley Road through the golden hills of northern California to the coast. It was breathtaking to come over the ridge and through the soft mist see the Pacific Ocean spread wide to the horizon where the ocean touches the sky. If you turn north on Highway 1, there is a magical cove called Shell Beach. I liked to stand on a rock outcropping at the water's edge, feel the gentle breeze on my face, and chant to call the sea lions. Standing at the edge of the continental landmass, a tiny speck within a vast, unbroken panorama, I felt at peace in my insignificance and could have perished without a problem. At such moments, self and other disappear; even life and death lose their meaning. Could it be that our fear of dying is a reflection of our fear of living, and that to live well is to die well—not physically, but metaphysically—to die to our ego-identification again and again, like waves surrendering upon the shore? Perhaps this is the lesson we are fated to learn. The moment we are born we begin falling to our death … *aah!* but to be like a skydiver in freefall, enjoying the ride, is where freedom and fulfillment are found.

Which brings us to the gates of The Mystery.

▲▲▲▲▲▲▲

In brief:

We typically consider surrender a sign of weakness. Yet it is only through surrender that we can enter the richness of the present moment and partake of its pleasure. The existential paradox of desire and surrender is analogous to the particle-wave duality of quantum mechanics. Simultaneously, we are a discreet self whose desires and ambitions compete with and bounce off other selves; and a wave that interpenetrates and merges with waves in the vast ocean of life. When fearful, we contract into a particle; when in love we expand into a wave. The trick is to bring these two aspects of our being into balance, at which point we are in the optimal flow of the Tao, which is the ultimate art of living well.

Considerations:
- Observe how your sense of self (I, me, mine, myself) ebbs and flows and even vanishes at times!
- Practice letting go for an instant into an experience.
- Listen to the sound of rain, look at the moon, smell the coffee so intently that you disappear into it.
- Notice how you feel when you are in the self-conscious, particle mode.
- Notice how you feel when you in the merged, wave mode.
- Which feels better?

Part 4: **The Mystery**

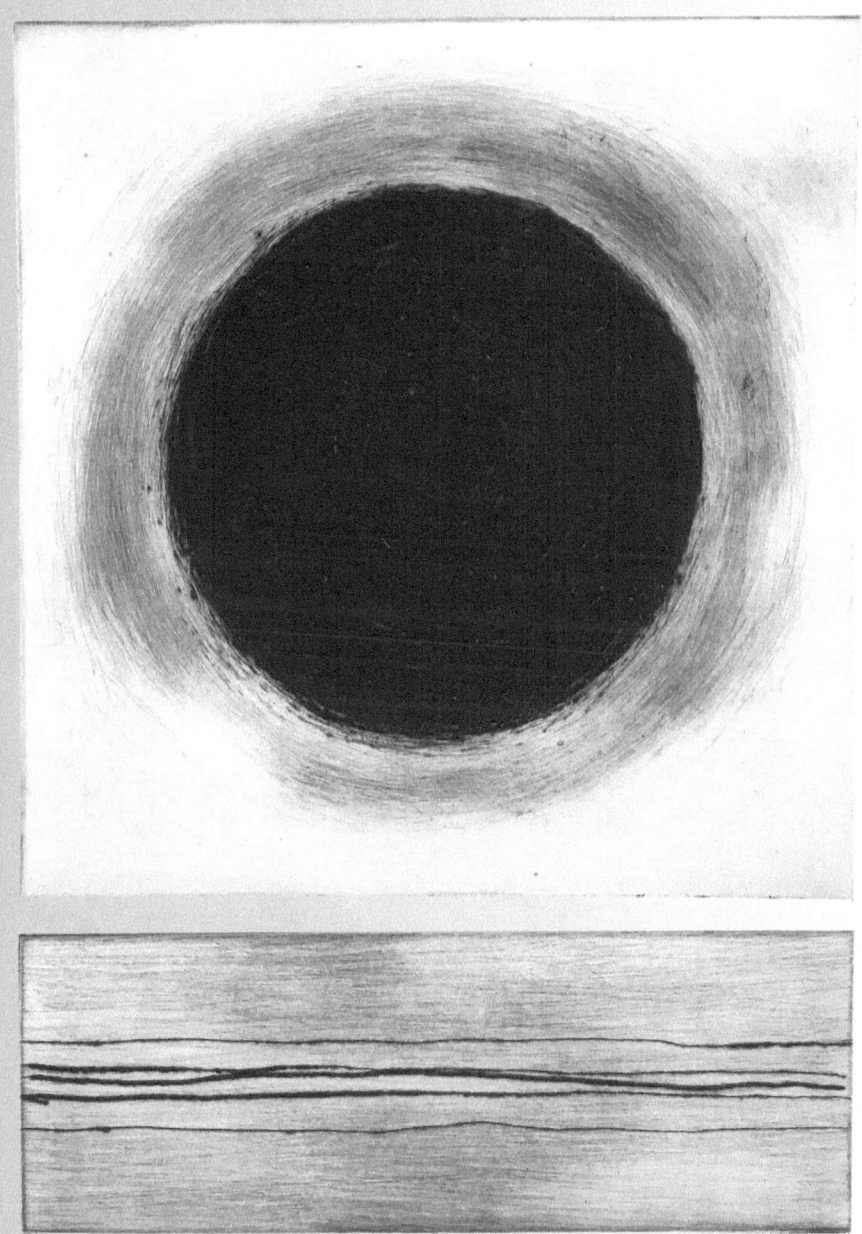

CHAPTER 17

Paradise Now

*We are already
within Paradise
but for the delusion
of a separate self.*
—JG

BEFORE WE DIVE INTO DEEPER WATERS, A FEW PRELIMINARY REMARKS WILL BE helpful to keep us from running aground on the shoals of skepticism or stumbling over the edge of blind faith. We live in a scientific world where the measurable (objective) is taken as fact and our personal, subjective experience is dismissed as mere opinion. We look outward to our scientists for truth rather than inward to our poets and mystics. As a result, our interior world seems somehow less real, and our intuitive powers have become stunted from lack of use.

Up to this point in our journey, we have analyzed pleasure from a scientific perspective—its evolution, anatomy, and natural history. The objective approach is appropriate for understanding how our physical body works, but that's not the kind of knowledge we're after here. Using our scientific understanding as a foundation, in the next three chapters we'll do some base jumping and leap into the subjective experience of pleasure beyond the limits of science, language, and conceptual thought. Just because our inner experience cannot be measured and reduced to numbers and equations doesn't make it any less real. After all, you don't need a weatherman to know if it's cold outside.

Here's the thing: *While we participate in an objective reality, we live in a subjective reality.* We can all agree to stop on red and go on green, but each of us experiences a different red and green; each of us lives in our own personal *umwelt*, perceptual niche, known only to us. Existentially, our embodied experience (subjective reality) is actually *more* real than objective reality, yet impossible to verify. This is particularly true of pleasure.

To navigate these subjective realms, you'll need to exercise your deep mind—your reptilian and limbic brains—the part of you that knows through direct experience, intuitively before words. Of course, I'll be using words but don't take them too literally. Hold them lightly, poetically, like signposts pointing to something beyond.

That said, *my* truth, born of my own perceptions and experience, need not be *your* truth. In the subjective realm, there are as many truths as there are people. If what I say doesn't make sense, no problem. But please keep an open mind; someday it may. As Aristotle said, "It is the mark of an educated mind to be able to entertain a thought without accepting it."[1]

A personal truth

Meditation has long been my ground zero, a kind of bench mark from which I start my day. So shortly after my first daughter Ashani was born, who we called "Bungy," I arranged with her mother some special father-daughter time to meditate with her upstairs in the great hall.

I devised a way to wrap a folded woolen poncho lengthwise about my waist and then around Bungy to keep her warm and snug against me and placed a small pillow on my lap for her head. Babies love to be swaddled, and this freed my hands. If she became restless, I would deepen my breath with a whispering sound and she would drift back to sleep. We spent many a peaceful and intimate morning this way.

And then the inevitable happened. While meditating in the luminous predawn darkness, Bungy began to cry inconsolably. It was like an alarm bell going off demanding something be done! But what? She had just been fed and diapered. All I could do was hold her closer to me to comfort her.

Such crying is often called "colic," suggesting an intestinal origin, but no one really knows the cause. The usual advice is to put the colicky baby in their crib and shut the door so that the child can learn to soothe herself. This seems counterintuitive, if not cruel. In a "primitive" society, such abandonment would be unthinkable and dangerous.

Before going on, I need to dispel a common misunderstanding about meditation. Although a meditator outwardly may appear to be like a stone Buddha detached from the world, inwardly a lot is going on. Meditation is a way to directly experience the raw datum of one's moment-to-moment existence free of habitual ego attachments and cultural biases. One withdraws from the distractions of the outer world to heighten the sensitivity of their inner world. The goal is not detachment, but rather non-attachment—to be fully present without grasping or pushing away. The Indian sage, Krishnamurti, described it as a practice of "choiceless awareness"—a conscious return to the naked awareness of an innocent child.

As I held Bungy close to me, her shrill cries cut through me like a serrated rasp. I felt overwhelmed with helplessness. When difficulties arise in meditation, the only thing to do is to breath and surrender more deeply. My chest felt heavy like being smothered from the inside. The stifling sensations grew more intense, when suddenly an unspeakable sorrow erupted in my core. Bungy's plaintive cries awoke in me a forgotten longing for when I was a child lying in my mother's lap, at peace, wrapped in her scent and warmth.

As we sat there, tears streaming down our cheeks, the door opened, and Mommy began to slowly climb the creaking, knotted-pine steps. She was following her instincts, as warm milk leaked from her taut, engorged breasts. She sat down next to us and began to weep. At that instant, Bungy and I stopped crying and bore silent witness to Mommy's tears of longing.

That's when I realized my personal truth: that my mother had been the representative, living embodiment of "The Mother," Mother Nature. I realized that within each of us, at the heart of every spiritual pursuit, every relationship, every heartbreak, and every desire is the longing to return to "Mother," the Source, the Absolute. We long to re-experience life before words, before ideas, before self-consciousness. We long to return to our original nature, to our Original Wholeness. This pull toward the Absolute is one of the most tender and profound forces in all of human life. It is the longing to return to the lost innocence of Paradise and lay our head in Mother Nature's lap. Indeed, *to return to the Garden is our ultimate, inescapable destiny, and every desire and pleasure is in some way a movement toward it.*

Paradise

We have now arrived at the highest frequency of the Pleasure Prism: the clear-white, *äsis* light where ecstasy, bliss, and equanimity shine forth. In classical literature, this realm is often referred to as Paradise. The word comes from the ancient Indo-Iranian *pairi* (around) and *daeza* (wall); hence, "the walled garden," a term that entered the Hebrew Bible after the Babylonian Captivity in the sixth century BCE, when Jewish intellectuals came in contact with Zoroastrian theology. It evokes images of a lush, primeval garden surrounded by a weathered, moss-covered wall.

But it is no ordinary wall that encloses this heavenly Garden. In the fifteenth century, Cardinal Nicholas of Cusa wrote, "The wall of the Paradise in which Thou, Lord, dwellest, is built of contradictories, nor is there any way to enter but for one who has overcome the highest Spirit of Reason who guards its gate."[2] If his words sound cryptic, it may be because he lived during the 700-year reign of terror known as the Inquisition, when he could have been burned at the stake for stepping out of line. At the same time, the realm of which he speaks is beyond logic (the highest Spirit of Reason). Writing as a mystic and a mathematician, the good Cardinal expressed his ideas with the brevity of a mathematical proposition, which requires a bit of unpacking to comprehend.

At this point in our inquiry, Niels Bohr would say, "How wonderful that we have met with a paradox. Now we have some hope of making progress."[3] Every theory, every paradigm, frays into contradictories at its edges; it is precisely at this ragged edge that anomalies appear and new theories are born. Logically (in the highest Spirit of Reason), a proposition (*A*) and its contradiction (*not-A*), cannot both be true. A cat is either alive or not; there is no third option. But as we saw in quantum mechanics, sometimes there is a third possibility (known as Schrödinger's cat paradox) where an elementary particle is in an indeterminate state, both a particle *and* a wave until a measurement is made. Bohr put it this way: "There are trivial truths, and there are great Truths. The opposite of a trivial truth is plainly false. The opposite of a great Truth is also true."[4] Well, we have come upon a True paradox!

One of the clearest descriptions of the paradoxical nature of Truth is summarized in the thin volume of the *Xin Xin Ming—Inscription of the Perfect Mind*, attributed to the Third Zen Patriarch Sengcan:

> The Great Way is not difficult
> for those who have no preferences.
> When love and hate are both absent
> everything becomes clear and undisguised.
> Make the smallest distinction, however,
> and heaven and earth are set infinitely apart.
>
> If you wish to see the truth
> then hold no opinions for or against anything.
> To set up what you like against what you dislike
> is the disease of the mind.[5]

The mind is originally perfect. The act of judging our experience prevents us from seeing the plain truth of it due to our biases. Discernment is different than judgement, hence the saying that *an object is most clearly seen the first time*. Bias error is particularly problematic in judgments about ourselves, which tend to be either overly harsh, in denial, or both. For this reason, a nonjudgmental mind is essential for honest self-reflection.[6]

Beyond duality

The problem is, we are so deeply conditioned in duality that we have difficulty comprehending what lies beyond the wall of contradictories. As discussed in Chapter 9, our entire nervous system functions in terms of contrast and comparison and is therefore inherently dualistic. This is reflected in our language, which divides everything into subjects and objects connected by verbs. Language fragments reality into pieces—words and symbols—and thinking contrasts and compares these symbols to create meaning, which inevitably is but a partial rendering of the whole. Still, there is value in trying to describe the ineffable, if only to point a finger toward the moon.

But who's pointing the finger? As many mystics have noted, we miss Paradise (enlightenment) not because it is so far away, but because it is so near. The wall is not around the Garden but around each one of us—an ego-shell that defines our individuality and makes us feel special, and at the same time, separate, alone, and alienated. *The truth is we're already in Paradise, only we don't realize it because we surround ourselves with a wall of contradictories (judgments) to protect our fragile ego self-image.*

Thus, Paradise is entered from within—literally, from within your own body. We'll talk more about this later. For now, all you need to do is go beyond your dualistic thinking—your preferences, distinctions, opinions—and open the pores of your being to the mystery of the ever-present *NOW*. This is easier to do than you might think, or more precisely, beyond thinking.

Zeroing in on the balancing point

We now come to the crux of the matter, the pivot around which our lives turn. What makes human existence so challenging is that we, ourselves, are a paradox. We are both a particle and a wave—individuals with separate boundaries and non-self ripples in the sea of existence. This same paradox lies at the root of pleasure: we require *ego-desire* to seek pleasure, yet *egoless* surrender to enjoy it. To resolve this paradox, we must penetrate the deep meaning of emptiness, which is represented mathematically by zero.

Being an alumnus, I called the chairman of the math department at the University of Colorado to ask if I could speak with someone about the concept of zero. He agreed to meet me for lunch, he later admitted, out of curiosity.

"Why are you so interested in zero?" he asked.

"Well, it's such a strange number," I said. "Multiply it times any number, and the product is zero. It annihilates and swallows every number. Add it to any number, and you get the same number as though it were nothing. But try to divide a number by this nothing, and you get infinity. Nothing becomes everything! It's so weird, it doesn't act like any other number; maybe it shouldn't be considered a number at all?"

He was unimpressed with my musings, and had little to say about zero, except for one small, profound detail. "You can think of zero," he said, "in geometrical terms as symmetry about a point, a line, or a plane."

"You mean balance?" I asked.

"Yes, balance."

That got me thinking about zero in more practical terms and gave me something tangible to wrap my mind around.

It turns out I'm not the only one who is fascinated with naught. According to mathematician Tobias Danzig, "In the history of culture the development of zero will always stand out as one of the single greatest achievements of the human race."[7] Charles Seife's little book, *The Biography of a Dangerous Idea*, details how zero came into existence and why it matters. While other ancient cultures had the notion of zero as a placeholder, the modern concept of zero originated in India as *sunyata*, the void or emptiness. It then travelled to the Middle East along with the Hindu numeral and decimal system, from whence Arabic numerals and algebra came. The Catholic Church resisted the entry of zero into mathematics for hundreds of years, retarding the development of Western science because it's difficult to do calculations with Roman numerals, which lack zero. It wasn't until the Renaissance weakened the Church's political hold that zero entered Western civilization.

Why were the Catholic theologians so uptight about nothing? They astutely understood that if you admit the concept of zero, infinity comes with it, and if the cosmos were infinite, then it would have no center, in which case Rome could no longer claim to be the center of the universe. The term "catholic" means universal, from the Greek *katholikos*, *kata* (with respect to) and *holos* (whole). The Catholics, being monotheists, conceived of the whole as the universal, *uni* (one) and *vertere* (version), the one and only version.

The number one is indeed a "uni-que" and powerful number in its own right. Once you have one, you get all the other whole numbers by simply adding n + 1, which gives you the next number in the sequence: 1, 2, 3.... Multiply or divide a number by one, and you get the same number. The idea of unity—one world, one humanity, standing united, and being all one—is attractive and feels warm and cozy. But compared to the profundity of zero, one is a limited and limiting concept. After all, there may be more than one version of the universe, more than one version of the Truth and, God forbid, more than one version of God and religion. Philosophically, the problem is that monotheism is inherently dualistic: one implies two. You can't have *one* without the *other*. Christ implies an Antichrist. Simply put, *Western civilization is built around one. Eastern civilization is built around zero.*

A return to innocence

So how can we transcend our ego-wall of contradictories and enter the Garden?

Like the two ends of a stick, you can't transcend duality by taking hold of only one end, just as you can't "shun the darkness and seek the light," because the two ends—dark and light—always come together. In other words, you can't use dualistic thinking to transcend duality. "You can't wash blood with blood," as the Zen saying goes.

In the real world, the only way to transcend duality is through balance. You can, in a sense, grasp both ends of the stick simultaneously by taking hold of the middle—the balancing point where the two ends meet, where opposites coexist and paradox is resolved—much in the same way as zero stands at the midpoint of the number line and contains all the positive and negative numbers. The emptiness of zero contains everything, and everything is just another name for the whole, which is to say: *Zero = Balance = Whole.*

We have a lot of difficulty thinking about the whole. For instance, many people think of holistic medicine in opposition to conventional medicine, when actually holistic medicine includes conventional medicine. The whole contains everything, even duality. Concepts like the whole, infinity, emptiness, and zero are mind-bending because they go beyond the limits of our dualistic thinking. You can't think your way to wholeness because, as the word suggests, it has a "hole" in it. However, you can intuit it directly, as the math professor pointed out, and grab hold of it at the balancing point.

Nature offers many examples of balance. The center of gravity of an object is its balancing point, which in a physical sense contains the mass of the entire object. The pivot of a wheel, the maximum torque range of an engine, and the speaker balance knob on your sound system are all examples of balance. And then there is the mother of all "wholes," the black hole, where space-time collapses and matter becomes so infinitely dense that nothing can escape its gravitational pull, not even light. Like zero, a black hole annihilates everything that falls within its event horizon. Our entire galaxy is believed to revolve around a massive black hole where the normal laws of physics break down and may even contain wormholes to other universes. These invisible objects were first predicted when solutions to Einstein's general relativity equations came up with zero in the denominator of some of the terms, causing the equation to blow up to infinity and become uninterpretable—a situation known as a singularity. As comedian Steven Wright joked, "Black holes are where God divided by zero." Even though we refer to it as a singularity (perhaps in honor of the Big One, God), more precisely, it is a *zero*-larity, the Big Nothing!

Practically speaking, a lot of good things happen at the balancing point, which is just another name for the "sweet spot" where we find maximum power, efficiency, stability, and freedom. In any athletic activity, from martial arts to ballet, power comes from being in balance. Balance a refrigerator on a dolly, and it becomes relatively light. In Sanskrit the technical term is *sukham,* the round hole that allows an axle to turn smoothly. Patanjali describes the ideal yoga posture as *"sthira sukham asanam"*[8]—the balance of *sthira* (steadiness) and *sukham* (ease). You can experience this for yourself by standing with your weight equally balanced on both feet, stable *and* yet free to move in any direction.

It is also at the balancing point that we encounter the maximum pleasure of ecstasy, bliss, and equanimity. *It all comes down to the greatest number in the whole universe—zero—and the most powerful principle in the universe—balance.*[9]

As it says in the Bible, "Truly, I say to you, unless you turn and become like children, you will never enter into the kingdom of heaven."[10] If you wish to enter the Garden, you must return to the innocence of a child who has not yet tasted the bittersweet (dualistic) fruit of the Tree of Knowledge of Good and Evil. The most basic duality is self and other. Recall that Adam and Eve only became self-conscious and reached for fig leaves *after* they ate the forbidden fruit. Indeed, the ego-self is often the biggest obstacle to experiencing pleasure. Conversely, as we will see, when ego-desire is perfectly balanced with egoless surrender, the self momentarily disappears, the wall of contradictories vanishes, and we can slip through the crack between worlds to once again frolic in the Elysian Fields and lay our head in the blessed peace of Mother Nature's lap.

▲▲▲▲▲▲▲

In brief:

We *participate* in a consensual reality that can be objectively measured and verified, but we *live* in a subjective reality known only to ourselves. Of the two, our embodied subjective reality is existentially more real. From this personal perspective, much of our life can be understood as a longing to return to our original state of wholeness, the Garden of Eden. We are separated from Paradise by a dualistic wall of contradictories: ego judgments of self and other, right and wrong, good and bad, and what we like and don't like. However, at the balancing point, these contradictions paradoxically coexist and we return to Original Wholeness.

Considerations:
- How do you return to the Garden in your own life?
- Notice when you judge yourself and other people.
- What do you get out of passing judgment on others?
- Explore your inner world through an expressive art (draw, sing, dance, write a poem); an exercise (run, swim, cycle, stretch); or self-kindness (prepare a meal, enjoy a bath, remember a dream, take a nap).
- Practice using the language of *both/and* rather than *either/or*.
- Notice the empty spaces between being and not being, self and other, wanting and not wanting, tension and release.
- Honor your inner child!

CHAPTER 18

The 3 Gateways to Paradise

▲ 6. The Law of Desire and Surrender

> *Life is a balance of holding on*
> *and letting go.*
> —Rumi

WHEN I WAS AROUND TEN YEARS OLD, I RECEIVED A BIRTHDAY PRESENT THAT changed my life—a crystal radio kit that initiated me into the magical world of science. Opening the box, I found a collection of strange parts: a small resistor banded with candy-baked colors; a shiny aluminum cylinder capacitor; a spool of brown-lacquered copper wire; a cardboard tube to wrap the wire around; a short boom with an attached wire as fine as a cat's whisker; a pair of black Bakelite headphones; and most mysterious of all, a lump of glistening gallium crystal mounted on a metal ring. By evening, I had assembled all the components on the pre-punched cardboard circuit board and connected two wires: one to the cast iron pipe in the corner of my room for a ground and another to the bedsprings of my bed for an antenna. I put on the headphones and, per the instructions, dragged the cat-whisker slowly over the surface of the gallium crystal (the forerunner of the modern semiconductor) like a blind man walking with a cane over uneven ground. All of a sudden, out of thin air, the booming voice of a radio announcer, "WCFL Chicago," came in loud and clear.

Thus began my "nerd years." By the following autumn, I had built a makeshift miniature crystal radio that fit in my shirt pocket. I was the kid in the back of the class who reported the score of the 1959 World Series when the Chicago White Sox lost to the Los Angeles Dodgers, four games to two. During the summers, I took classes in math and science at the Illinois Institute of Technology (IIT), learned to use a slide rule, and studied Fortran, an early computer programming language that required feeding stacks of punched IBM cards into a mechanical reader.

If you had asked me back then why I chose to major in engineering physics, I would have told you I wanted to work in an intellectually challenging field where I wouldn't have to interact much with people. I was shy and awkward and deep into the scientific paradigm. I remember my freshman year walking across the Kittredge Hall patio, a Cartesian grid of sandstone squares and rectangular columns, and thinking physics could explain everything if we just knew all the laws and initial conditions. I took comfort in the belief that I was acquiring the keys to a logical, clockwork universe. Two years later I switched to arts-and-sciences physics to expand my social life and philosophical horizons.

Throughout all the twists and turns in my life, my insatiable curiosity to understand how things work has been a common thread, and I'm still at it.

Physics teaches that the universe is composed of two fundamental building blocks—matter and energy—and when they are arranged in a particular spatial configuration (like a crystal radio), they create a third phenomenon: information. It's difficult to say what information is, exactly. Radio waves, the gears of a watch, silicon crystals on a microchip, DNA, the food we eat, and the news we consume are all examples of matter and energy arranged in a particular way to hold and convey information. When the density of information becomes sufficiently complex, we recognize it as intelligence; when intelligence becomes sufficiently complex, we recognize it as consciousness. (Some would argue information, as consciousness, precedes matter and energy, but that's a discussion for another time.)

We live in an intelligent universe. I say this with great confidence because you and I are intelligent, and we are products of the universe. Moreover, our body, without the least exaggeration, is one of the most complex pieces of matter in the known universe and gives us a unique ability to consciously (in a self-aware way) tune into radio station LIFE. Among the frequencies available to us are a bandwidth of subtle higher frequencies called ecstasy, bliss, and equanimity.

▲ The Law of Desire and Surrender

Frequencies have to do with waves and oscillations. As we learned in Chapter 15, we can think of pleasure as a pendulum swinging over the Sensual Continuum, generating a Pleasure Cycle. Recall that when we push the pendulum toward greater intensity (through an act of desire), we experience active pleasure, and when we relax (surrender), the pendulum swings back toward lower intensity and we experience passive pleasure. At the midpoint in between is neutral pleasure.

We usually think of a pendulum as having a single balancing point at the plumb line where it comes to rest, but there are two additional balancing points at the ends of its swing where it turns around. At each of these *three* balancing points, we encounter the mystical zero where desire and surrender come into equilibrium. Using this conceptual framework, we can define three states of consciousness, or frequencies:

1. *Ecstasy* occurs at the extreme of active pleasure, where, in the midst of intense effort, we surrender.

2. *Bliss* occurs at the extreme of passive pleasure, where, in the midst of deep relaxation, we maintain a glimmer of desire.

3. *Equanimity* occurs midway between at the extreme of neutral pleasure.

In other words, *ecstasy, bliss, and equanimity are found at the points of the Pleasure Cycle where desire and surrender come into balance.* This is the Law of Desire and Surrender.

The *Taiji* symbol (written *T'ai Chi* using Wade-Guiles) provides a convenient way to visualize these relationships. Properly understood, the *Taiji* is in dynamic motion with the black (*yin*) and white (*yang*) crescents continuously swirling in a dance of expansion and contraction. The traditional image of matching black and white crescents with a contrasting dot within the head of each represents an instant in time when *yin* and *yang* are at the midpoint of the pendulum's swing, a snapshot of equanimity. When the *Taiji* has turned entirely white with only a black dot remaining (extreme *yang*), we see a snapshot of ecstasy. When it has turned entirely black and only a white dot remains (extreme *yin*), we get a snapshot of bliss.

Yin and *yang* are cosmic principles that are entirely equal and opposite complementary pairs and only have meaning in relationship to each other; that is, they are relative terms. For example, in Chinese medicine, the top half of the human body is *yang* and the lower half is *yin*, but the chest is

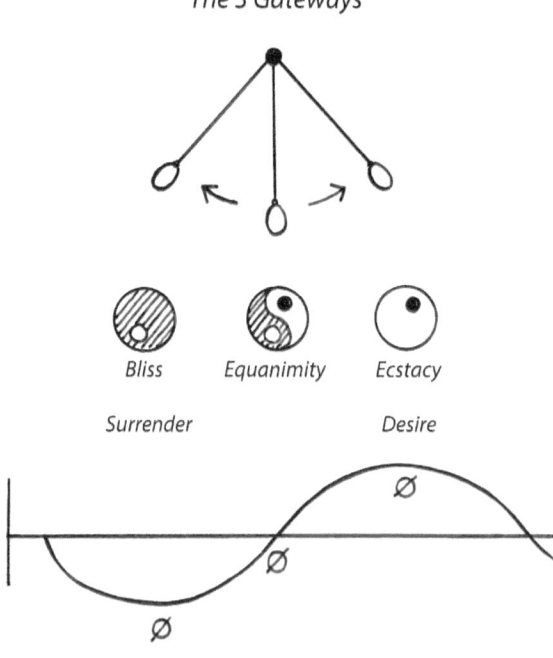

Figure 21: The balancing points of the pleasure pendulum, *Taiji*, and pleasure wave as ecstasy, equanimity, and bliss..

yin in relationship to the back. In their earliest formulation, *yin* is like the shady side of a riverbank, cool and damp, and *yang* is like the sunny side, hot and dry. *Yin* is earth, matter, substantial, and slow to change; *yang* is heaven, spirit, light, and quick. In terms of pleasure, *surrender is yin* (yielding and passive) and *desire is yang* (hard and active).

At each of the three extremes of the Pleasure Cycle, surrender and desire come into balance, paradox is resolved, and the walls of contradictories vanish. These then, are the three gateways to Paradise and each gate is approached from a different direction. Again, *pleasure is path-dependent*. The enjoyment you experience depends on how you get there. Ecstasy is approached through activity, bliss through passivity, and equanimity through balancing the two extremes at the midpoint. These relationships are summarized below:

Yin	Yang
Negative	Positive
Wave	Particle
No-self	Self
Passive	Active
Surrender	Desire

Now let's bring these abstract ideas down to earth by physically locating ecstasy, bliss, and equanimity within three "vital centers" of your body.

The ecstasy center

Ecstasy is an extreme form of active pleasure. American psychologist Abraham Maslow called it a "peak experience," an apt description that evokes the image of a ball tossed into the air reaching a peak of weightless suspension, where the upward force (desire) is perfectly balanced by the downward force of gravity (surrender). Leonard Cohen describes it poetically as "reaching for the sky just to surrender."[1]

Ecstasy comes from the Greek *ekstasis: ek* (outside) and *stasis* (to stand), literally "to stand outside oneself," outside one's ego-shell. Hungarian psychologist, Mihaly Csikszentmihalyi, calls it "flow," a state of focused effortlessness where we become so absorbed in an activity that self, time, and other vanish. Jazz players refer to it as being in the groove and basketball players as being in the zone. Lakers basketball great Kobe Bryant, who at the age of thirty-four became one of only five players to score over 30,000 points in NBA play, says, "When you get in that zone, it's just that supreme confidence that you know it's going in … things just slow down … when that happens, you really do not try to focus on what's going on because you can lose it in a second. Everything becomes one noise [and] … you have to really try to stay in the present … you know, not let anything break that rhythm."[2]

Bryant is a virtuoso of the zone. His supreme confidence comes from being in the sweet spot, the balancing point of efficiency, power, and freedom. Things slow down because in states of high concentration you perceive more details—more data points per second—literally stretching time. The statement, "You really do not try to focus on what's going on" sounds paradoxical until you realize that he is already in a state of extreme focus where his intense desire needs to be counterbalanced with a touch of surrender (the black dot in a sea of white). When this happens, *voilà*, the gateway to ecstasy opens. And yet, the balancing point is delicate, something that you can lose "in a second."

"Not let anything break that rhythm," illustrates several key elements. First, the zone is a wave; it has a rhythm that alternates between effort and non-effort, self and no-self, particle and wave. Second, at the moment of surrender, when you release your ego-desire, the reptilian brain instantly takes over. (Reptiles like repetition, which is just another word for rhythm.) Third, in an intense situation, you need to keep your emotional brain cool and not let the ego get in the way. This is done, not through denial, but by staying present, remaining open, and allowing the life-stream to flow through.

Where is the vital ecstasy center in your body? To locate the center of something is to find its source, its origin. Ecstasy, being the result of intense effort, is located at the origin of effort in the body. At the moment of maximum effort, we naturally exhale: boxers breathe out like a steam piston with each jab; tennis players make a guttural "ugh" when serving; and martial artists shout "*ki-ai*" as they attack.[3] Sharply exhaling galvanizes the body by integrating internal and external muscular contractions into a focused effort.

The exhale can lead us to the ecstasy center. Take a deep breath and exhale slowly, making a "*sissss*" sound between your teeth like the sound of steam from a boiling tea kettle. Breathe out fully until you have to squeeze out the last few drops. At the terminus of the outbreath, you will discover a muscular contraction deep at the bottom of your pelvis (Latin for bowl)—the pelvic floor muscles lift up and the lower abdominal muscles draw in like a purse string. The ecstasy center is at the epicenter of these contractions. It lies two centimeters in front of the lumbosacral junction at the level of the groin, deep within the pelvis. This is also the location of your physical center of gravity, your balancing point in the standing position. All physical effort is ultimately mediated through the center of gravity, which is why core strength—lower abdominal and pelvic support—is so critical for optimal physical performance.

When I meet an avid golfer or tennis player whose sport requires a vigorous whipping action, I sometimes ask them, "So, where's the handle of the whip?" If they answer, "It's the club or racquet handle," I ask, "What about the arms, shoulder, and spine?" Then, working our way back through the kinetic chain, we arrive at the actual handle of the whip: the sacrum, deep in the pelvis, the center of effort and ecstasy. (It's also the center from which we aim.)

The pelvis corresponds to the reptilian tail of the sphinx. The pelvic floor muscles (sometimes referred to as the pubococcygeus or levator ani muscles or the pelvic diaphragm) are, in fact, vestigial tail muscles. Effort is motivated by desire, which is a function of the reptilian brain, thus bringing us full circle to the ecstasy center. If you have any doubt as to the location of your ecstasy center, simply observe the epicenter of your next pelvic-thrusting orgasm.

The bliss center

Bliss is the mirror image of ecstasy and is born of surrender. It is an extreme form of passive pleasure at the other end of the pendulum's swing. We enter bliss by maintaining a glimmer of conscious awareness within the midst of deep relaxation. In a yoga workout, bliss is practiced at the end, lying symmetrically on your back in *shavasana*, the corpse pose, completely relaxed, yet aware. As such, bliss isn't something we *achieve*; it's something we *receive*. Like gravity, it is continually attracting us. All we need to do is let go. Each night, we surrender into bliss when we fall asleep, but aren't aware of it because we lose consciousness. Nonetheless, we experience its aftereffects when we awaken the next morning rested and refreshed.

Locating the vital bliss center is—pardon me—a big *yaahn* ... A yawn is a deep core release and can lead us to the bliss center. Give it a go: take a big, toothy yawn, and as you breathe in, you'll hear an *aah* sound. Follow the inhale to its epicenter and you'll be led to a spacious emptiness (zero-point) at the soft palate in the back of your throat. As the name suggests, the palate is a palatial, domed structure. The bliss center is located at the highest expanse of the dome above the soft palate, just beyond the uvula, the fleshy appendage that flutters in the wind when you snore. In the poetic language of the ancient yogis, it is said that a pool of *amrita* (nectar) lies at *talu chakra,* the palate center.[4] When the palate is released, the *amrita* drips down like dew, nourishing the petals of the lotus blossom of the heart, which turn upward to receive the moisture and spread open, radiating *ananda* (pure bliss) in all directions.

Now, take another big, *aah*some yawn, and this time, observe where your mind is. "No place in particular," is how one person described it. Teachers have long known that when students are *yaahning*, they're not learning (but they are absorbing bliss). This experiment demonstrates that the soft palate acts like an energetic cork. When the palate relaxes, the cork is released, the body-stream flows unimpeded, and the mind-stream instantly ceases. When thinking ceases, ideas, preferences, ego and desire also vanish, at which point bliss floods in to fill the void of *sunyata*, emptiness, like air filling a vacuum. The more the palate releases, the greater the relaxation, which can vary from a sigh to a smile to laughter to the awe of a spiritual epiphany. It is a subtle palatal release that makes Mona Lisa's smile so captivating. If you wish to see what pure bliss looks like, check out the face of an infant after breastfeeding.[5] The ability to release the palate and suspend thought is one of the secrets of tuning in to the higher pleasure frequencies.

The equanimity center

If bliss is like dropping a marble in a bowl and letting it roll to the bottom, and ecstasy is like turning the bowl over and rolling the marble up the side to balance precariously at its top, then equanimity is like placing a marble on a table where it can roll freely in any direction. Of the three gateways, equanimity is the most subtle and easily missed, which is why the Zen master Ummon called it the "gateless barrier."

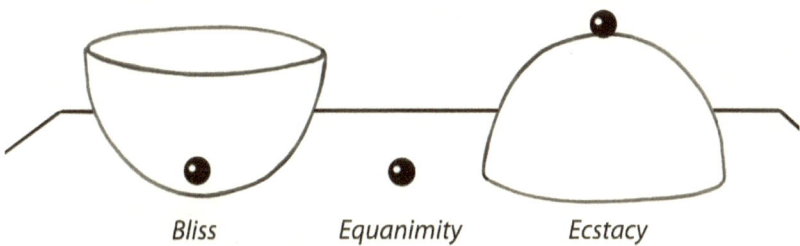

Bliss   Equanimity   Ecstacy

Figure 22: Ecstasy, equanimity, and bliss in three dimensions as two bowls and three marbles on a table.

The word "equanimity" comes from the Latin *aequus* (equal) and *animas* (spirit/mind, as in "animal" and "animated"). Hence, equanimity means "equal-minded, even-spirited, a place of balance, or equipoise." It is found at the extreme of neutral pleasure.

Equanimity dwells in the gaps that punctuate the rhythm of our lives, where one desire leaves off before the next one arises. It's present when you're lazing in bed in the morning, going on a stroll to nowhere in particular, waiting in line, or looking vacantly out a window. It arises quite naturally after a wave of active and passive pleasure streams through the body and we float back to baseline. Notice that as the pendulum's amplitude decreases, the three balancing points eventually converge into an equanimous vibration about the plumb line.

You might think that the very notion of neutral pleasure is an oxymoron. Doesn't the nervous system require contrast and comparison to perceive anything? To many, a life without highs and lows sounds incredibly boring and monotonously flat, as flat as the Great Plains where I grew up, where the cornfields stretch as far as the eye can see, where, as they say in North Dakota, "you can watch a dog run away for three days." But *what one person calls boring, an Epicurean calls ataraxia, peace of mind.* Equanimity is an acquired taste weaned on the bitter rind of life. We frequently don't appreciate it until we have known suffering. This may explain why the cycle of war often skips several generations.[6]

Epicurus understood the futility of chasing after empty pleasures and our "thankless nature of the soul that makes the creature endlessly greedy for variations in its lifestyle."[7] He was aware of habituation, which leads to an endless turning up the volume to higher levels of intensity. Epicurus recommended turning up the *sensitivity* instead. To be sensitive requires a healthy nervous system, which is why he advocated simple, clean living. When we turn up our sensitivity, we see that the Great Plains aren't actually flat but textured with ravines, dells, bluffs, and rolling hills.

As you might expect, the equanimity center is located midway between the ecstasy and bliss centers. To find it, inhale deeply and feel the sides of your rib cage lift as the skirt of the diaphragm spreads open. At the center of this expansion you can feel a subtle contraction at the highest point on the dome of the diaphragm. As the diaphragm contracts, the dome draws downward, gently tugging on the heart that rests upon it (the heartstrings). At the epicenter of this contraction lies the equanimity center.

Equanimity can be experienced at all four levels of the Pleasure Prism. Physically, equanimity arises when pain and discomfort are absent. Emotionally, it abides calmly in the present moment, free of past regret and future anxiety. Mentally, it is a state of open awareness. And at the *äsis* level, it is the mystical emptiness of the gateless barrier. When our appetites—for food, drink, sex, possessions, status, enlightenment, or anything else—have abated, we are undisturbed and free to simply enjoy life as it is.

The human *āsis* field

When these three vital centers are well aligned, something extraordinary happens. The ecstasy and bliss centers define the plus and minus poles of our body-tube, which acts as an inductor (a coil of wire that stores magnetic field energy). In between the plus and minus poles, the equanimity center acts as a capacitor (charged parallel plates that store electrical field energy). When our Light-body is properly aligned, we become like a crystal radio, tuned to resonate with the higher vibrations of the Pleasure Prism.

The Human āsis Field

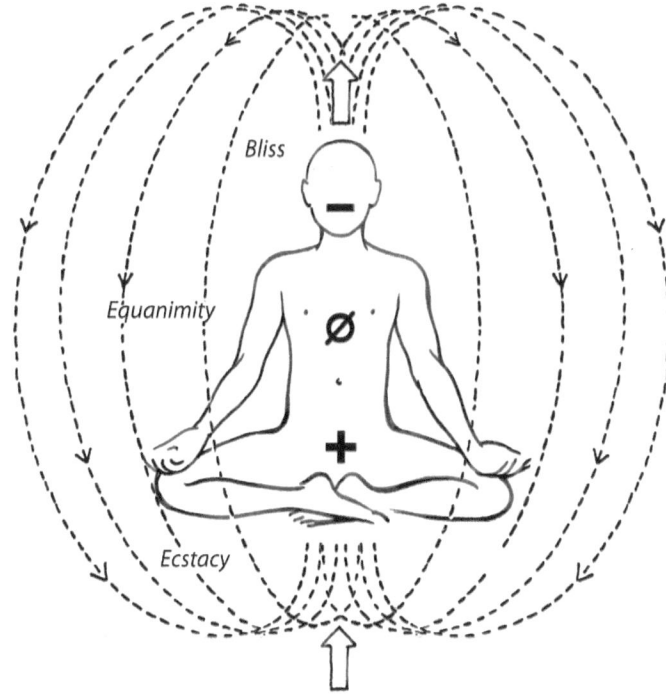

Figure 23: The human āsis field.

Resonance is a unique property of waves and is the second most powerful principle in the cosmos right after balance, with which it is intimately related. If you push a pendulum with just enough force at a precise moment in its trajectory (like pushing a child in a swing) the amplitude of the pendulum will get larger and larger and eventually swing all the way around its pivot. When the frequency of the push is perfectly matched to the natural frequency of the pendulum, the two oscillators are said to be in resonance. Every object has a resonant frequency, which is why a singer who hits a note that matches the resonant frequency of a wine glass can shatter it and why soldiers marching over a bridge at a particular cadence can cause it to collapse.

Just as a pendulum oscillates between storing potential energy when it swings upward and releasing kinetic energy when it swings downward, a crystal radio oscillates between storing magnetic energy in the inductor and electrical energy in the capacitor. When you tune in a station on your radio, you are matching the frequency of the inductor and capacitor with the electromagnetic frequency of the radio-wave signal. Most mysterious is that *things that resonate at the same frequency attract each other*. They cohere from the Latin *co*, "together" and *haerere*, "to stick." The radio antenna *attracts* the radio station. That's why pendulum clocks hanging on a common wall synchronize with each other, women living together have their menses at the same time and, I suspect, why we resonate (feel a good vibe) with some people more than others. It is this coherence that makes laser light so powerful.

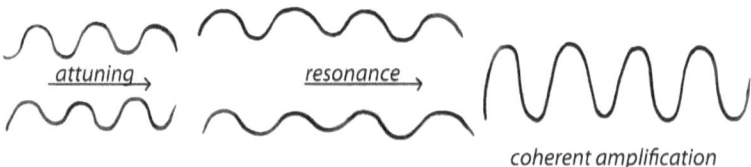

Figure 24: Resonant waves attract and amplify.

When we tune our Light-body to resonate with the higher frequencies of ecstasy, bliss, and equanimity, we attract these energies. This tuning, or more precisely attuning, is accomplished by aligning the vital centers of the three diaphragms (domes) of the body—the pelvic diaphragm, the respiratory diaphragm, and the soft palate diaphragm—along the central axis of the *sushumna*.

For this reason, posture is important. Aligning the outer body is just the first step that must be further refined by aligning the inner Light-body. Adjusting the tension of the Light-body requires a delicate balancing of desire and surrender, as delicate as a cat's whisker. If all this seems vague and murky when you look within, don't be discouraged. The sense of internal touch (*vedana* in Sanskrit) never feels as clear as touching something with your fingertip or looking at a pine needle in the sunlight. It is mysterious, like gazing through pine branches at a hazy moon, and the more you look, the more you see. In the end, it is a mystery that you never get to the bottom of. Like anything worthwhile, tuning into these higher frequencies takes patient, persistent practice, and an abiding trust that the lotus blossom will eventually spring forth from the dark, turbid water. When you get it right, you will feel light in every sense of the word. You will be coherent. And you will discover that *within ecstasy is a drop of bliss; within bliss is a drop of ecstasy; and within equanimity is a drop of both*—just like the black and white dots in the *Taiji*.

There are many ways to practice attuning yourself to the higher frequencies. One of the most simple and direct is to use *äsis* as a mantra: intoning *aah* as you breathe in, and *siss* as you breathe out. The mantra replaces the mental chatter of the discursive mind with a more wholesome object, like giving a bone to a dog. You might intone *äsis* out loud at first and then inwardly once you get the hang of it. After the *äsis* sound and breathing are synchronized, the next step is to tune into the associated body sensations as a kinesthetic mantra.[8] Notice that when you inhale, the chest and palate naturally expand with a pleasant felt sense of open receptivity and surrender ... *aah*. When you exhale, the chest, lower abdomen, and pelvic floor naturally contract with a subtle feeling of effort and desire ... *siss*. By focusing on these body sensations of expansion and contraction (surrender and desire), you can connect with your primal kinesthetic source—your genesis—and ride these waves into sublime realms of ecstasy, bliss, and equanimity, which we will explore next. (For further details on practical ways to develop your pleasure awareness and capacity, please see the Afterword.)

▲▲▲▲▲▲▲

In brief:

The Pleasure Cycle can be visualized as a pendulum with three balancing points: one at either end of its excursion and one in the middle. These correspond to the crest of active pleasure, the trough of passive pleasure, and the plane of neutral pleasure. Each of these balancing points is a gateway to Paradise where desire and surrender come into equilibrium and we can experience ecstasy, bliss, and equanimity. Anatomically, these balancing points correspond to three vital centers in the body: the ecstasy center in the pelvis, the bliss center at the palate, and the equanimity center in the core of the heart. When these three centers are properly aligned, our Light-body acts like an antenna, allowing us to tune into and resonate with the higher *äsis* frequencies of the Pleasure Prism and experience moments of Original Wholeness.

Pleasure Cycle	Gateway	Vital Center
Active	Ecstasy	Pelvis
Neutral	Equanimity	Heart
Passive	Bliss	Palate

Considerations:
- What lifestyle changes can you make to tune-up your Light-body?
- Notice how your sensitivity and state of being varies according to your lifestyle choices.

- What is the effect of eating heavy versus light? A good night's sleep? The vibrational level of the people you associate with?

- Take the *äsis* mantra for a test drive and tune into your ecstasy, bliss, and equanimity centers.

CHAPTER 19

It's a Fractal Thing

> *Strictly speaking, there is no such thing as
> an enlightened person.
> There is only enlightened activity.*
> —Shunryu Suzuki

So, if we're living in the midst of Paradise and the pendulum of the Pleasure Cycle is endlessly swinging back and forth through the gateways of ecstasy, bliss, and equanimity, why aren't we experiencing more ecstatic peaks, blissful valleys, and broad plains moments? This is an important question and answering it will help us zero in on the higher, *äsis* frequencies of pleasure. But first, it will be helpful to understand something about fractals.

When my family lived on the north shore of Lake Tahoe, I loved to wake up, grab my yoga mat, a small cushion, and blanket, and walk out to the end of the old wooden pier to meditate. The calmness of the lake in the morning made it easy to quiet the waves in my mind and slip below their surface. At the end of the meditation, I practiced expanding my consciousness by opening my eyes very slowly and raising my gaze across the glimmering expanse of water to the misty-blue mountains on the distant shore. Then returning to the shallows lapping languidly against the fissured, waterlogged pilings, I studied the surface of the lake heaving like a slumbering beast. Atop the broad undulations were shifting patchworks of wavelets, and on top of these rode still finer ripples breaking in delicate crests. The morning sun penetrated this play of waves and cast a luminous lacework on the furrowed sandy bottom. Gazing into the depths of this dizzying kaleidoscope of light and shadow, I sensed that I was witnessing a profound mystery beyond my comprehension, that I was witnessing the very nature of nature.

Fractals—from the Latin *fractus,* meaning broken or fractured—are repeating patterns that display self-similarity at different scales. For instance, a photograph of waves on a lake would appear similar whether seen from twelve feet above the surface or twelve inches. We would need an object like a leaf or the prow of a ship to gauge the height. Similarly, the branching of a tree repeats itself at every scale (distance). From a hundred yards, we can see the branching form of the trunk and limbs. As we get closer, we see that the limbs are also branching, and so on down to the level of twigs and the veins within a leaf.

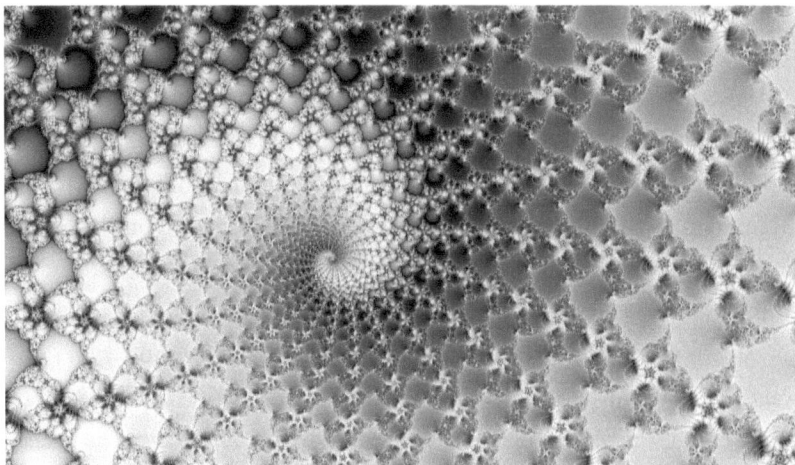

Figure 25: Mandelbrot fractals.

Before Benoit Mandelbrot discovered fractals in 1975, we had no way to mathematically describe or think about such complex irregular patterns. We lived in a tidy Euclidian world of lines, circles, triangles, squares, and other regular polygons in which the sun and moon were spheres, the mountains cones, and snowflakes star-shaped hexagons.

Fractal beauty

Once you become sensitized to fractals, you'll see them everywhere—the scattering of leaves on a rocky path, the stippled crowns on a head of cauliflower, waves breaking on a shore, the grain in marble and wood. Have you ever noticed that Mother Nature never makes an aesthetic mistake? We never look at a mountain range and think, "that's ugly," or feel like the boulders in a creek need to be rearranged or that the clouds overhead are misshapen.

Nature is always perfectly beautiful because nature is fractal, and so are we. The proportion of the segments of our fingers, limbs, torso, and the branching of our arteries and veins are fractal. *Our nervous system is tuned to resonate with fractals, and whenever we are in the presence of fractal phenomena, we experience beauty.* Artists intuitively know this. We see it in the fractal placement of color and form on a canvas like Hokusai's *Great Wave* and the intricate pattern of mosaic tiles in a mosque. We hear it in the variation on a theme in a symphony and in the rhythmic structure of a poem, and we "feel" it (with our mirror neurons) as our eye moves over the smooth proportions of a bronze sculpture. *Beauty is fractal.*

Look deeper still and you'll see that within chaos, there is often hidden fractal order and within order, there may be chaos, from the crystalline structure of snowflakes to swirling weather patterns to the rings of Saturn to the planets twirling around the sun. Mandelbrot demonstrated that

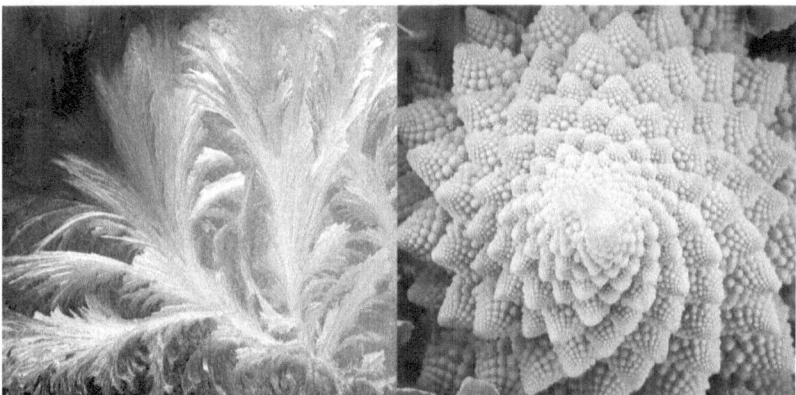

Figure 26: Natural factals—ice crystals and Romanesco cauliflower

complex fractals arise from the iteration of very simple mathematical relationships. Thus, there can be simplicity in complexity and complexity in simplicity.

Fractal pleasure

Beauty is just another word for pleasure, which itself is fractal. Every pleasure is composed of self-similar waves of sensual intensity that propagate through the body-mind continuum over different time scales and intensity. I described this earlier in terms of the body-stream and mind-stream. Take, for example, the pleasure of eating ice cream. Each lick sends a wave of stimulation from our taste buds and olfactory receptors to the brain, releasing a shower of dopamine in the N. accumbens. This in turn triggers a surge of electrical activity through the hippocampus (memory) and the prefrontal cortex (thinking). Simultaneously, pleasurable sensations spread throughout the body to give us a familiar, cozy feeling (physical and emotional) of receiving a sweet reward, and we think, "Mmm … this ice cream tastes good!" The pleasure wave moves from the level of molecular vibrations at sense organ receptors to body sensations to undulating waves of emotional feelings and thoughts. I suspect the rich, milky mouthfeel of ice cream arouses ancient memories of breast feeding. If you look at a breastfeeding baby you can see waves of pleasure ripple through their body, curling their toes with delight. Zoom out to a longer time scale, and ice cream may be merely the finishing touch to a sumptuous meal, which itself is just one of many waves in a pleasant evening and a pleasant life.

A pleasurable experience is made up of wave upon wave of smaller pleasures, each rising, cresting, and falling in self-similar cycles of desire, surrender, and reward, often repeating and overlapping at different time scales and levels of intensity to form a multi-wave of pleasure. In other words, *pleasure is a fractal wave of desire and surrender that washes over our lives.* The next time you get a chance to savor a fresh raspberry, notice how each of its coiled, crimson beads holds a bud of expectation and a microburst of tangy-sweet pleasure.

To take this a step further, each instant of pleasure functions as a "holon"—an experience enjoyed as a whole unto itself and at the same time as part of a larger pleasurable experience. You can think of a holon as a kind of "organizational" fractal in which each unit functions as a semiautonomous whole at various scales within larger wholes, like Russian dolls nesting inside one another. We see this in biology when cells form tissues, tissues form organs, organs form organisms, organisms form colonies, colonies form communities, and communities form ecosystems. In much the same way, subatomic particles, atoms, molecules, planets, stars, solar systems, and galaxies—the whole cosmos—constitute a grand hierarchy of holons (known as a "holarchy"). In a holarchy, information flows bidirectionally, from top down and from bottom up. The entire system depends upon the functioning and integrity of each part. Political organizations operate best as holarchies when change is driven both from the leadership and grassroots.

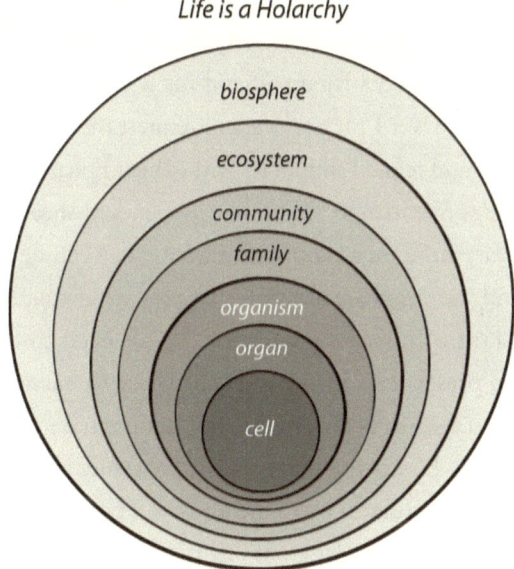

Figure 27: The universe is a holarchy of wholes within wholes.

Within the ethical sphere, there is a crucial lesson to be learned here. As Chief Seattle reminds us, we are but one thread in the web of life. If we don't—as individuals and as a species—expand our consciousness beyond crude hierarchies based on domination and submission (winning and losing) and learn to live together cooperatively as holons within a holarchy—if we don't get with the cosmic program—we will be eliminated from it.

Scaling pleasure

Fractals by definition are eminently scalable. As the ancient Hermetics observed, "As above, so below." The implications are huge. It means that *a change at one dimension is a change at every dimension.* In other words, we can learn everything we need to know about ecstasy, bliss, and equanimity from everyday, low-amplitude pleasures. Balancing five pounds of desire and five pounds of surrender is essentially the same process as balancing 500 pounds of desire and 500 pounds of surrender, only at a different scale. Micro and macro pleasures are holonically related.

A true Epicurean savors countless *extra*ordinary moments of micro-ecstasy, micro-bliss, and micro-equanimity throughout the day. In a letter fragment, Epicurus asked a friend, "Send me a little vessel of cheese, so that I can feast whenever I please," a small request that gives us a glimpse into the humility and refined simplicity with which Epicurus lived his life.[1] Biting into a juicy, ripe mango can be an experience of sheer micro-ecstasy, laying your weary head on a pillow after a long day can be a moment of micro-bliss, and the simple realization that you are alive in this moment can be an instant of micro-equanimity. All we need to create an *äsis* moment is the presence of mind and sensitivity to balance desire and surrender. When I go to bed at night, my last conscious act often is to murmur, "*aah* … " Loosening my muscles, I surrender to the river Lethe, whose waters of forgetfulness carry me away to Hypnos's cave of sleep.

Indeed, the moment we let go of our judgments and contradictories, the ego-filter falls away from the Pleasure Prism and the red, green, and blue colors of our Light-body spontaneously merge into the clear-white, *äsis* light. A gentle summer breeze caressing your cheek, a sip of water, a child's smile, a sigh of relief, holding the hand of someone you love, a bird taking flight—it's all so simple, really. Like child's play.

Our lives, for the most part, are made up of a series of very ordinary moments, and to enjoy life is to extract delight from these moments. I'm reminded of a cartoon of an old monk and a young novice monk walking through a park. They sit down on a bench. After a while, the young monk turns to the older monk and asks, "So, now what?"

And the older monk replies, "This is it!"

Missing in action

This brings us to the final and most mysterious piece of the pleasure puzzle. Technically speaking, at the instant of equilibrium—when desire and surrender come into balance at the zero-point of the present moment—self, the thinking that creates the self, and the world as object, vanish. *At the moment of ecstasy, bliss, and equanimity, no one is there to experience it.* Li Po in eighth-century China described it this way:

> The birds have vanished into the sky.
> Now the last cloud drains away.
> We sit together the mountain and me,
> Until only the mountain remains.[2]

To be precise, the mountain also disappears. That's why no one ever experiences enlightenment, and *anyone who claims to be enlightened, isn't.*

But in the next moment, self and other reappear: I am me and the mountain is the mountain. If you watch carefully, you can observe your *self* flickering in and out of existence, oscillating between the dualistic and merged states, flipping back and forth between particle and wave. In the time it takes you to read this paragraph, your ego-self will have gone through several cycles, appearing and disappearing. It's like watching a celluloid film clip. Usually, the individual frames are moving so quickly that they create the illusion of continuity and we're not aware of the gaps between the frames. But when the speed slows down, as with an old-fashioned silent film, the flickering becomes noticeable.

Time is based on the perception of passing events. The introspective practices of yoga and meditation are a way to slow down the flow of the life-stream by cultivating high states of concentration. When you pay close attention to your moment-to-moment existence, the density of perceived data points per second increases, and like a slow-motion camera, time is drawn out. Slow down the life-stream enough, and you enter the ecstatic flow-state described in Chapter 18, where high performance athletes, musicians, and artists become fully absorbed in their activity. Many people report similar high-concentration, slow-motion experiences during a dangerous event like an accident. I remember watching the hood of my car crumple like an accordion when my car slid into another car on a snowy street at an intersection.

To reiterate, *it is not possible to directly observe the gap between frames because there is no observer*. However, it is possible to observe the arising of self when "I" re-emerges as a separate entity in the subject-object mode. Looking back, I can infer by my *absence* that the merged state just happened. In fact, the existential contrast of coming back into ordinary consciousness (for instance, when I opened my eyes and gazed across the lake) is a gauge of the distance I have travelled and the depth of my meditation. With practice, you may be able to dwell in the merged state for perhaps an entire breath or even several minutes. During these *extra*ordinary moments, the ego is absorbed into the experience and vanishes like breath into air.

Although there is no one there to observe (objectify) the merged state, it does leave a distinctive aftertaste. Thus, *äsis* experiences of Paradise, ecstasy, bliss, equanimity, zero, emptiness, and enlightenment are, properly speaking, an acquired aftertaste, a *re*-cognition that can be cultivated with practice. Angelus Silesius, a seventeenth-century physician and Catholic priest, expressed this well:

> God, whose love and joy
> are present everywhere,
> can't come to visit you
> unless you aren't there.[3]

As a result of this subtle "absence," enlightenment, or *samadhi*, is frequently misunderstood. In Japan, for instance, there are two main schools of Zen: Rinzai and Soto. The Rinzai school has the reputation of being the rough and tough generals who believe that if you train hard, you may experience enlightenment in this lifetime. In contrast, the Soto school, which was traditionally for landowners, teaches that you are already enlightened and that to try to become enlightened is already a mistake. Soto practitioners sit in meditation as an acknowledgement and expression of their enlightenment. The truth is, both schools are correct.

Alan Watts describes Zen instruction as playing a game with a child where you pretend to hold something precious in your closed fist, say a piece of candy. The child struggles to pry open your fingers with eager anticipation only to discover that your hand is empty. In this sense, there is nothing to achieve. *We are already enlightened, only we aren't aware of it.* Enlightenment, like Paradise, is immanent, mundane, and quite ordinary. We flicker in and out of it thousands of times a day, but so rapidly that we don't notice it unless we slow down the oscillations, hence the value of introspective practices.

Practice teaches us that when we disappear, nothing terrible happens. In fact, these are often the moments when we feel most alive, fulfilled, and refreshed. Once we comprehend this, we can loosen the grip of our ego-fears and enjoy life, surfing the waves of self and no-self. When life requires us to perform in our role of wife, husband, mother, father, doctor, baker, tinker, or candlestick maker, we can show up fully as a self, and when these roles are not required, we can relax and bask in the pleasure of being nobody, going nowhere.

The converse is also true. The more egocentric, narcissistic, and self-absorbed we are, the more disconnected and fearful we become and the more difficult it is to surrender. Pleasure pales, kicks get harder to find, and pleasure seeking, as a result, becomes more extreme. Tragically, many a famous rock star and extreme athlete has fallen into this deadly trap.

The supreme irony is that the more we get things just the way we want them, the more inflated our ego becomes, the more demanding our expectations, the greater our sense of entitlement, and the *less* we actually enjoy what we have. Alas, this is the curse and malaise of the First World and our selfie-obsessed iGeneration.

I once attended a Christmas party in the remote hills of northern Thailand with a group of Westerners who had donated money to build a residential grade school for the indigenous, hill-tribe children. In addition to learning how to read and write, the students learned how to raise pigs and chickens and cultivate the land. After being welcomed with a group song (attempted in English), we toured the hog stalls, chicken coops, and the two-room school house. At the center of the compound was a concrete playground with a bare basketball hoop at one end. A long wooden table had been set up and we sat down to a modest dinner of rice and thin soup, ladled from big pots. Fifty kids sat on the ground in a large square around us, eating, talking, and watching us with curiosity.

Once dinner was over, the party began in earnest. The table was cleared and a boombox with a mix of Thai and Western music filled the chilly late afternoon air. Each of us had brought along several small gifts—hats, scarves, socks, writing supplies, and other practical items—that we handed out to the kids, who received them with immense anticipation and enthusiasm. In one corner, stood a small tree with more gifts, wrapped in plain paper, hanging from its branches like Christmas tree ornaments. The students were invited by age to come up and pluck a present from the tree, the youngest students first. The excitement and joy of opening their gifts was infectious, and afterwards, we—teachers, students, and Western guests—all danced in celebration. Without doubt, it was the merriest Christmas party I've ever attended.

The path from here

At this point in our journey, we have reached the end of "scaling" the Pleasure Prism's mystical heights. Along the way, we have seen how the infinite emptiness of zero resolves the contradictories of paradox at the balancing point; how the three gateways of Paradise are to be found within the three vital centers in our body; and how by aligning them, we equilibrate desire and surrender and return innocent and naked to the Source. And lastly, we have seen how all of this can be accomplished whenever we wish, in the blink of an eye, by simply attuning to the micro-gaps that are ever present. From here, we will turn our attention to the practical application of these insights.

The good news is, once you humble yourself and kneel at the Pierian spring and drink deeply its refreshing waters, you will never again want for thirst, for you will always know how to find your way back to the Source. In my experience, it's something like living beneath a thick blanket that, from time to time, is pierced by a brilliant shaft of sunlight, offering a glimpse of wholeness. With practice, you can become more aware of these egoless, illuminating beams of micro-ecstasy, bliss, and equanimity. Eventually, the blanket becomes so shot through and tattered that a radical shift of foreground and background takes place (like wearing out holes in your socks). The merged state now becomes the baseline level of reality, punctuated with moments of self-conscious separation. At that point, you're just going about your day when suddenly self arises, and you notice, "Oh, here I am … driving the car; talking to a friend; cooking dinner; reading a book; being a hero or a scoundrel." Kabir, a fifteenth-century Indian mystic, expressed it most beautifully as a poetic holarchy:

> Between the conscious and the unconscious,
> > the mind has put up a swing:
> > all earth creatures, even the supernovas, sway
> > between these two trees,
> > and it never winds down.
> Angels, animals, humans, insects by the millions,
> > also the wheeling sun and moon;
> > ages go by and it goes on.
> Everything is swinging: heaven, earth, water, fire,
> > and the secret one slowly grows a body.
> Kabir saw that for fifteen seconds, and it made him
> > a servant for life.[4]

▲▲▲▲▲▲▲

In brief:

We live in an irregular universe where objects and processes tend to repeat themselves in self-similar patterns at different dimensions and scales. We find this in everything from the way ice crystals form on a window to the texture of tree bark to the sound of raindrops. These natural patterns are a reflection of underlying fractal processes called holons—semi-autonomous functional units that are both a whole and part of a larger whole—which together constitute a holarchy (a hierarchy of holons). In a holarchy, the integrity of the whole depends on every part.

Pleasure is also fractal and is made up of self-similar waves of desire, surrender, and reward that interweave and overlap at different scales of time and intensity. The fractal nature of pleasure means that sublime pleasures can be experienced in *extra*ordinary, low-amplitude moments of micro-ecstasy, bliss, and equanimity when for an instant, desire and surrender come into balance and we are absorbed into the mystery.

Considerations:

- Notice the irregular beauty that is all around you when you open your fractal eyes. What do you see?

- Practice with small, ordinary pleasures and then scale what you learn to more intense pleasures.

- Savor micro-moments of ecstasy, bliss, and equanimity whenever you wish.

- *Re*-cognize when you have vanished.

- When Kabir wrote, "The secret one slowly grows a body," who is this secret one?

Part 5: **The Art and Practice**

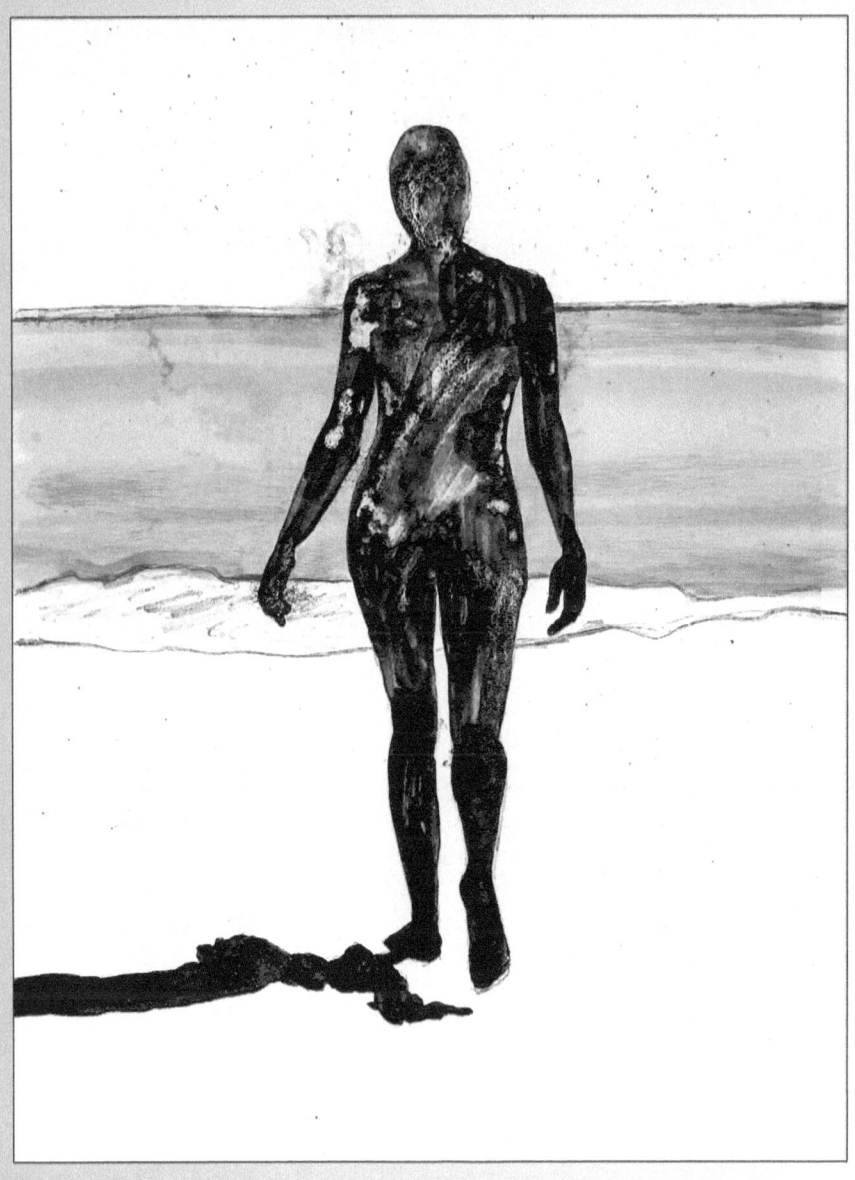

The following field notes are gathered from my own experience and that of my friends, family, and patients. I offer them as data points to stimulate your own exploration. While each person and situation is unique, the basic Laws of Pleasure remain the same and I will point them out along the way.

In my experience, *life is a required pass-fail course where you keep taking the same course over again until you either pass or run out of time.* Hopefully, these notes will save you some retakes.

The Seven Immutable Laws of Pleasure

1. **Original Wholeness**—*You were born from pleasure and you are born for pleasure. It is your origin, source, and birthright.*

2. **Colors**—*Pleasure comes in four colors: red (physical), green (emotional), blue (mental), and white (spiritual).*

3. **Contrast and Comparison**—*Pleasure is relative and continually changes.*

4. **Thresholds**—*Pleasure is separated from pain by a threshold of intensity.*

5. **Cycles**—*Pleasure comes in waves.*

6. **Desire and Surrender**—*Pleasure is an inner dance of effort and relaxation.*

7. **Renewable Pleasure**—*The highest quality pleasure is that which you exchange with another being.*

CHAPTER 20

Make Relationship

*There is no love greater
than Love with no object.
For then you, yourself,
have become Love itself.*
—Rumi

By the time I met Dr. Ben Weininger, a well-known Santa Barbara psychiatrist, he was a wizened old man with a shock of white hair that radiated from his bald pate like a wild corona and a matching pair of untamed eyebrows. His spirit, unencumbered with flesh, was light and animated, and he spoke plainly with a glint of mischievousness in his eyes that gave him the unmistakable bearing of a Hasidic sage.

At the completion of my four-year journeymanship, I returned from China and had the good fortune to be his house guest. Our meeting was one of those synchronistic encounters too perfect to be mere coincidence. Like joining two ends of a circle, he was at the end of his career just as I was beginning mine. He would complete my formal training with one final lesson.

We had both gone to medical school in Chicago, and in between playing chess, we swapped war stories about our clinical rotations at the legendary Cook County Hospital.

Despite his advanced age, he was still seeing a few patients at his home. One day I asked, "So, Ben, what do you talk about with your patients for an hour? Could I sit in and observe?" He would have nothing of it.

"Much too personal and intimate," he muttered in his crusty voice.

I persisted, "Well, how do you do psychiatry?"

He paused, peering into my eyes to plumb my sincerity, and then with the brevity and directness of a man who could see the end of his life approaching, he answered matter-of-factly, "Make relationship."

And with that, our conversation ended.

His words, "make relationship," lodged inside me like a Zen *koan*, an existential plum pit that I could neither swallow nor spit out. That week, at the local urgent care where I was working, I tried to make relationship with my drive-through patients by listening more carefully to who they were as people, rather than just seeing them as a disease I needed to diagnose and treat. It took more time, but the encounter was much more satisfying and impactful for both of us. After a few weeks of chewing on his pithy advice, I was ready for my second and final lesson.

"So, Ben, I've been thinking a lot about making relationship … How *do* you make relationship?" He paused and then answered as abruptly as he had the first time: "Be present."

That was it. In those two terse statements—*be present* and *make relationship*—he had transmitted the essence of his forty years of psychiatry. Being present and making relationship with my patients allowed me to see beyond their medical diagnosis to the root of their suffering: their dissatisfaction with work, the long hours, the bills piling up, their kids' trouble at school, the sleepless nights. *To be truly present is to give someone high-quality attention, which is an act of love!* In time, I would discover Ben had given me more than just the key to psychiatry; he had given me the key to the good life (Aristotle's *eudaimonia*)—something all of us once knew well.

The true masters of being present and making relationship are young children. Look into their eyes and you can glimpse humanity's vast potential. I'll never forget the first time I saw my five-month-old daughter, Ashani, sitting up on her own, perfectly erect and poised, regally surveying her surroundings like a sovereign. She had no past to regret, no future to fret, no words or images to distract her. She was a baby Buddha, completely present and engaged in the moment, yet non-attached, without the need to judge or evaluate. Her gaze graced all that lay before her with equanimity and perfect concentration, a living embodiment of pure consciousness.

Children make relationship effortlessly because everything is an extension of themselves. Theirs is an enchanted world of wonder and oneness. From this undifferentiated oneness, it is but a short distance to zero. Like a breeze ruffling a curtain, they drift easily between unity and emptiness. Some might call it a state of grace; I prefer to call it true Love.

True Love

When we utter the words, "I love you," we are speaking from a dualistic perspective in which "I" is the subject, "love" is the verb (the action performed), and "you" is the object that receives the action. Notice that the rules of our grammar (syntax) powerfully structure the way we think and the meaning our words convey (semantics).

Typically, the emphasis is on the subject "I," and "you" is objectified (reduced to an object). We refer to this as conditional love because in order to receive love, "you," the love-object, must fulfill certain conditions: "I love you as long as it benefits me and you service my needs," as with any useful piece of equipment. And if the love-object fails to perform adequately, we either try to change it or replace it with a better model. This can lead to disposable relationships—a common occurrence these days with 50 percent of marriages ending in divorce and lasting an average of seven years.[1] But if two people who voluntarily come together and publicly swear their love and allegiance to each other can't make it, what hope is there for the rest of us? What hope is there for world peace?

Karl Marx called this kind of objectification *verdinglichung*, "thingification." Although humans have objectified one another as slaves and serfs throughout history, thingification accelerated sharply in the thirteenth century when the first mechanical clocks were placed on bell towers, marking the entry of the "clockmind" into human consciousness. From then on, our lives became less organic, less like a growing forest and more like a mechanical clock that never varies. Previously, communal life was regulated by ringing church bells to mark the liturgical day. Clocks in the home were uncommon prior to the eighteenth century, and as recently as 1950, most people didn't own a watch. When you said you would meet someone at a certain time, it was a much looser affair; nothing ran "on time."

The first engineers were watchmakers because they understood how to regulate time and motion with mechanical gears.[2] Hence, the first machines were called clockworks. If you think about it, an assembly line is nothing more than a kind of human/machine clockwork. (This was brilliantly depicted in Charlie Chaplin's classic *Modern Times*.) Put a number of assembly lines together, and you get a company. Put a number of companies together, and you get a corporation, which, despite the legal fiction, is not a corporeal body but a huge clockwork. But here's the thing: as we build machines in our own image to extend our abilities, our machines become more like us and we become more like our machines. Robots and AI are just the next evolutionary turn of the clockmind, and if we aren't careful, we may become enslaved droids in the process.

What we look for in a good clock is uniformity, reproducibility, efficiency, and replaceable parts. These form the foundational ethos of every corporation, such as McDonald's, which produces a hamburger from order to delivery in 112 seconds (42 seconds to grill the beef patty), whether you are in New York, London, or Tokyo.[3] While such efficiency may be great for fast-food restaurants and building cars, it's not exactly what you want when you see your doctor. Unless, of course, you're in a hurry and only have time to drive through a "doc-in-the-box."

Over the course of my medical career, I have seen medicine go from my childhood doctor (who had a small office upstairs next to the local cinema and kept his notes on 5x8 inch index cards stored in a long cardboard tray) to a multi-specialty medical practice in a modern light industrial complex of human suffering where the median doctor visit is 15.7 minutes (five minutes devoted to the main issue and 1.1 minutes spent on each remaining issue).[4] A 2018 *Forbes* study found the average time a doctor listens to a patient before interrupting is 11 seconds.[5]

The "corping" of modern medicine is just one example of the corporatization of society as a whole. The problem is that *when we objectify others, we objectify ourselves*. Human relationships are becoming mere object-object relationships. Take, for example, the prevalent practice of sexual objectification. In order to use a person as a sexual object, we must first objectify our own sexuality, that is, we must first disconnect sexual pleasure from emotional love; disconnect our pelvis from the heart in the same way that you might disconnect an amplifier from a stereo receiver. People become replaceable, interchangeable cogs. Mothers and fathers have been reduced to "parental units." Ghosting is commonplace. As my friend Steve likes to say, "In a perfectly efficient society, people are redundant." (Press 1 for reservations; press 2 for departures; press 3 for ….) Today, we live "on the clock," where time is money and we never seem to have enough.[6] As we will see, objectified living greatly diminishes our ability to experience pleasure.

Less common, but often praised, is unconditional love where the focus is on the object rather than the subject. Unconditional love says, "I love you no matter what you do." In this case, the subject "I" is thingified, as illustrated in the following German fairy tale my father told me:

> A young man fell in love with a beautiful woman in a neighboring village. As proof of his love, she demanded he cut out his mother's heart and bring it to her. His desire for her was so great that he did her bidding, cut out his mother's heart and wrapped it in a cloth. Running through the forest to his love, he tripped over a log and dropped his mother's bleeding heart on the ground. From beneath the blood-clotted cloth came a tender cry, "Are you hurt, my son?"

Conditional and unconditional love are both dualistic, which I will refer to as love with a small "l." Generally, this kind of love occurs at the first three levels of the Pleasure Prism with physical, emotional, and mental love objects. It is only when we get to the *äsis* level that we experience true Love with a capital "L." The Christian term for such exalted Love is *agape*. To be agape is literally to be slack-jawed with your mouth open in a state of awe. Have you ever wondered why medieval churches have such tall towers and frescos painted on their vaulted ceilings? Churches were built to inspire awe. When we look heavenward, our mouth naturally gapes open, releasing our palate and putting us in the proper relationship to God and, by extension, the authority of the church. Government buildings are designed to have a similar effect.

In true Love, the subject-object duality is *recollected* into Original Wholeness (the first Law of Pleasure).[7] We arrive once again at the limits of language where "ideas, language, even the phrase 'each other' doesn't make any sense," as Rumi wrote.[8] For this reason, true Love can never be a personal love, because as with *samadhi*, there is no person, no individual subject, no I who is doing the loving, nor an object receiving the love. In the moment of true Love, "I love you" makes no sense because there is only the activity of Love. When we awaken from our self-centered delusion of I, me, mine, and myself that objectifies and separates us from the world, we become a Buddha (an honorific title for one who is "awake") and realize that the entire cosmos has been Loving and supporting our existence since before we were born. Indeed, we are nothing other than a living expression, a star child of the cosmos. Therefore, we cannot try to Love, just as we cannot try to surrender. Rather, the moment we let go of fear, the walls of duality vanish, and we are *in* Love, or more precisely, we disappear into the activity of Love and become *Love itself*.

Intimate relationships

Of all our relationships, perhaps the most challenging is an intimate relationship with another human being, for to truly fall in Love is to die to the illusion of a separate self. There is hardly anything more frightening. It takes courage to awaken from the trance of separateness and surrender to the wholeness of reality without the protective delusion of a self. In the

Hindu tradition, it is to take up the life of a *sadhu*, a renunciate, which is not appropriate for those of us who choose to have families and live as householders. But we can touch into it for moments.

As we have seen, emotional pleasure exists on a continuum of intensity, which, like other pleasures, is limited by a Pleasure-Pain Threshold (the Law of Thresholds). When love crosses the threshold, we experience fear, anxiety, anger, jealousy, and other existential insecurities. It is at this boundary that the power struggles of relationships are waged. As we become more intimate with each other, we also become more vulnerable and sensitive to our partner's energy, moods, facial expressions, and words. Our fear of abandonment grows greater and our feelings can be more easily bruised.

Because the Pleasure-Pain Threshold is continually shifting, it can be tricky to synchronize our needs and capacity for intimacy with those of our partner. This is particularly true when coming together after a period of separation, such as when returning home from a hard day at work or after a long trip. What could be taken as an innocent jest on a good day might push us over the edge on a bad one, causing tempers to flare and feelings to be hurt. Near the emotional threshold, we may feel the confusion of "I love you, but I don't like you." At higher levels of intensity, the pent-up pressures can lead to an emotional explosion, rupturing the bond of trust that holds the relationship together, and love turns to hate. It happens all the time.

Some relationships fall apart from a lack of intensity, others from too much. There are basically two kinds of relationships: those of "similars" and those of "dissimilars." Each has its advantages and disadvantages. Similars can enjoy great friendship, but lacking contrast, they may be short on excitement and passion. Dissimilars, on the other hand, can enjoy great passion and excitement, but may be short on companionship.

If the emotional threshold is not approached with sensitivity and skill, the whipsawing between love and hate can fatigue and eventually break even the most ardent relationship. Indeed, the more passionate the relationship, the more violent the whipsawing may be, and the more intense the contrast of joy and suffering. In this case, fear of intimacy can easily become a self-fulfilling prophecy.

Fortunately, you can increase your emotional capacity for intimacy in the same way an athlete increases aerobic capacity and strength—through training. It begins by cultivating self-intimacy, which means getting in touch with your reptile, limbic, and cortical aspects. It takes skill and awareness to dance at the edge of your emotional threshold (knowing when to lean in and when to lean back to give your partner space) and a willingness to be vulnerable. For some couples, space may require withdrawing to separate bedrooms, and for others, separate houses or even different states. In this way, you can avoid slamming into the wall with painful, destructive outbursts and instead build a virtuous Pleasure Cycle of trust and emotional safety.

That most love is self-referential is no great moral indictment. Self-interest (desire) is an essential aspect of our human nature, and there is never a need to apologize or feel guilty for being a human being. What's important is that we embrace our humanness, refine it, and bring it into harmony. A relationship built on mutual respect and kindness can overcome the greatest obstacles. The emotional trust creates an alchemical crucible with the power to transubstantiate love into true Love. In the end, to be *truly present* is to make *true relationship*.

▲▲▲▲▲▲▲

In brief:

When we say, "I love you," we usually mean I love you as long as you satisfy my needs—a *conditional* love where "you" is objectified. The objectification of human relationships was accelerated by the introduction of clocks on church towers in the thirteenth century. At that moment, we became enslaved to the clockmind, which paved the way for the corporatization of humanity. In *unconditional* love, the subject "I" is objectified. Both of these forms of love are dualistic and limited by a Pleasure-Pain Threshold. The success or failure of a relationship often depends on how this threshold is handled—with kindness and respect, or fear and anger.

In *true* Love, subject and object ("I" and "you") merge and disappear into the activity of Love, which is a form of *samadhi* (recollection). The key to experiencing true Love is to be present and make relationship.

Considerations:
- Practice being present and making relationship when you pick up a piece of paper, turn a door knob, feel a body sensation, notice a thought or anything else that catches your attention.

- Imagine your attention is like a dart that pierces a target, quivers for an instant, and then releases, free to focus on another object.

- Try spending a day off the clock without a time piece.

- Notice how your intimacy ebbs and flows along a continuum with an emotional Pleasure-Pain Threshold.

- Take opportunities to stretch your capacity for intimacy—with another and with yourself. What does it feel like to be intimate in relationship? What does intimate aloneness feel like?

- Commit to treating your partner (and yourself) with respect and kindness.

Chapter 21

The Myth of Discipline

> *Don't ask what the world needs.*
> *Ask what makes you come alive*
> *and go do it,*
> *because what the world needs*
> *is people who come alive.*
> —Howard Thurman

DISCIPLINE IS ANOTHER ONE OF THOSE WORDS, LIKE PLEASURE, GOOD, AND ethics, whose original meaning was once pure and profound, but then was perverted with a moral twist and fashioned into a tool of social control. The value of reclaiming its original meaning is that in the process we reclaim a part of ourselves and become more whole.

The word comes from the Latin *discere*, by way of the Greek *dekhesthai* (to receive), as in a disciple who receives the teachings of a master or studies a discipline like music. In its original sense, discipline implies humility, because a worthy disciple must first empty their cup before she or he can receive instruction with openness and gratitude. Humility, however, should not be mistaken for Original Inadequacy. One can bow deeply without losing self-esteem. In fact, the ability to do so is the mark of a developed person.

Words are a living medium of exchange that take on the values and meanings of those who utter them. By the Middle Ages, discipline had been twisted into a short crop of knotted-leather strands called *la disciplina* with which Christian monks beat themselves to mortify their flesh and subdue their bodily desires. At an institutional level, a would-be disciple had to first kneel and submit to the authority of the church to receive its orthodoxy (Greek *ortho*, "right" and *doxa*, "opinion"). Those who refused would be disciplined, often cruelly, hence the darkness of the Dark Ages. The notion of the willing disciple had been perverted to serve the needs of the willful disciplinarian.

Discipline, we're told, is essential for self-mastery and success. It makes us stronger, more effective, and a better person. We should pride ourselves for having it, pity those who lack it, and scorn the lazy who neglect it. But discipline is a false concept based on the belief that part of "me" wants to do something while another part doesn't. The good-self must use discipline to make the bad-self do what's "good" for it, creating an internecine struggle of biblical proportions. But *in a war with one's self, there can be no winners.*

And so, when we think about doing something good for ourselves, like exercise, dieting, or homework, we reflexively reach for *la disciplina*. Each January, millions of penitents flock to health clubs, whip in hand, to make good on New Year's resolutions, grunting "no pain, no gain." They torture themselves on geared mechanical racks and hire personal trainers to "kick ass." All the while, just beneath their pained grimaces is a conceit that they can "take it," at which point the tyranny of the disciplinarian has been internalized. But their resolve soon grows thin and so do the crowds. By May, 80 percent have quit. (Commercial gyms expect one out of five sign-ups to become regulars; their business model depends on it.)[1] When we fail in our attempt to whip ourselves into shape, it's easy to feel inadequate. Ironically, we berate ourselves for not having enough discipline when it was the myth of discipline that defeated us.

St. Francis of Assisi referred to his body as Brother Ass. It's true; the sting of *la disciplina* can motivate short-term results, but as any mule skinner worth his salt knows, the carrot works better than the stick. You can only throw yourself against the wall of the Pleasure-Pain Threshold so many times before giving up and saying, "To hell with it." And with each failure and broken promise, the thwarted penitent spirals deeper into a vortex of shame, guilt, and self-loathing. The harder you flog yourself, the more divided and the less capable you are to effect positive change. Some $2.5 billion is spent annually on weight loss to achieve in the best programs a mere 3 to 5 percent decreased weight at twelve months (that's 6 to 10 pounds for a 200-pound person).[2] Discipline is not only ineffective, it is debilitating. We don't get to pleasure through pain; pleasure is the way—but not just any pleasure. In the case of losing weight, for instance, one must realize that "nothing tastes better than healthy feels."[3]

There are, of course, exceptional individuals who swear by discipline and have the trophies to prove it. But I suspect what they are calling discipline is just a more refined approach to the Pleasure-Pain Threshold. For instance, one of the biggest differences between elite runners and good amateurs (besides the number of training hours) is that elite runners continually monitor their time, effort, and body sensations while amateurs resort to discipline and denial to gut it out. When my friend Lorraine Moller, an Olympic marathon runner, comes up on a male jogger during a training run, she speeds up and flies past them so quickly they have no chance of catching her. She does this out of compassion because it pains her to see these men torture themselves trying to keep up with a woman.

In a 1993 landmark study of hundreds of exceptionally gifted people, Anders Ericsson demonstrates that the so-called "gifted prodigy" possesses, for the most part, neither extraordinary innate talent nor a genius-level IQ, but something much more mundane—ambitious parents fiercely dedicated to their child's training and discipline.[4]

There is ample evidence that, were it not for Amadeus Mozart's father, Leopold (a violinist and noted musical pedagogue who devoted himself to young Wolfgang's career), the world would never have had "The Marriage of Figaro" or "The Magic Flute."[5] The same can be said for countless other famous musicians, mathematicians, chess players, scientists, and athletes. Take for example, the notorious Asian "tiger mom" who begins training her budding concert pianist with a half-hour daily practice at three or four years of age. By the age of five, the child is moving fluidly on the keyboard and logging three hours a day, ratcheting up to four to six hours as their skills increase. In the highly competitive world of concert pianists, a child who begins at age six is already at a serious disadvantage. Ericsson discovered it takes roughly ten years of hard practice for a child to reach a level of excellence and another ten years to attain a level of mastery to make a significant contribution to the field.

But what of the countless siblings and would-be prodigies who fell by the wayside, the shooting stars who burned out early, and the lost childhoods and missed adventures of living life on one's own terms beyond the hothouse conservatory? Books have been written about the discipline—some would say abuse—these children endure, which may include threats, intimidation, spanking, shame, and other forms of coercion, as well as lavish praise for success. In one striking anecdote, a mother threatens her seven-year-old daughter, who has been struggling for days to syncopate a two-handed rhythm: "If the next time's not perfect, I'm going to take all your stuffed animals and burn them."[6] Yo Yo Ma, who began the cello at age four, admitted it wasn't until he turned forty-nine that he thought playing the cello was cool. In a *New York Times* interview, he said, "Since I always played, as far as I can remember, I never said, 'This is what I want to do.'"[7] As a result, he always wondered who else he might have become.

Tennis legend Andre Agassi began his training when his father, a former Iranian Olympic boxer, taped ping-pong paddles to his wrists to swat at brightly colored tennis balls in a mobile suspended over his crib. By the age of six he was forced to hit 2,500 balls a day, spat out by a machine that his father built called the Dragon, at speeds up to 110 miles per hour. Despite his induction into the Hall of Fame, winning an Olympic Gold Medal, and being lauded as one of the greatest tennis players of all time, Agassi confessed in his autobiography, "I play tennis for a living even though I hate tennis, hate it with a dark and secret passion and always have."[8]

We admire and celebrate these individuals for their extraordinary skill, and the matrix holds them up as role models, but does "success," defined in such a narrow bandwidth, constitute a good life? As Agassi demonstrates, being successful in one's career is not the same thing as being successful in one's life, particularly when it comes to satisfaction and personal fulfillment.

The confusion around discipline increases as we near the Pleasure-Pain Threshold. It is here that willfulness—the desire to push harder—and the willingness to surrender to greater intensity meet in a delicate dance. It takes experience and skill to apply the Law of Colors and tease out the physical (red), emotional (green), mental (blue), and *äsis* (white) threads of enjoyment that exist in any worthwhile activity, rather than to whip ourselves to achieve some imagined goal. For instance, when my swim workout gets intense, instead of just pushing through, I sometimes take a break and hang off the edge of the pool, stretching my legs on the wall, and breathe into the intensity as I surrender into a moment of ecstasy.

If you love something, what need is there for discipline? As Joseph Campbell advised, "Follow your bliss." In the next chapter, we will discuss how.

▲▲▲▲▲▲▲

In brief:
"Discipline" is another word that was conflated with morality and then twisted into a tool of social control. The notion of a humble disciple acting from love was perverted into a domineering disciplinarian acting in fear and then released into the meme stream like a communicable disease. Once infected (internalized), it turns people against themselves. Just as Original Sin causes feelings of inadequacy, discipline disintegrates the psyche into a war with one's self. Fortunately, there is an effective vaccine for this contagion.

Considerations:
- How do you motivate yourself?

- When you use the word "discipline," notice how you feel. Listen to which part of you is talking and which part of you is resisting.

- Instead of willfulness, try surrendering to an activity.

- Practice using the language of "I want to," "I love to," and "I choose to," instead of "I have to," "I should," or "I must."

- Trust your natural intelligence to seek quality pleasure.

CHAPTER 22

For the Love of It

> *When I was 5 years old, my mother always
> told me that happiness is the key to life.
> When I went to school, they asked me
> what I wanted to be when I grew up.
> I wrote down 'happy.'
> They told me I didn't understand the assignment,
> and I told them they didn't understand life.*
> —John Lennon

We are all familiar with the grim, work-hard, fear-centric approach to life, spurred on by *la disciplina*. But what would it look like to live an *aah*-centric life, motivated by the things we love? Here are a handful of stories—ranging from the mundane to the extreme—to illustrate, inspire, and perhaps remind you of your own successes pursuing pleasure.

Child's play

I heard a woman play an incredibly moving viola piece at a memorial service. She was the aunt of a young nineteen-year-old man who had tragically died on the streets of Puerto Vallarta, Mexico, trying to protect his mother from a petty theft. After the service, I asked the violist how she had learned to play so beautifully.

"I was good at the viola in high school," she said, "so I decided to study music at a conservatory. But by my second year practicing four, sometimes six hours a day, I found myself getting more and more discouraged."

"Was it the long hours?" I asked.

"It wasn't the practice so much; it's that they kept pushing me. The moment I managed to play a piece, they gave me a new one. It was an exercise in endless frustration. It got so bad I finally quit and changed my major to psychology."

"Did you find any answers in psychology?"

"I did, in a way. To make ends meet, I gave violin lessons to young kids, which meant that for a couple of years all I played were children's songs. The amazing thing is, I started to enjoy them. Even a simple piece of music can be really beautiful when played well. I discovered the immense satisfaction of mastering a piece of music. I fell in love with music again, or maybe, for the first time."

"What about psychology?"

"I learned there wasn't any book thick enough to explain how I felt when I played the viola. I learned that I played not to be perfect, or to get approval, but because I loved it. So, I returned to the conservatory, only this time I approached each piece of music like a children's song, aiming for that feeling of ease, enjoying each note. It changed everything. I'm now a violist with the North Carolina Orchestra and can truly say that I love my work. Like they say, *"choose a job you love, and you'll never have to work a day in your life."*

I never did catch her name, but she taught me that mastery is Love, not in the sentimental, possessive sense, but in the transcendent sense of pure attention, like a young child absorbed in play.

An unknown artist

On a lovely autumn day, my friend Lais and I were walking through the grounds of one of Kyoto's many beautiful Buddhist temples. As the heat of the afternoon sun passed and the day's activities were winding down into a pleasant lull before evening, we came upon an elderly Japanese man who was standing at a card table. He wore a dark blue beret over his close-cropped silver hair. He had been demonstrating his painting at a festival and was packing up. A stunning picture of a snake on his table stopped us in our tracks. Its shimmering scales were so alive, it looked as though it might slither away. But it was just a series of segmented, spare black ink brush strokes painted on an ordinary sheet of paper.

Sumi-e is the traditional Japanese brush painting that is closely related to Chinese calligraphy. A *sumi-e* artist learns by practicing precise, individual brush strokes that serve as elements of a visual alphabet. When painting, however, one works quickly and spontaneously. The aesthetic is to find the balance between structure and freedom (the Law of Desire and Surrender) and to capture, in a flash of intuition, not the form but the spirit of the object.

Lais had studied *sumi-e* and was captivated by the snake. With my newly learned Japanese, I asked, "*Kore wa oikura desuka?*" How much does this cost?

After a few mangled attempts, he understood that I was trying to buy the painting for my friend, and he handed it to her. It took her a few awkward moments to realize that he was giving it to her, at which point her eyes opened wide and her shoulders drew up like a child thrilled to receive the unexpected gift.

"*Arigato, arigato gozaimasu!*" Thank you very much, she said, bowing deeply with gratitude. He was unfazed, maintaining the reserved formalism that is so much a part of Japanese culture.

Admiring her treasure, she then gestured for him to sign it. He looked away, waving his outstretched hand in obvious refusal. A true *sumi-e* artist never signs their work. To do so would be considered crude. Then to make his point, he set his ink-stained bottle on top of a stack of snake pictures that he had on his table and used the next one as wrapping paper, as if to say: If you think the picture is valuable, you are mistaken. The true value is unseen and not some "thing" to be possessed, nor to be sold. He had given us a profound lesson in *sumi-e* that we would never forget, all without uttering a word.

There is a saying in Japanese: "*Ware, o wasu reru,*" when I forget myself. The true work of art is how you live your life. The painting that hangs on the museum wall, the *objet d'art,* is merely a by-product that stands in silent testimony to what the artist saw and resonated with—the wood shavings on the shop floor, so to speak. Artists often live lives of poverty, without acknowledgement. We might wonder why anyone would choose such a life. I believe it is because an artist receives an uncommon reward: they forget themselves in their work and in the process, remember their true Self, which is something no amount of money or recognition can buy.

Baby steps

In 1985, two young men—Joe Simpson, then twenty-four years old, and his climbing partner, Simon Yates, aged twenty-one, made the first ascent of the west face of the 21,000-foot *Suila Grande* in the Peruvian Andes. The following day, on the descent, Simpson fell through a cornice, jamming his tibia into his knee joint and shattering it. Yates lowered the pain-wracked Simpson down the ice face for nine hours, when the rope suddenly went taut over an overhang. Yates knew by the weight on the rope that Simpson had slipped off the face and was dangling helplessly in the air, but they were unable to communicate over the howling blizzard that was closing in. Exhausted, his fingers growing numb with frostbite and his snow anchor loosening, Yates made the agonizing decision to cut the rope and send his partner to his death. Shaken, he dug a snow-cave to weather the storm. The next morning, he discovered the yawning crevasse Simpson fell into, concluded he obviously died, and made his way back to base camp.

Miraculously, Simpson survived the fifty-foot fall, landing on a narrow ledge of snow and ice. After regaining consciousness, he had no choice but to descend deeper into the crevasse with the hope of finding an opening back onto the slope, which he did. For the next three-and-a-half days, against all odds, with a broken leg, no food, and very little water, he hopped and crawled six miles over glaciers and boulder fields to arrive back at camp just as Yates was preparing to leave.

When asked how he kept himself going, Simpson said he thought he would likely die on the mountain but his survival instinct (reptilian brain) wasn't about to call it quits. He knew he had to keep his head together, so he broke down the immensity of his ordeal into doable baby steps within the limits of his physical and emotional capacity (the Law of Thresholds). He focused on immediate goals and time limits in which to accomplish them: twenty-five yards to a particular rock in fifteen minutes, then make it to the next outcropping in thirty minutes and so on, hour after hour, day after day. Setting up achievable goals rewarded his limbic brain and kept him from falling into hopeless despair. Discipline, with its self-conflicted ambivalence, would not have been able to keep him going. Baby steps enabled Simpson to live to tell his extraordinary story in his book *Touching the Void*.

Two simple agreements

Some years ago, I had an unusually vivid dream which I took to be a shamanic communication. In the dream, I was playing a *shakuhachi* (an end-blown, five-holed Japanese flute fashioned from the gnarled root end of a bamboo stalk) in front of a large audience. Years earlier when I lived in Japan, I had seen one of these flutes but never thought much of it. Traditionally, it was played by the monks of the Fuke sect of Zen Buddhism in lieu of chanting sutras, a practice known as *suizen*, blowing meditation.

A few days later, a patient who worked in the import business was leaving for a buying trip to Japan, so I asked him to pick up a *shakuhachi* for me. Soon I had a flute in hand but no one to teach me. Then, a professional violinist in need of a medical consult happened to be passing through town and arranged an introduction with her friend Robin Harteshorne, a mathematician at the University of California in Berkeley, who gave me my first lesson.

With an already overflowing plate and a busy medical practice, it seemed unlikely that I would have time to take up a musical instrument (notice I didn't say discipline). So, I made two simple agreements with myself: I would pick up the *shakuhachi* and blow into it for an unspecified amount of time each day, and, given its reputation for being a difficult instrument, I would give myself ten years to decide whether the first agreement was worthwhile or not. Two doable baby steps. And, just to cut myself some slack, I took one day off a week.

Several months later, Cory Sperry, another doctor in town, heard that I was playing and came over for a lesson. He had picked up a *shakuhachi* when he lived in Hawaii. Of course, I didn't have much to teach him, but at the end of the lesson I shared with him my two agreements. The next thing I heard, Cory had travelled to the small town of Bissei-Cho in Japan to attend the first World Shakuhachi Festival in 1994. At the end of the festival, everyone was in high spirits and discussing where to hold the next one in four years, when Cory stood up and said, "Why not Boulder, Colorado?" Oddly enough, Boulder had recently received some press in the Japanese media as a beautiful city to visit. By the time he returned home, he had half a dozen emails waiting for him to begin planning.

In 1998, Boulder hosted the second World Shakuhachi Festival with fifty of the top *shakuhachi* players in the world and over 350 participants. It was not only a phenomenal success, it was the largest event in the history of the instrument. As people were saying farewell at the closing ceremony, I found myself on stage at the mike pleading for a *shakuhachi* teacher to move to Boulder. One of the festival organizers, David Wheeler, who was living in Tokyo at the time, subsequently did move to Boulder and launched an annual local *shakuhachi* summer camp, bringing in top-notch teachers each year.

The most famous teaching of the Bhagavad Gita is *to act without being attached to the fruits of one's actions*. Baby steps are an easy way to do just that. How often are we defeated not by the immensity of the task, but by the immensity of our expectations and impatience? How often do we fall short of our ambitious goals (or not even attempt them) because we believe we lack the necessary talent and discipline, lose interest, and give up? Acting without being attached to the fruits of one's actions is just another way of stating the Law of Desire and Surrender. Balancing desire (action) and surrender (non-attachment) liberates us from discipline and the tyranny of achievement and failure. Like the saying goes, *if you stand in line long enough, eventually it's your turn*.

Surfer babe

When my first born, Ashani, was four years old, we had to literally drag her screaming and kicking up the trail on a hike. Even at an early age, she could be stubborn when she wanted to. Try as I might, I couldn't get her involved in any of the usual sports—gymnastics, soccer, basketball, running, ballet, martial arts. We even tried fencing, but nothing took. Part of the problem was that she grew so quickly she had difficulty coordinating her long limbs and keeping up with her shorter peers. Finally, exasperated, just before she entered high school, I said, "Ash, you've got to do some kind of sport. What would you really like to do?" It was not the first time I had asked this question, but this time she had a definite answer.

"I'd like to surf," she replied. In retrospect, this should have been obvious since her email handle was "surferbabe."

"Well, if you want to surf, you're going to need to be a strong swimmer," I said. I arranged for her to take swim lessons with a swim coach who checked her out in the pool and said, "If you give me six months to a year with her, I could get her ready for the swim team." Her assessment was not far off.

Stubbornness cuts both ways, and to Ashani's credit, she joined the freshman swim team under a terrific coach, Bob Smartt, who took her under his wing, as he had done with many girls, which explains why his team has a roster of over sixty swimmers and is top ranked in the state.

At her first swim meet, the noise and activity in the echo chamber of the pool took a little getting used to. Ashani swam freestyle in the lane next to the bleachers. It was painful to watch her clawing through the water as the other girls quickly left her in their wake. But she stuck with it, and four years later she had the sixth fastest time in the state championship finals against girls who had been swimming since they were five years old. She went on to swim for the University of Northern Arizona, a Division 1 school, on an athletic scholarship. That meant four years of being in the water at five thirty every morning for two hours before class and another two hours in the afternoon.

I never would have had the focus and drive to do what she did when

I was in college. I had a hard time just getting to my eight o'clock classes. Ashani graduated with honors and easily became the best athlete in the family. These days, when I find myself getting tired and gasping for breath as I swim laps, I slow down, think of her, and am inspired to keep going, not with discipline but with curiosity to push the intensity envelope.

▲▲▲▲▲▲▲

In brief:

Each of these stories illustrates how willingness can accomplish more than willfulness. Where discipline divides, Love integrates, allowing us to overcome obstacles that otherwise would seem impenetrable. Baby steps are a way to skillfully work with the Law of Thresholds and the Law of Desire and Surrender to accomplish our goals without discipline. There's a saying that the hardest part of a workout is turning the doorknob. If you set high expectations, you may not even turn the knob at all. But if you tell yourself, "I'll just have a light workout," then getting out the door is easy. Never underestimate the power of baby steps and how they can make even the most daunting, awful task *aah*some!

Considerations:

- Choose something that you'd love to do but believe you can't for lack of time, opportunity, or talent.

- Decide on a modest, doable step (an appropriate baby step) in the direction of your goal.

- Give yourself a leisurely time frame in which to reach your goal.

- Take the baby step and keep taking it on a regular basis without being attached to results. If you find yourself getting frustrated, doubting yourself, or losing interest, observe these thoughts and feelings with non-attachment.

- Surrender to the process. You may be pleasantly surprised!

CHAPTER 23

Freedom from Addiction

> *Original sin left him wounded and blind*
> *so that he is easily deceived by appearances*
> *and chooses an evil*
> *which has disguised itself*
> *as good.*
> —The Cloud of Unknowing

GETTING HIGH, BLITZED, HAMMERED, RIPPED, SMASHED, AND WASTED ARE ALL apt descriptions of the roller-coaster ride of drug intoxication. As we discussed in the Law of Cycles, it's not just the amplitude (intensity) of the stimulus but how fast you get there. If a natural high is like an airplane that takes off and then touches down with a soft landing, a drug high is like firing a missile that peaks, flames out, and then craters.

Addiction is the quintessential "pleasure disorder" caused by artificial stimulation of the reward system. For many, it is the unintended consequence of an attempt to self-medicate an underlying spiritual malaise. When intoxicated, one often feels more connected. Sights, sounds, tastes, and smells seem more vivid compared to one's sober state. Drugs become a way to access *äsis* pleasure. But this heightened sensitivity proves illusory and the side effects, devastating. If your ordinary state is already sensitive and connected, then being drugged feels unpleasant. *If you're standing at the North Pole, every direction is South.*

Much of what I've learned about addiction has come from my own struggles. It started when I was sixteen, that vulnerable age of surging testosterone when young boys make their first awkward steps to find their place within the herd. After surveying the social landscape, I thought it would be cool to be a sophisticated intellectual, which meant ditching the white socks, wearing turtlenecks, and smoking a pipe. After all, my father smoked a pipe and so did Hugh Hefner, that bigger-than-life icon of *Playboy* magazine.

I bought my first pipe at Iwan Ries, a high-end tobacconist on Wabash Avenue in downtown Chicago where my father bought his smoking supplies. The narrow storefront opened into a long room lined with dark, wood-trimmed, glass display counters in an old-world style, redolent with the smell of tobacco, leather, and a dash of bourbon. The store had pipes for every mood and lifestyle, from a rustic bowl fashioned from a branch of cherry wood to a fine meerschaum, smooth as porcelain. The salesmen indulged my naïveté and outfitted me with a couple of pipes, a suede tobacco pouch, a fancy lighter, a tin of house blend, and a bag of pipe-cleaners. My favorite was a long-stem churchwarden that offered an exceptionally cool, contemplative smoke.

I found the smell of tobacco appealing but the smoke was harsh and distasteful—the "bite," as it's called. This, I was assured, would go away once the pipe was broken in or, more likely, my taste buds were broken down. I would just have to man up, which I was determined to do, and pretended to enjoy it.

The young developing (reptilian) nervous system learns quickly and is particularly susceptible to the influence of role models and habit formation. Ninety percent of adults who smoke cigarettes started smoking as an adolescent.[1] Similarly, teenagers who start drinking by age thirteen have a 43 percent chance of becoming an alcoholic, whereas people who start drinking at twenty-one have only a 10 percent chance.[2] I told my girls in middle school, "Someday you may want to experiment with drugs, but please wait until you get to college, after your brain has had time to develop." I also exposed them to lots of authentic pleasures to establish healthy reward pathways and a clear point of reference.

When my father discovered I was smoking, he confiscated all of my pipes. That's when I got started on cigarettes. It was 1965, the peak of cigarette smoking in the United States—the culmination of a carefully laid marketing plan that began in WWII with the American Red Cross handing out free smokes to GIs. Back in the States, newly liberated women learned to smoke on the job at the weapons factories. At that time, about half of men and a third of women smoked cigarettes.[3] By the time I got to college, I had a pack-a-day habit. The stench of cigarettes permeated every aspect of my life.

"I'm really quitting this time," I'd tell myself as I flushed the last few cigs down the toilet or tossed a half-smoked pack in a garbage can. As I became more desperate, my attempts became more dramatic. The most memorable was on a night train, highballing from Bali to Djakarta on New Year's Eve. At the stroke of midnight, standing between two jostling train cars, I hurled my last pack of smokes into the humid, moonlit jungle that was rushing past, but all to no avail. It was always the same story; a few hours later I'd be bumming smokes or digging through ashtrays looking for butts. I was hooked. With every failure my resolve grew weaker, and so did I.

Compared to other drugs of abuse, nicotine has a relatively mild stimulant effect on the dopamine reward system. Its addictive power comes from the ease of administration and repetition. (Baby steps work in both directions.) The small tickle of current to a head-wired rat repeated frequently is as effective as an infrequent, intense jolt. It was not until pre-rolled cigarettes were invented in 1881 that smoking began to take off, yet another example of technology enabling the abuse of artificial pleasure.

The summer after my first year of medical school, I came down with a horrendous cold. I was laid out flat in a boarding house on the Hill in Boulder, sweating with a fever and coughing up thick clots of yellow-brown phlegm. The lining of my lungs and throat burned so badly I couldn't bear to smoke. In the pathology lab, I had seen lung specimens of smokers floating in formaldehyde jars speckled with carbon-black and fungating cancerous growths or blown out with paper thin, emphysematous cysts. I had to quit. There was just no way I could call myself a doctor and smoke cigarettes.

When I recovered from my cold, I resolved to kick the habit by getting in shape. Each morning I jogged uphill toward Baseline road. It was rough. After a couple of blocks, I'd be gasping for breath, chest burning, and hacking up phlegm as the ciliated cells lining my lungs came back on line. That's when I struck a deal with myself: I could smoke as much as I wanted, but for every cigarette I smoked, I'd have to run an extra block. I had stumbled upon my own aversive conditioning program. Within a couple of days, the burning in my lungs from that extra block just wasn't worth it, and by the end of the week I had quit smoking for good.

Getting high

Getting high is never a trivial event. Addictive drugs are supernormal stimuli that hijack the pleasure-reward system and flood the N. accumbens with supra-physiological levels of dopamine. Each time a person gets high, they are training their reward system to orient toward the drug, which corrupts the exquisitely tuned internal guidance system we are born with. What starts out as a casual flattened grass path through the brain reward circuits soon becomes a well-worn dirt trail and eventually a deep rut.

At a biochemical level, the increased dopamine levels reach down into the neuron's DNA and direct the manufacture of proteins that change the shape and function of the dopamine receptors. This is called neural plasticity, and it actually remodels the neuron's architecture. Like remodeling a house, these "architectural" changes—knocking down walls, rewiring, and plumbing—can last a lifetime.

Once addicted, you never forget. When an alcoholic walks by a bar, sees a billboard of a glass of scotch, or just has a stray thought about alcohol, it can trigger a trickle of dopamine and craving in the pleasure circuits, even years later. The old well-worn neural pathway acts as a fixed reaction pattern much like a Graylag goose returning an egg to her nest. Recall from Chapter 6 that the problem with addiction lies not in quitting, but in not starting again. As one young patient, Owen, who had abused every common street drug by his early twenties, said, "I have a whole cornucopia of receptors just waiting to get turned on."

Emotional stress can also be a powerful kindling event. I remember once, during a painful breakup, a sudden urge to smoke a cigarette came over me—something I hadn't felt for over a decade. I watched myself with perverse curiosity as I drove to a nearby liquor store and bought a pack of Marlboros. The familiar feeling of the cigarette between my fingers and the act of lighting up and blowing plumes of smoke was surprisingly comforting, like slipping on an old pair of shoes. It was as though I had never quit. I furtively followed the first cigarette with a second. It would have been so easy to become a smoker again, except for one thing: I'd have to change my whole scene. I'd have to abandon my nonsmoking friends, give up exercise, and turn my back on my identity as a health-conscious person. Peer pressure is a powerful force, for good or ill. Fortunately, the momentum of my healthy lifestyle habits kept me from sliding back into my former nicotine-addicted self.

The cruel irony of addiction is that what begins as a euphoric rush ends in a desperate compulsion that yields little satisfaction. The neurobiology that underlies this uncoupling of desire and pleasure is subtle and important to understand. The stimulation of the reward system goes through two phases. Initially, when we encounter a novel pleasure, the VTA (desire-center) drenches the N. accumbens with dopamine. However, with repeated exposure, this initial surge fades, as we would expect with habituation, but it doesn't go away. The dopamine response merely shifts earlier in the process to the anticipation of receiving pleasure.[4] The desire for a fix—the expectation of receiving a reward—becomes more powerful than the actual enjoyment of it. (Wanting and liking uncouple.) As many smokers will confess, "It's just a bad habit." But one that they can't stop. Craving by definition is an unquenchable desire.

The supernormal stimulation of *hedonic* drugs eventually exhausts the reward system and disrupts the integrity of the triune brain, resulting in *anhedonia*, an inability to feel pleasure, which is also a common feature of depression, schizophrenia, and PTSD. Addiction is a weed that takes root in the fault line between cortical reason, limbic pleasure, and reptilian desire, fracturing the psyche, the same fault line St. Augustine cleaved with his wooden cross of Original Sin.

Brain imaging studies demonstrate that in the late stages of addiction, the inhibitory impulse control of the prefrontal cortex is markedly impaired, and the greater the impairment, the worse the clinical outcome as measured by drug usage and the likelihood of relapse.[5]

Phenomenologically, the psyche is split in two, as we saw in the case of the fallen Pastor Ted Haggard (Chapter 13). On one side of the fault line is the "good boy" (good-self) who wants to be strong, healthy, and respectable and do what's right. On the other side, the "bad boy," (bad-self) who desires immediate satisfaction, is self-indulgent, childish, devious, and could care less what others think. The good boy would just as soon get rid of the bad boy but can never quite manage it. Instead, he lords over the bad boy and shames him with guilt, calling him weak, lazy, stupid, undisciplined, self-destructive, evil, and so on. When the good boy is in the driver's seat, the bad boy hides in the shadows of the unconscious, biding his time. The two selves are careful to never occupy the same time and space, which is how people get blindsided by their own hypocrisy. The irony is the "gooder" the good-self, (the more the good boy represses the bad boy), the "badder" the bad-self (the deeper the denial); *the brighter the light, the darker the shadow.*

We assume the bad boy has the problem, and if he could just be whipped into submission or eliminated, the problem would be solved. "Just say no!" fails because it ignores that the good boy also has some serious problems.

The first step to resolving any conflict is to get both parties in the same room at the same time. For this to happen, the threats of annihilation and bullying on the one side and the underground guerrilla warfare and sabotage on the other must give way to an attitude of mutual respect and a willingness to listen to what the other side has to say—in other words, a suspension of judgments. As Sengcan reminds us:

> If you wish to see the truth
> then hold no opinions for or against anything.
> To set up what you like against what you dislike
> is a disease of the mind.

Only a mind free of prejudice can perceive reality as it is and see ourselves as we truly are, in all our glory and depravity. The good boy needs to recognize the tyranny of his fascist tendencies, his overcontrolling obsession with perfection and achievement. He needs to drop the arrogant facade of moral superiority that he hides behind to keep from feeling vulnerable and inadequate. At the same time, the bad boy needs to see through the folly of his adolescent pleasures, grow up. and step into the light of day to claim his birthright to enjoy life without shame. He needs to learn what authentic pleasure is and realize that reckless, artificial pleasures will ultimately lead to his own destruction, at which point the party will be over for everyone. He needs to appreciate the hard work, diligence, and dedication of the good boy, without which the food, shelter, and other logistics to enjoy life would not exist. By the same token, the good boy needs to realize that without the fun-loving zest of the bad boy, life would become an efficient but dreary mechanical affair. They need each other to be whole.

This was why the aversive training program I stumbled upon to quit smoking succeeded. The bad boy could smoke as much as he wanted, and the good boy could exercise his need for control and run farther. A successful deal aligns the self-interests of both parties. Both could agree that life is more fun being healthy and in better shape. Moreover, the physicality of running and the burning in my chest ensured that the message, "hey, a new cooperative administration is in charge," was sent down the line to my emotional and reptilian selves. My inner reptile rejoiced at rekindling the pleasure of running, and my limbic brain was emotionally inspired to be doing something healthy for a change. By giving myself permission to smoke as much as I wanted *and* running uphill every morning, I regained my Original Wholeness. After a short while, it was obvious that there were better ways to have fun and I had quit smoking forever.

The biggest challenge with quitting is getting all the selves in agreement. Once aligned, stopping is relatively easy, which is why when we finally quit, we wonder why it took so long. Like Dr. Seuss says, "It is fun to have fun. But you have to know how," and knowing how begins with knowing and embracing *all* of *your selves*.

While I believe each of us is responsible for the choices we make, from a public health perspective, addiction is a societal disorder. I once gave a lecture on mind-body relaxation techniques to a group of about thirty Colorado judges at the Breckenridge ski resort. (It turns out, judges also need continuing education credits.) As I looked around the circle, at one point I said, "The War on Drugs is not about whether we should be taking drugs or not—we're a huge drug-taking society. The war is on who should be in control of access and distribution." About half the judges nodded in agreement and this was long before medical marijuana was legalized. Addiction, whether to coffee, chocolate, alcohol, binge watching serials, sports, gambling, or the habit-forming drugs dispensed by your doctor, is built into the matrix and one of the ways it keeps us distracted and the money changing hands.

▲▲▲▲▲▲▲

In brief:

Addiction is a common pleasure disorder where the reward system gets hijacked by supernormal stimuli with an artificially heightened experience of empty pleasure. Like a weed that takes root in the crack between what the good boy *should* do and the bad boy *wants* to do, addiction splits the psyche, weakening our ability to act with integrity and wholeness. Freedom and self-efficacy occur when all of our selves are moving together in the same direction, which is antithetical to the objectives of the matrix.

Considerations:

- Be honest with yourself about your addictions. No shame, no blame.

- When you find yourself hankering for some unwholesome habit, feel into it. Notice the loss of control, the bargaining, the self-deception, the disintegration.

- What emptiness, what genuine need, are you trying to fill with your addiction?

- To answer the above question takes honesty and the courage to feel your pain.

- The truth shall set you free.

CHAPTER 24

Erotica

We are angels with monkey organs.

—JG

MY INTRODUCTION INTO THE MYSTERIES OF THE OPPOSITE SEX HAPPENED ONE fresh spring day when I was twelve years old. I bolted out of the house after lunch to meet my best friend Scott and walk back to school as we usually did. The moment we got out of earshot, he could barely contain himself. "Did you hear? Fred found some nude magazines near the playground!"

Right before the afternoon bell, we found Fred, sprinted across the street to an old brick walk-up apartment, and ducked beneath the gray painted wooden stairs. The air was damp with the sweet smell of rotting garbage, and on the stained concrete floor were a couple of woven peach crates piled high with girlie magazines. We grabbed a handful and stuffed them under our shirts, exhilarated with our plunder, and planned to return for more after school.

But the authorities had been tipped off, and just as school was letting out, a troop of four eighth graders, decked out in chalk-white cadet straps slung across their chests, cinched at the waist, marched through the schoolyard two by two, carrying the crates of the seized booty between them like prisoners, led by Mr. Brown, the gym teacher. They took the confiscated magazines to the towering smoke stack at the back of the school and burned them (a fitting way to rid young minds of evil).

That afternoon, and for quite a few afternoons afterwards, Scott, Fred, and I sat on a secluded garage roof devouring the glossy images of barely clad, full-breasted women standing or lying in suggestive poses, while I felt an inexplicable thrill swelling intermittently between my legs. For the first time, we saw breasts and nipples and studied them with keen interest. In those days, the token fig leaf of lace panties or a discreetly crossed thigh was the norm and what lay beneath remained a dark mystery.

Among our loot were several magazines printed on cheap newsprint with black and white photos of ordinary people of all shapes and sizes—couples and families walking in nature, picnicking by a lake, playing volleyball or lounging by the pool side, sipping drinks—all without a stitch of clothing. I didn't know what to make of these nudist colony enthusiasts with their darkly tanned bodies and naked casualness. Somehow, they were more disturbing to my suburban sensibilities than the glossy, posed pin-ups.

In retrospect, those rooftop sessions made a deep impression in my innocent pubescent mind, like a chisel gouge in an uncarved block of wood. Despite being forbidden, or perhaps because of it, these images defined not only what was desirable, but in a twisted way, what was "normal."

Turn ons

The ancient Greeks described several forms of love. They called sexual love *eros*, distinct from *philia* (friendly love), *storge* (family love), and *agape* (selfless love). They considered *eros* a kind of *theia mania*, a divine madness from the gods that seemingly out of nowhere could transport a person beyond the bounds of ordinary life. The Romans depicted erotic love as a chubby, winged Cupid, armed with a torch, a bow, and an arrow to pierce one's heart and inflame it with desire. Being shot with an arrow captures the sense of helplessness that arises when sexual lust takes hold of us at the root of our limbic and reptilian brains. You may recall that it was this helplessness that Saint Augustine attempted to explain with his doctrine of Original Sin. *Eros* is indeed a powerful force and, at the same time, a highly individual one that results from a complex interplay of culture and biology that has as much to do with what's between our ears as what's between our legs.

In the next three chapters, we will use the principles we've developed to reveal the mysteries of erotic pleasure. (If you skipped ahead to this section, you'll get more out of it if you start at the beginning of the book, as knowledge, like pleasure, is path-dependent. When it comes to erotic pleasure, slowing down will get you much further.)

Searching for the elusive erogenous zones

In the 1950s, dermatologist R. K. Winkleman attempted to solve the mystery of the erogenous zones once and for all by performing detailed microscopic studies of the skin and nerve supply of the glans penis, clitoris, perianal skin, lips, and other sexually sensitive areas. He was looking for special "erotic" nerve endings, but all he found was that these areas possessed a higher than average density of ordinary nerve endings. As mentioned before, pain receptors have been well described, but curiously, no pleasure receptors have ever been found.

Half a century later, a distinguished neuroscientist, V. S. Ramachandran, resumed the hunt, hypothesizing that an area is erotic not because of its anatomic proximity to the reproductive organs on the surface of the body, but because of its proximity to sexual regions on the surface of the brain. This can be seen with a homunculus, a little cartoon man, draped over the sensory cortex with its body parts drawn in proportion to the associated cortical innervation. Foot fetishism, he reasoned, can be explained because sensations from the feet project to an area on the sensory cortex adjacent to sensations received from the genitalia, and therefore could, presumably, stimulate the genitalia by proximity.

To test this hypothesis, 800 participants from the British Isles and Sub-Saharan Africa were asked to rate the erogenous intensity of forty-one body parts.[1] A high level of agreement was found among participants and the results were independent of age, nationality, race, sexual orientation, and even gender. As expected, the glans (acorn head) of the penis and the clitoris (*kleitoris* or key) topped the list. Feet, however, came in twenty-eighth, disproving Ramachandran's hypothesis.

I suspect that peripheral areas like the nape of the neck (ranked fourth), inner thigh (ranked seventh) and ears (ranked ninth) are erotic in part because of their associated vulnerability. Whatever the case, the high level of agreement among participants in this cross-cultural study suggests that *erotic touch is primarily biologically determined.*

In contrast, shifting tastes about the ideal body type, dress, accessories, and hairstyle suggest that *visual erotica is more symbolic and therefore culturally determined.* For instance, all the fuss we make about women's breasts must have

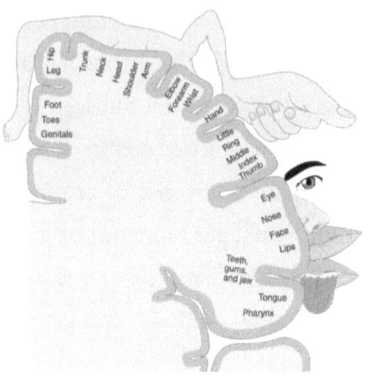

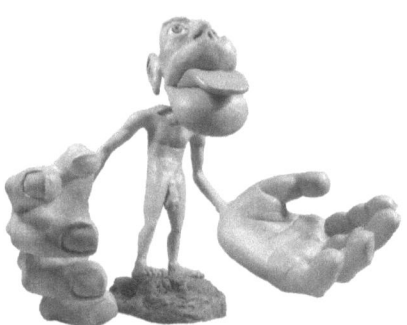

Figure 28: (Top) Mapping of the sensory cortex. The relative size of the illustrated part corresponds to the area of the cortex devoted its function. (Bottom) 3D model of homunculus.

seemed bizarre to the Hawaiian islanders when Captain Cook arrived in 1778. Women wore skirts made from the soft inner bark of the mulberry tree, wrapped several times about their waist similar to a hula skirt, and were bare-chested like the men. Female royalty wore skirts that rose higher, to just beneath their breasts.

Protestant missionaries arrived soon after Captain Cook, and their good wives insisted all women on the island cover their chests. For this purpose, they created the *holoku*, a modified "Mother Hubbard" garment consisting of a long straight dress attached to a yoke with a high neck (basically a sack with long sleeves). Beneath this garment, women wore another looser fitting sack, the *muumuu*, which eventually became the accepted informal dress.

In eighteenth-century Europe, when woman's bodies were hidden in long skirts and sleeves, a nicely shaped wrist or ankle was an object of erotic interest. Similarly, in ancient Japan, the exposed nape of the neck from a low-slung kimono was the risqué equivalent of today's plunging cleavage—an example of coinciding visual and tactile erotic stimuli. As noted in Chapter 14, women in other parts of the world spend millions every year on skin-lightening products because light skin indicates not having to toil in the sun and is associated with the upper class. Ironically, their pale Western counterparts lie on beaches or in tanning beds to burnish their tans. In the West, it is the privileged who can afford the leisure of an oceanside vacation.

The old adage, *beauty is pain*, illustrates just how bizarre the biological-cultural interface can get.[2] This was certainly true of the cruel Chinese custom of foot binding, which lasted nearly a thousand years into the early twentieth century. (My grandmother refused to have my mother's feet bound.) The practice began among the wealthy but soon spread to the lower classes. The ideal foot size was reckoned to be the length of an extended index finger (about three inches). The crippled feet were adoringly referred to as "golden lotuses" and forced women to walk on their heels in small, swaying, child-like steps described as "walking lightly as a lotus blossom." Poetic odes extolled their delicate beauty and their musty, perfumed odor was considered highly erotic. A Qing dynasty sex manual described forty-eight ways to fondle the golden lotus. Lest we dismiss bound feet as a barbaric Oriental relic, conceptually it is not far removed from its modern equivalent, the five-inch heel, which also visually foreshortens the foot and infantilizes the gait. It is also possible that the use of scarification among some African tribes and the recent fascination with tattoos and skin piercings such as tongue and nipple rings in the West are more than visual stimuli. They communicate a person's willingness and ability to endure high levels of sensual intensity (pain) that push the limits of the erotic Pleasure-Pain Threshold similar to other sadomasochistic practices.

We can understand fashion as a cultural artifact designed to arouse sexual attention through the creation of supernormal stimuli. A stylish hairdo, mascara, and lipstick, or a tight pair of jeans, pointed boots, and other accoutrements may be the human equivalent of Tinbergen darkening the horizontal lines on a butterfly's thorax or applying black magic marker to the breast feathers of a barn swallow.

Henry Kissinger said, "Power is the ultimate aphrodisiac."[3] As herd animals, we are naturally attracted to status and power because it defines a person's position within the herd and by association their reproductive fitness. This likely explains why celebrities, athletes, politicians, religious leaders, and other uber-males are prone to sexual misconduct and why sex goddesses like Marilyn Monroe and Angelina Jolie command oversized cultural influence. Male rhesus macaques in a pay-per-view experiment, given the option of a sweet drink or viewing female hindquarters and the faces of high-status monkeys, will choose the images, indicating the value of information about the social hierarchy.[4]

The reproductive advantages of power are not to be underestimated. Genghis Khan, whose empire was twice that of the Roman Empire, is the direct progenitor of 0.5 percent of the world's men, according to genetic studies.[5] Benito Mussolini reportedly had sex with a new woman every day for the fourteen years of his reign (some 5,000 women), earning him the title among the Italian cognoscente as the Phallus in Chief.[6] Could it be that increasing a woman's vulnerability by mimicking infantile features, such as cosmetically enlarging the eyes or having a dainty gait, exaggerates the power differential with men, and through enhanced contrast and comparison acts as a supernormal stimulus? Might this play a role in other forms of sexual domination such as rape, pedophilia, and sadism?

What's normal

Every culture assumes the sexual mores of its cultural matrix are normal, but a study of history and anthropology demonstrates that "normal" is a malleable concept. In ancient Greece, pederasty—the sexual relationship between a man and an adolescent boy—was a common practice. A boy's father often selected the older male who would then be responsible for training the young boy in warfare, the arts, and other manly skills. We find the same practice among the Japanese samurai. In some Polynesian societies, pubescent boys are initiated into sex by the older women of the tribe. This is certainly a more humane, if not effective, approach to sex education compared to high school health classes or masturbating with pornography.

In their groundbreaking book, *A Billion Wicked Thoughts: What the Internet Tells Us About Sexual Relationships,* cognitive neuroscientists Ogi Ogas and Sai Gaddam analyze the viewing habits of half a billion male and female internet porn users, providing a unique window into human sexuality. Their methodology represents a major advance over the 1950s Kinsey Reports that were based on 18,000 interviews of participants self-reported sexual activities. Ogas and Gaddam found some interesting gender differences:

- Men overwhelmingly prefer visual erotica—photographs and videos—while women prefer to read romance novels.

- Men form their sexual preferences in adolescence and rarely change; women's sexual preferences can easily change throughout their lives.

- Men approach sex like reckless pilots with a joystick; women take a more cautious approach like that of fighter pilots in a cockpit with numerous gauges, switches, and warning lights.

Of course, the data gleaned from cybersex is hardly the same as real sex. In fact, some men prefer the supernormal stimuli of cybersex where they can click through dozens of willing fantasy partners. By comparison, ordinary, vanilla sex has fewer choices and is far less exciting, as evidenced by an alarming epidemic of impotence among young men who use porn.[7] This trend toward artificial sex is likely to accelerate with the development of customizable, AI-enabled sex robots that are already on the market.

Gender math

These gender differences have a simple mathematical explanation when viewed through the lens of evolutionary biology. If we assume an organism's primary goal is to reproduce and project its genome into the future, then a man has roughly a million shots on goal with each and every ejaculation for the better part of six decades. A woman, on the other hand, produces only one ovum a month, or about 400 eggs over the course of the three decades of her reproductive life span (generally fifteen to forty-five years of age). Consequently, a man can easily afford to broadcast his seed far and wide and play the odds. He can also see at a glance all that he needs to know about the genetics of a potential sexual partner, as revealed by her facial symmetry, the straightness of her teeth, the luster of her hair, the size of her breasts, her waist-to-hip ratio, and overall conformation. His genetic investment could be as little as a one-night stand.

A woman's investment is significantly greater. She has far fewer shots on goal, as each ovum can be fertilized only during a narrow seventy-two-hour window, and should a pregnancy occur, she will be anovulatory (without menstruation) for at least nine months and even longer if she breast feeds. It makes sense that a woman needs to be more selective about whom she mates with and requires more information up front. It is in her best genetic interest to partner with a man who has not only superior physical genetics—strength, good bone, and stature—but also superior intelligence, character, honesty, sincerity, status, and financial means.

When a woman asks, "Do you love me?" she is seeking, consciously or unconsciously, reassurance that the potential father of her child will stick around to protect and raise their offspring. The technical term for this commitment is "parental investment." It behooves a woman to choose a man who is willing to make as big a parental investment as she is. From a purely numbers perspective, the hesitancy many men have toward commitment reflects the tension between the relative genetic advantages of making a singular, high-parental investment versus multiple, albeit superficial, investments.

▲▲▲▲▲▲▲

In brief:

Human sexuality exists at the boundary where the tectonic plates of biology and culture collide. At this erogenous impact zone, the eroticism of touch appears to be more biologically based while visual eroticism is more culturally mediated. (In the bedroom, it's the difference between having the lights on or off.) For women, assessing their partner's investment in parenting requires an additional cultural calculation. The image of a single ovum surrounded by a swarm of eager sperm cells is apt: men pursue and women choose. Although erotic desires are highly idiosyncratic, when it comes to actually consummating our sexual desires, pleasure follows a more predictable trajectory firmly guided by our biology, as we'll discuss next.

Considerations:

- How were you introduced into the mysteries of sex?

- What exactly do you find attractive in an "attractive" person?

- Notice your personal style choices and the messages you are communicating.

- Be curious about your erogenous zones. Tell your partner and have fun exploring them.

- If you have been unlucky in love, you may want to reconsider the kinds of erotic cues you're attracted to.

CHAPTER 25

Orgasm 1.0

> *An orgasm is the cosmos shuddering with ecstasy and bliss.*
> —JG

MOTHER NATURE TAKES NO CHANCES WHEN IT COMES TO PERPETUATING THE species. She drenches every aspect of sex in pleasure, the ultimate pleasure being orgasm, the divine paroxysm that the French astutely call *la petite mort*, the little death. Given all the interest, money, and effort devoted to sex, you'd think we'd take more time to enjoy it. And perhaps we would if it weren't so laden with anxiety on both sides of the gender divide. As the German actress Marlene Dietrich observed, "In America, sex is an obsession, in other parts of the world it's a fact."[1] The fact is that for the vast majority of couples, sexual intercourse is a brief, fleeting event.

According to a multinational population study based on stopwatch measurements, sex for the average man, from the time of vaginal penetration to orgasm, lasts a mere five to seven minutes, about the time it takes to smoke a cigarette.[2] Other studies have found that on the far end of the bell-shaped curve, roughly one in three men suffer from premature ejaculation, spilling their seed within seconds of, or in some cases even before, penetration.[3] (Note that in sexual pleasure, the Pleasure-Pain Threshold and orgasm are synonymous.)

The disconnect between sexual desire and performance—as if sex needed to be performed rather than simply enjoyed—is particularly disappointing for many women. While three out of four men orgasm during intercourse, only a third of women consistently do, half sometimes, a fifth seldom, and 5 percent never.[4] Yet 95 percent of women can achieve orgasm easily and quickly with masturbation. According to the Kinsey Reports, nearly 50 percent of women orgasm within three minutes of masturbation (similar to men) and 70 percent within five minutes.[5] The reason for the dramatic disparity between intercourse and masturbation is that women typically masturbate by stroking their clitoris, the primary source of pleasure that the ancient Greeks (over 2,500 years ago) clearly recognized was "the key," *kleitoris*. In this case, "the key" was not lost in translation but ignored, which is the real meaning of ignorance.

Contrary to popular belief, women get turned on as quickly as men. They just don't realize it. Using highly sensitive thermal-scanning cameras, researchers at McGill University found that the genitalia of both men and women became sexually aroused within thirty seconds of viewing sexually evocative images and reached their peak arousal within ten minutes (665 seconds for men and 743 seconds for women, a statistically negligible difference).[6] Whereas men are immediately aware of something stirring between their legs, women, as a result of their internalized genitalia, take longer to recognize it.

The biggest disconnect between men and women has to do with the anatomy of intercourse. For the man, the head of the penis is at the center of action, while the clitoris, the equivalent female structure, is at the periphery. It doesn't help that many men (and some women) aren't quite sure where the clitoris is even located. Despite readily available medical illustrations, it's not the same thing as visually inspecting the female genitalia in the light of day. Still, the part of the clitoris that can be seen is only the proverbial tip of the iceberg. Few people, including doctors, realize that the clitoris is an extension of two corpora cavernosa, *crura* (legs), and vestibular bulbs that wrap around the vaginal opening and constitute an internal pelvic system of erectile tissue that rivals that of the male penis by volume.

It was not until the mid-twentieth century that anatomists began to study the female genitalia in detail, and controversy remains to this day concerning such things as female ejaculation (some women discharge a viscous fluid from Skene's glands, the female counterpart of the male prostate), the G-spot (an area located five to eight centimeters within the anterior wall of the vagina), and vaginal orgasm. What is clear is that a fetus will develop female genitalia unless exposed to high levels of testosterone, which externalizes the genitalia into the male form. You can think of the vagina's anterior wall as corresponding to the base of the male penis and having similar erogenous sensitivity. If a couple is willing to engage in twenty minutes of foreplay, sexual satisfaction is significantly increased and 90 percent of women can reach orgasm.[7]

The term "foreplay" suggests the nature of the problem and its solution. Foreplay presumes that the purpose of sex is orgasm, which is like saying the purpose of eating is to get full. While true biologically, there's a world of difference between wolfing down your food like a dog and savoring it like an Epicurean. Again, as discussed in the Law of Cycles, the quantity and quality of pleasure we enjoy depends on how we get there and is a function of the net pleasure—the area under the pleasure-time graph curve (Chapter 15). Orgasm signals the end of pleasure. Slowing down and enjoying the ride not only increases our overall satisfaction, it prepares the nervous system for a more full-bodied climax, which as we will see, is the key to multiple orgasms in both women and men.

Great sex, then, is less a matter of technique and more a matter of attitude, specifically shifting one's focus from goal to process, from arriving to approaching, and from thinking to being. That's why thinking about baseball or other forms of distraction doesn't help men with premature ejaculation. They are already thinking too much and overwhelmed with anticipation.

You can't think your way out of thinking. The way to get out of your head is to get into your body. When the sensual doorways to consciousness are flung open wide, there is nothing left to fuel thinking. *The way to stop thinking is to go deeply into feeling.* The life of the body is always in the present moment, and when we surrender to the sensations in the body, we're there. Paradoxically, the fellow with premature ejaculation needs to become more in touch, more sensitive to his body sensations, not less. How else will he know how close he is to the edge of the ejaculation threshold? The cure for premature ejaculation is to stay present in the moment, riding the fractal waves of desire and surrender.[8]

The sexual Pleasure Cycle

My father never sat me down for the birds-and-the-bees talk. Instead, when I was a junior in high school, he handed me a book in a shiny dust jacket and said, "Here, I think you should read this," and then never spoke of it again. The title of the book was *The Human Sexual Response*, by Masters and Johnson, which had just been released in 1966.

It was groundbreaking because it stripped away the fig leaf of taboo that had shrouded sex for over 2,500 years and illuminated it with the stark light of science—literally. One of their scientific probes was a dildo equipped with a small camera and light to film the physiological changes in the vagina during intercourse.

Masters and Johnson's research identified four distinct phases in the human sexual response (Pleasure Cycle): excitement, plateau, orgasm, and resolution. The excitement phase begins with priming the N. accumbens/VTA pleasure-reward circuits with anticipation, that delicious tension between what is and what is coming—the tease. During this phase, we are actively making our way up the sensual continuum along with our partner, layering fractal wave upon wave of desire and surrender, building the tension for the coming tidal wave of orgasmic release.

As active pleasure increases, we enter a state of sustained, heightened sexual arousal—the plateau phase—a sensitive sweet spot where each caress sets off an exquisite wavelet of delight. One of the hallmarks of the plateau phase, along with an increase in blood pressure and a quickening pulse and respiration, is a generalized increase in muscle tone. Like tightening a violin string and then plucking it, waves of muscular contractions quiver through the system, causing toes to curl, hands to clench, and throats to moan with pleasure. The contractions converge at an epicenter in the pelvic floor muscles (the ecstasy center), which begins to rhythmically grip the root of the genitals, causing them to throb with desire. We have entered an altered state of heightened arousal and perception.

As the intensity builds further, the waves of pleasure grow more insistent and the pelvis becomes like a vortex, drawing in tendrils of pleasure from erogenous zones throughout the body, tuning our lust to an exquisite, almost unbearable pitch. Our pelvis begins to thrust and arch wildly with mounting urgency. Our muscles become rigid and tense; we breathe in tight gasps or hold our breath, gripped in the throes of excruciating pleasure until at last we reach a point of inevitability, suspended at the peak of desire and surrender, as we are drawn helplessly over the event-horizon into a swirling *zero*-larity. As one woman describes it: "I flush, my pelvic muscles tighten and loosen repeatedly. I moan, and at the peak, my body tightens to the point where I'm paralyzed and I usually say something like, 'Don't stop!'"[9]

Physiologically, an orgasm is a convulsion, a series of rapid muscular contractions and releases, that shakes the body like a fig tree in a violent wind, causing it to shed its fruit. In fact, much of what we know about orgasm is based on epilepsy research. Some epileptics at the onset of a seizure report a pre-orgasmic aura and feeling of inevitability. Recent neuroimaging studies demonstrate that at the moment of orgasm, there is marked decreased activity in the prefrontal cortex. The amygdala (fear-aggression center) also ceases, abolishing our survival instinct and fear of death. Simultaneously, the N. accumbens/VTA reward circuit lights up in a way that is indistinguishable from a heroin or cocaine rush. Because the prefrontal cortex inhibits the more ancient limbic and reptilian brains, when it goes offline, we are quite literally out of control, and our usual rational Apollonian persona is overtaken by a fit of Dionysian madness.

At a phenomenological level, an orgasm represents a rapid oscillation of the pleasure pendulum between ecstasy and bliss—between extreme desire and surrender—as the body shudders with spasms of intense muscular contraction and profound relaxation. Each person has their own orgasmic signature just as they have their own distinctive laugh or sneeze. Orgasms tend to fall into one of two types. The most common and quickest is a single, brief series of tonic-clonic (rhythmic muscular) contractions. The second, less common pattern begins with a burst of contractions followed by a number of random contractions that can occur over the course of many seconds to several minutes. It is this second pattern of "multiple" orgasms that we will explore next.

▲▲▲▲▲▲▲

In brief:

Human sexuality is complicated by a number of disconnects: the desire is long, the pleasure short; men are aware of arousal quickly, women slowly; the penis is at the center, the clitoris at the periphery. These differences work against mutual satisfaction but can be overcome. Sexual pleasure follows a unique Pleasure Cycle of excitement, plateau, orgasm, and resolution. As excitement builds, the senses sharpen and converge at the pelvis. Orgasm is a violent swinging back and forth between ecstasy and bliss—extreme desire and surrender—when we are shaken into Paradise for a few brief moments.

Considerations:
- Sex is an excellent place to explore how pleasure works.
- Practice staying present in the moment by focusing on sensations and ignoring thoughts.
- Letting go of expectations and judgments will help.
- Engage in and become absorbed in the process, not the goal.
- Experience the mystery of self, other, and the cosmos unfolding moment by moment.

Chapter 26

Orgasm 2.0

*The orgasm has replaced the Cross
as the focus of longing and
the image of fulfillment.*
—Malcolm Muggeridge

For many of us, orgasm is the one place where we can reliably experience ecstasy, bliss, and equanimity, which may explain why something lasting a mere ten to twenty seconds can command such importance in our lives and why multiple orgasms are so intriguing. Still, no one's counting how many orgasms you're having with a stopwatch and the logic of "more is better" doesn't apply. Multiple orgasms are merely an interesting variation, and if you never happen to experience one, there's no need to feel deprived or inadequate. Of course, any attempt to trivialize multiple orgasms doesn't play well in a marketplace that commodifies sexuality, and the confusing media hype doesn't help.

To clear up this confusion, we need to understand the biology of the resolution phase of the human sexual response—what happens after an orgasm—which is not the same for men and women. In men, what goes up must come down. After ejaculating, a man's erection withers quickly and, along with it, his sexual interest. He enters an erotic no-fly zone, an absolute refractory period where genital stimulation is irritating, even painful, and he is incapable of an erection. In a twenty-year-old man, this post-orgasmic crash may last a mere two to five minutes before he can spring back to attention, while in a sixty-year-old man, it could last twelve to twenty-four hours or more. After the absolute refractory period, he then enters a relative refractory period where his sexual interest (as well as general energy) may be sluggish for hours to days. As one fellow described it, "Monday morning, after a big weekend, I hardly notice women on my way to work. By Wednesday I see an occasional attractive woman, and by Friday I notice all sorts of attractive women."

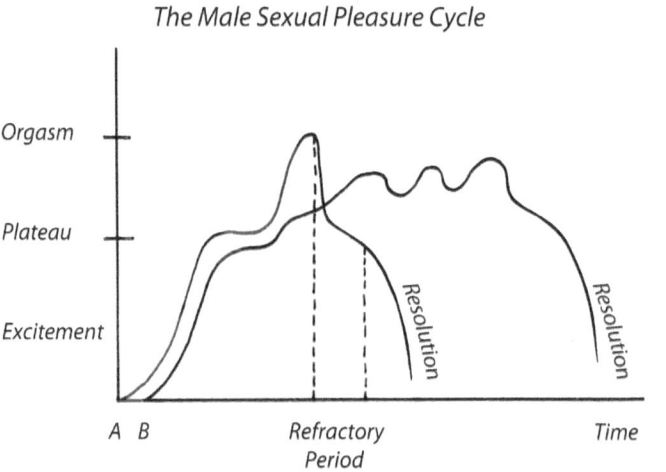

Figure 29: The Pleasure Cycle of the human male sexual response. A: typical 1.0 orgasm. B: multiple, 2.0 valley orgasms.

A woman follows a different trajectory. After an orgasm, her swollen internal genital structures do not immediately detumesce nor does her sexual desire. She experiences a brief absolute refractory period just long enough to catch her breath, and with further sexual stimulation may quickly return to her pre-orgasmic plateau of heightened sexual arousal. From there, she can re-summit the erotic continuum and may have six or more orgasms, each one successively easier to achieve and more intense.

Although only 15-20 percent of women are multiorgasmic, every woman has the potential to be. Men, on the other hand, due to a longer absolute refractory period, cannot have these kinds of multiple orgasms, but they can experience something closely related. As mentioned in the previous chapter, people typically have one of two types of orgasm: a burst

Orgasm 2.0

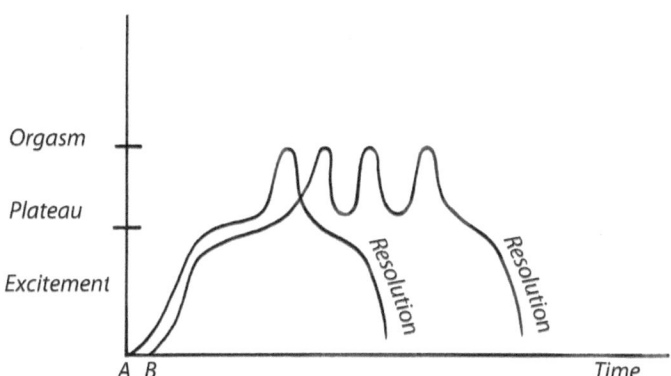

Figure 30: The Pleasure Cycle of the human female sexual response. A: typical 1.0 orgasm. B: multiple, 2.0 orgasms.

of spasms or a burst of spasms followed by random brief convulsions, which last only a second or two and gradually fade out. This second type occurs when the body-tube is so open that the orgasmic release continues to reverberate through the system as a kind of aftershock. In some people, however, the discharges are more like a light beam reflecting between parallel mirrors that can continue almost indefinitely, a condition known as persistent genital arousal syndrome.

More is not necessarily better. This debilitating condition primarily affects women and some men as a form of priapism. Afflicted individuals have uncontrolled, prolonged episodes of genital arousal without sexual feelings and may experience spontaneous orgasms triggered by such ordinary activities as crossing their legs, sneezing, or going to the toilet. The intrusive sensations may or may not be relieved with orgasm and can severely impact one's life. In Chinese medicine, this condition falls into a category known as disorders of *qi* and in the yogic literature as disorders of *kundalini*.[1]

During states of deep meditation, it is not uncommon to experience spontaneous movements such as grimacing, shaking, sudden jerking, or twitching, as tension patterns spontaneously release. According to yogic subtle physiology, at the root of the spine lies a sleeping serpent of primal *kundalini* energy. When aroused, it rises upward through the *sushumna*, central energy axis of the body. However, should this awakening occur prematurely before a person's Light-body is ready to receive it, the energy can short circuit, causing aberrant energy rushes, abnormal movements, and disordered states of consciousness.

For this reason, it is important to explore subtle phenomena such as multiple orgasms and other esoteric energy practices with humility and a sense of wonder. In the fifteenth century *Hatha Yoga Pradipika*, it is said that training the *prana* is like taming a lion, elephant, or tiger. If not approached with care, it can turn on you and kill you.[2] There is also a danger of using these techniques to adorn one's ego. Mature spiritual systems have ritualized, humbling practices to prevent such self-aggrandizing hubris. By delighting in the joy of discovery and not taking yourself too seriously, you can avoid the pitfalls of spiritual materialism.[3]

How to have multiple orgasms

As discussed in Chapter 12, pleasure is path-dependent. The intensity of an orgasm depends on the path by which the system is charged. It's like drawing a bow—literally drawing taut the body with sexual tension. If done hastily, the resulting release is shallow and not fully developed. Eugen Herrigel describes how to draw a bow in his classic *Zen in the Art of Archery*: "You must learn to wait properly ... By letting go of yourself, leaving yourself and everything yours behind so decisively that nothing more is left of you but a purposeless tension."

Herrigel is speaking of (you guessed it) the Law of Desire and Surrender. To draw a bow requires an act of will (desire). You must grasp the bow and pull the string taut. The only way to create a "purposeless tension" is to balance the drawing of the bow with relaxed surrender. Usually we think of a muscle as being either in a state of contraction or relaxation, but there exists a third state of relaxed contraction. I studied this form of relaxed muscular effort in the martial art of *aikido*, which is distinguished by its smooth, flowing, powerful movements.

The most difficult technique to master in Zen archery is the release of the arrow. For this purpose, the archer wears a special glove to pluck the bow string from the nock, the slotted end of the arrow. When the arc of tension across his chest, pulling his hands apart is maximally stretched and perfectly balanced, he plucks the string and lets the arrow fly like snow slipping from a leaf.

In much the same way, drawing the bow of your partner's desire (and your own) and "waiting properly" for the tension to build is the art of making love. A way to do this is to bring your partner to the thin edge of the Pleasure-Pain Threshold and then back away, easing the tension, only to approach it again, as though flexing a bow of desire. With each repetition, the bow becomes more pliable and can be drawn tighter, making it possible to store more potential sexual energy, which results in a stronger, more satisfying orgasmic release. As every child knows, if you want to build a higher sand pile, you need to start with a broader base. It's just how things work.

As with Zen archery, the most subtle technique occurs at the moment of orgasmic release. When desire is perfectly balanced with surrender, there is no resistance in the body-tube and the energy can flow unimpeded—the optimal condition for multiple orgasms. In the language of physics, it is a kind of superconductivity where the resistance to the flow of electrons abruptly drops to zero.

The valley orgasm

As the erotic bow is repeatedly flexed, the lines begin to blur and things can get confusing. The waves of tension and release build fractally and can grow so intense they create a "valley orgasm." This type of orgasm is based on a unique feature of male physiology. Orgasm and the ejaculation that follows two to three seconds later are two distinct physiological functions. Orgasm is primarily a cerebral event that happens between the ears. It involves the three brains in differing proportions at different times, which is why some orgasms are quick reptilian affairs and others are more deeply emotional and spiritually profound.

Ejaculation, in contrast, is a simple spinal reflex that happens from the waist down, no brain required. It originates in a region of the lumbosacral spine called the spinal-ejaculation center. The existence of this center was first discovered in WWII veterans who had suffered spinal cord injuries and limb paralysis.[4] A number of these men were still able to achieve erections and ejaculate with direct genital stimulation and in some cases by stimulating the peripheral erogenous zones of their ears, neck, or nipples. Some spinal-cord-injured men actually have more frequent erections due to the interruption of the normal inhibitory control the brain exerts on erections.

Valley orgasms require uncoupling orgasm and ejaculation. It's something like holding back a sneeze—not an unsatisfying, muffled sneeze, but a much more interesting and challenging "valley sneeze." You feel it coming on, you tip your head back, your mouth opens, the soft palate widens, but instead of exhaling sharply, you remain suspended in that moment of inevitability as the urge to sneeze fills your body like a wave that gathers at the tip of your nose and then passes. You have the energetic experience of a sneeze without the explosive release.

Some valley sneezes arise spontaneously like the "almost" sneeze described above. With sufficient presence of mind, any ordinary sneeze can be transformed into a valley sneeze by easing the impulse to sneeze gently over the edge. The same technique can be used as you approach the orgasmic Pleasure-Pain Threshold (see line B in Figure 29). Learning how to generate and surf valley orgasms can be very satisfying for both partners and a great way to prolong intercourse while building intimacy and trust. As one man described it: "It's like I'm about to be tumbled by a huge wave, but if I relax and don't panic, I can play the edge of it and then ride it out over and over again. When I hit the edge, my body trembles from deep inside. I feel like I'm coming, but I'm not."

At times, this approach is called "peaking," which is an unfortunate choice of term as one does not actually reach the peak of a typical orgasm. Energetically, it's more like falling back into an orgasm rather than madly rushing toward a climax. Unlike the dissipating feeling of an external discharge, a valley orgasm has a quality of internal release and accumulation. Because there is no ejaculation, there is no refractory period and

Orgasm 2.0

the process can be repeated as many times as one wishes. At the same time, oxytocin, the "cuddle hormone," along with endorphins (an internal opiate) and prolactin (a satiety hormone) flood the body, diminishing the emotional distance between partners and bonding them together, perhaps for a lifetime.

Every erotic touch is at once an invitation to desire and to surrender. The key is balance. Since we generally have an overabundance of desire, it boils down to developing our ability to surrender. That's why an orgasm of any type comes most easily when we let go of our attachment to having one. All that is required is a willingness to die. *Vive la petite mort!*

Like moths drawn to a flame, nature conspires to strip us naked and merge us with the destructive-creative force of the universe, returning us to the Garden where it all began.

▲▲▲▲▲▲▲

In brief:

Both women and men are capable of multiple orgasms, but of a different sort. Women have a brief absolute refractory period and can orgasm again within moments. Men, because they have a longer refractory period, are unable to have multiple *peak* orgasms but can have multiple (non-ejaculatory) *valley* orgasms. Whether it is a single robust, full-body orgasm or multiple orgasms, the sexual encounter is more satisfying if you focus on the process of accumulating net pleasure rather than on the goal of achieving an orgasm. As with surfing, it's all about the ride!

Considerations:

- The first step to enhance your orgasmic pleasure is to prepare your Light-body.
- This requires clean living and engaging in authentic pleasures with high-intensity Pleasure Cycles that invigorate and increase your sensitivity and Pleasure Capacity.

- With practice you will develop the experience and skill to play at the orgasmic edge of the Pleasure-Pain Threshold.

- Set aside a special hour or two to enjoy exploring the erotic realm with your partner through intimate sharing, massage, and playful exploration.

- The key is to go slowly and practice breathing and relaxing into high intensity pleasure rather than grasping.

- Take turns giving each other pleasure.

- Give up (surrender) your attachment to orgasm.

CHAPTER 27

Living in the Sweet Spot

> *Wealth is the ability*
> *to fully experience life.*
> —Henry David Thoreau

One of Leonardo da Vinci's most iconic images is a small sketch known as the Vitruvian Man that was found among his notes. He created it to study the symmetry and proportion of the human form (think balance and fractals) and to illustrate man's relationship to the cosmos.[1] Being the genius he was, he based his drawing on measurements taken from various subjects using a large wooden compass and then overlaid upon it the sacred geometry of a circle and a square.

His drawing also provides us with a convenient way to remember the six essentials of a well-proportioned, good life. The left leg represents nutrition and the right leg exercise; together they form an equilateral triangle, the physical foundation upon which we stand. The navel, which is the central point from which the limbs extend, represents sleep, through which we recharge our mind and body each night by plugging into the mainframe and downloading the dream wisdom of the collective unconscious. The left arm represents relationships and the right arm work, the two ways we reach out to the world. The head represents our *äsis* connection to the Source. When these six essentials of nutrition, exercise, sleep, relationships, work, and *äsis* connection are well proportioned and balanced, we can stand securely in the world, take hold of our life, and bring forth our highest potential. Da Vinci's sketch also reminds us that the *objet d'art* is merely a testimony to the artist's life and that the greatest artistic expression of all is a life well lived in which we are at once the subject, medium, and creator.

The sweet spot

Balancing the six essentials can be challenging because we are easily distracted by the demands of daily life. The solution, as Aristotle observed, is to find the golden mean between the extremes. Think of it like stringing a tennis racquet. When the tension between nutrition, exercise, sleep, relationships, work, and *äsis* connection are well strung, they form a sweet spot.

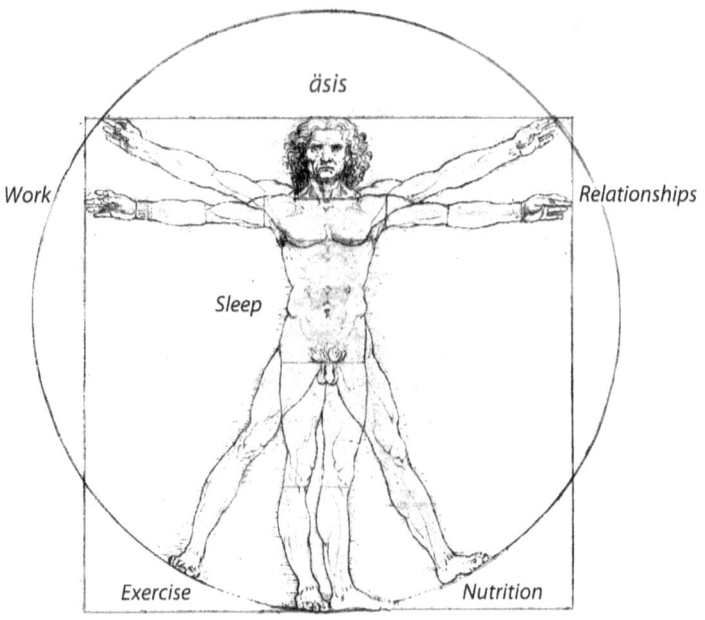

The Six Essentials

Figure 31: The Six Essentials of a good life.

You can tell when you hit the sweet spot because it feels great. You move through your day with ease; you accomplish tasks smoothly and efficiently; you feel well rested, alive, confident, and in control of your life. *The sweet spot is just another word for the zero point where we find maximum power, efficiency, control, freedom, and pleasure* (which is why it's sweet).

But like any balancing point, the sweet spot is not something you can possess or hold on to. It is an activity, a quality of being that you move in and out of, through and around. Applying the **Seven Immutable Laws of Pleasure** will help you hit the sweet spot more consistently:

▲ 1. **Original Wholeness**—Our natural state is like the original joy of a young child: fresh, alert, and present.

▲ 2. **Colors**—Pleasure is composed of three primary colors—red (physical), green (emotional), and blue (mental)—which combine to form clear, white (*äsis*).

▲ 3. **Contrast and Comparison** – The nervous system functions through contrast and comparison.

▲ 4. **Thresholds**—Our physical, emotional, mental, and spiritual lives unfold along continuums of intensity, each limited by a Pleasure-Pain Threshold.

▲ 5. **Cycles**—Pleasure cycles through active, passive, and neutral phases.

▲ 6. **Desire and Surrender**—When our desire and surrender (effort and relaxation) come into balance, our life-stream flows optimally in alignment with the Tao and the gates to ecstasy, bliss, and equanimity open.

▲ 7. **Renewable Pleasure**—Feeling good is a vital natural resource that resides within the warmth of our human heart.

Ultimately, hitting the sweet spot is a feeling that requires sensitivity, timing, and lots of practice. Here are some tips to help you get started.

Nutrition

Despite all the hype and controversy, nutrition need not be complicated. Every animal in the wild knows what to put in its mouth and what not to. Deer know what part of a plant to eat by the smell of a berry or the taste of a leaf and what time of the year to eat it. Obesity is rare in the wild.

We are born with the same natural intelligence (the Law of Original Wholeness). This was demonstrated in a famous study conducted in 1939 by a pediatrician named Clara M. Davis, who wanted to get to the bottom of all the dietary dogma of her day.[2] She convinced unmarried, teenage mothers and widows who were financially strapped to place their infants in what amounted to an experimental eating orphanage in an affluent lakeshore suburb of Chicago. A total of fifteen newly weaned, six- to eleven-month-olds were enrolled. At each meal, these children were presented with thirty-four different minimally processed foods from which to choose, ranging from water and sweet milk to tomatoes and spinach, from raw liver and fish to bananas and barley. Care was taken not to influence the child's choices. Portion size, nutritional content, and body weight were all carefully measured and recorded. At the outset of the study, four of the children were poorly nourished and underweight, and five had rickets. Yet over the six-year study, all of the children self-selected a nutritionally balanced intake of calories, maintained a normal weight, and thrived.

Of course, we don't live in the wild. Most of us hunt and forage at the grocery store, where unhealthy food options outweigh healthy ones and corrupt our *sense*-abilities. A nationwide study found that 60 percent of calories for an average American come from processed foods, which tend to have more fat, sugar, and salt than less processed food.[3] Fortunately, there's a simple way to make healthy food choices, which we touched on in Chapter 15. I call it **WAC** for short:

> **W**hole – Select whole foods which naturally have a balance of nutrients.
>
> **A**live – Eat fresh foods whenever possible.

Clean – Buy organic to minimize your exposure to toxins.

Whole. Alive. Clean. As Epicurus advised: keep it simple, and you won't get confused.

Exercise

The body is built to sweat, a unique ability among mammals that allowed Paleolithic hunters to run down large, furry game on the savannah until the animals collapsed from heat exhaustion. Sweating is also an important way to eliminate toxins. The body's primary detoxification enzymes are present in the skin, lungs, and liver—the three places where we interface with the outer world.

One of the best indicators of overall fitness (and predictor of longevity) is how well you breathe. In exercise physiology, this is called the VO2 max, which measures the maximum volume of oxygen your heart, lungs, and muscles can effectively utilize. It is an indirect measure of how well your mitochondria "breathe," the tiny powerhouses that oxidize glucose into ATP to run your cells, known as cellular respiration.

When it comes to increasing your VO2 max, the intensity of exercise is as important as the duration. The amplitude is measured from the peak of exertion to the trough of relaxation. The body responds optimally to a blend of sustained, low amplitude (aerobic) activity and intense, high amplitude (anaerobic) activity.[4] This is consistent with the Law of Contrast and Comparison and the Pleasure Cycle. The greater the delta in intensity between active and passive pleasure, the more life we can channel and the higher our Pleasure-Pain Threshold. Even brief bursts of intensity like bounding up the stairs or walking fast have a significant cumulative effect that can help keep your muscles toned and your mitochondria tuned.

Another important aspect is muscular strength. There's no substitute for real strength. But not all strength is the same. Weight machines isolate specific muscle groups and make you stronger in a piecemeal way. Lifting free weights is more integrated but can still lead to an unbalanced, muscle-bound physique if not done correctly. The most balanced resistance training uses your own body weight. Pull-ups, push-ups, squats, running, swimming, and gymnastics engage the entire body in an organic, integrated way and develop intelligent strength.

There are also functional and aesthetic considerations. Each form of exercise develops a particular musculature: dancers are light and graceful; body-builders, compact and dense; and yogis, long and flexible. Our bodies respond to the demands we place on them, and this includes our intentions. Male dancers, for instance, have well-defined chests and arms, not from lifting weights or ballerinas in tutus, but through the expression of intention in their gestures. In other words, the quality of the awareness we bring to our exercise is as important as the amount of exercise, which is why watching television while running on the treadmill misses the point.

One of the easiest ways to keep fit is to work hard. I knew a window-washer who ran up and down ladders all day washing and squeegeeing with both hands. He was in terrific shape. My father, who never went to the gym, undertook chores with vigor and was physically active well into his eighties. Working hard has the additional benefit of getting a lot done. If you keep your blood moving and sweat every day, you'll stay in shape and live longer.

Sleep

aah ... sleep, sweet sleep, is a tender mercy and, like nutrition and exercise, fundamental to good health. But alas, for many, a mercy denied, an unintended casualty of modernity. Even though sleep is the navel of the Vitruvian Man (at the center of the six essentials), half of American adults are sleep deprived and get less than the recommended seven to nine hours.[5] A third of Americans complain of insomnia.[6] The expectation of sleeping a solid eight hours and then awakening rested to start the new day, however, is an artifact of industrialization. Once the mechanical clock was placed on the bell tower (Chapter 20), it was only a matter of time before it would be placed at the bedside to alarm us. Industrialization necessitated the consolidation and compression of sleep to regiment workers into factory life. Biology is not easily changed. What we call "insomnia" is, for the most part, a disorder of our own making, a natural response to an unnatural situation.

For most of human history, sleep was a more fluid and intermittent affair. Hunter-gatherers slept as other animals do—when they felt like it. At night, a communal tangle of women, men, and children gathered around a fire pit. Snoring, conversation, crying babies, sexual activity, and getting up to tend the fire were commonplace. People did not sleep in a single eight-hour stretch. In the 1700s, people often slept for four hours, were awake for an hour or two to enjoy some quiet personal time (known as the watch or vigil), and then went back to sleep again.[7] Any residual sleepiness the following day could easily be accommodated with a nap.

Napping is uncommon in our frenetic, caffeine-driven workplace. We are the only creatures on earth who voluntarily deprive themselves of sleep (otherwise known as the Protestant work ethic in Western culture). Most people of the world nap after lunch, as is common throughout China, India, Latin cultures, and tropical climes.[8] While we might pride ourselves on our "moral superiority," tampering with the reptilian sleep-wake cycle comes at a high cost.

Indeed, the circadian rhythm (Latin *circa*, "around," and *dies*, "day") synchronizes virtually all our physiological functions from digestion and energy production to hormonal secretions and cognitive ability. When this cycle is disrupted, with jet lag or a bad night's sleep, the different functions come back on line at different times, which adds to our feeling out of sorts.

The health consequences of inadequate sleep are massive. Sleep deprivation is associated with an increased incidence of breast, colon, and prostate cancer, prompting the World Health Organization in 2007 to declare night shift work a probable carcinogen.[9] At a cellular level, insufficient sleep causes transcription errors in the genome and decreases natural killer cell activity by as much as 70 percent.[10]

For teenagers, early school start times not only lead to lower test scores, they also increase motor vehicle accidents, the leading cause of death in this age group.[11] On the other end of the age spectrum, merely advancing the clock one hour during daylight savings time increases the rate of heart attack 24 percent in the spring and turning the clock back in the fall decreases it 21 percent in the days after the change. Short sleep is also associated with an increased risk of Alzheimer's. Impaired sleep is a common finding in practically every psychological disorder including anxiety, depression, schizophrenia, PTSD, and suicide.[12] The bottom line is that the "you-can-sleep-when-you're-dead" ethos is a self-fulfilling prophecy. If you run on less than seven hours of sleep, you probably won't live as long.

Unlike taking a loan from a bank, you can't pay back the sleep debt with more sleeping on the weekends, nor is there a pill solution. "Sedation," as Mathew Walker, neuroscientist and director of the UC Berkeley Center for Human Sleep Science, makes clear, "is not the same thing as natural sleep."[13] Sleeping pills, alcohol, and other sedatives disrupt the natural brainwave sleep architecture, which unfolds in a precise sequence of sleep cycles of about 90 to 120 minutes. Each sleep cycle, in turn, is composed of five phases that repair the body, store memories, and process emotions. It's hard to improve on 3.5 billion years of evolutionary trial and error. What the drug companies don't tell you is that the benzodiazepines (Xanax and Restoril) and the hypnotics (Ambien and Lunesta) only increase total sleep time by twenty to thirty minutes.[14] The downside is these drugs interfere with memory and alertness the next day and are highly habit forming—a euphemism for addictive. Once you start taking them, they can be very hard to get off of. What's more, many drugs, particularly psychoactive ones (including alcohol and cannabis), interfere with REM sleep, the rapid eye movements associated with dreaming, an important part of our emotional well-being.

Dreaming is another casualty of modernity. When sleep was more fluid, humans sojourned between the waking and dream worlds more easily, blurring their distinction. In many cultures, dreams occupy a reality (ontological status) on par with waking life and the two inform and support each other. This is more reasonable than you might think. Ordinary consciousness and dreaming use identical neural pathways and have indistinguishable brain wave patterns, prompting neurologist Oliver Sacks to say, "Waking consciousness is dreaming—but dreaming constrained by external reality."[15] Zhuangzi, the Taoist sage, pondered the same question: "I dreamt I was a butterfly, flitting around the sky; then I awoke. Now I wonder: Am I a man who dreamt of being a butterfly, or am I a butterfly dreaming that I am a man?"[16]

Relationships

Of the six essentials, personal relationships are the most challenging because they depend so much on others. The most important relationship is with our self because *we do unto others as we do unto our self.* Sigmund Freud was the first to describe this psychological process. He called it "projection," borrowing a term from the budding movie industry of his day. Like a film projector projects images on a screen, we project our thought-images onto people and the world. As Carl Jung described it, "We naively suppose that people are as we imagine them to be ... projecting our own psychology into our fellow human beings. In this way, everyone creates for himself a series of more or less imaginary relationships based essentially upon projection."[17]

In other words, we live within a bubble, a psychological *umwelt* of our own making, that is based on our personal experiences, biases, and perceptions. Even worse, we tend to attribute to others the desires, motivations, feelings, and impulses that we cannot accept in ourselves (what Jung called the "shadow") as an ego defense against seeing our own wickedness. For instance, a fearful person experiences a threatening world; a person with low self-esteem, a world of victimhood and failure; and a distrusting person, a world of deceit.

Projection is what makes self-righteous people so dangerous because they cannot see their own shadow. (I imagine Hitler looking at himself in the mirror in a spiffy uniform, thinking himself rather dashing.) Seeing only their positive aspects and believing themselves to be morally superior, the self-righteous cast their shadow onto a scapegoat. (During Yom Kippur, the high priest symbolically laid the sins of the Israelites upon the head of a goat, which was then banished into the wilderness, a role the Jews would often tragically play themselves.[18])

This sort of negative projection can be extremely toxic. As Jung noted, "All projections provoke counter-projection when the object is unconscious of the quality projected upon it by the subject."[19] The trading back and forth of negative counter-projections can easily destroy a relationship.

This brings us to the problem of anger. If kindness and respect are essential for a healthy relationship, how are we to deal with negative emotions? At the psychotherapists's conference with Thich Nhat Hahn, mentioned in Chapter 13, the topic of anger came up repeatedly, as did the question, "Isn't it better to express anger than to keep it pent up inside?"

Thich Nhat Hahn observed, "Beating the pillow with a tennis racket doesn't get you in touch with your anger. You aren't even in touch with the pillow. If you were, you wouldn't be beating it.... You're not working out your anger; you're rehearsing it!" Anger arises when we don't get what we want or feel we have been slighted. As an emotion, it inflames the ego and morally elevates the "offended" party, who therefore feels entitled to lash out at the "guilty" party.

A more skillful approach is to radically open ourselves to the energy of our anger and allow it to flush the detritus from our Light-body and transform the self. Beneath anger are often tender feelings of vulnerability and pain. Getting in touch with and acknowledging these feelings ("bringing forth what is within us") is the only way to address and resolve them. But please remember, the radical acceptance of our emotional experience is entirely an *internal* process. How we choose to express these feelings in the *external* world is another matter, requiring the utmost skill and compassion. This is where honesty, kindness, and respect come in. At the close of the conference, Thich Nhat Hahn offered these words as a parting gift:

> You are me and I am you
> Together we inter-are.
> You cultivate the flower in yourself
> So that I will be beautiful.
> I transform the garbage in myself
> So that you do not have to suffer.[20]

Projection can also work the other way around. A positive projection can bring forth the best in the other person, initiating a virtuous Pleasure Cycle of reinforcing positivity. If it weren't for this "honeymoon" phenomenon of mutual positive projections (infatuation), we might never be able to overlook our partner's shortcomings long enough to couple. Through projection, we create and are created by the social world in which we live. As novelist Wallace Stegner writes, "There is a sense in which we are all each other's consequences."[21]

Lastly, when it comes to love, it is important to know that you are the source of love in your life. While you may receive kindness from others, your experience of love comes from within. Just as the sun can't see its own light without the moon to reflect it, we can't experience our love without a love object. For this reason, pets are so endearing because they make excellent reflectors. (I had a Chow/Blue Heeler mix, Mooli, who, without a doubt, opened my heart and made having a family possible.) So please remember, should you lose your love object, though it may be extremely painful, you have not lost love. Love is still within you if you are willing to open yourself to it.

Work

Roughly half of our waking life is devoted to our job. Yet, according to a 2015 Gallup poll, only a third of people are actively engaged in their work, half are not engaged, and a fifth are actively disengaged.[22] Overall, two out of three people derive little meaning from their work beyond a paycheck. Spending one's life chasing reward pellets in a maze hardly seems a worthy use of what poet Mary Oliver calls "your one wild and precious life,"[23] as the following parable illustrates:

> Juan grew up in a small fishing village. Each morning he went out on his skiff along with the other fishermen but would return by midday. One afternoon, his friend Felipe saw him tying up his boat at the dock and offered him some advice: "You know, Juan, if you stayed out longer, you could catch more fish."

Juan paused thoughtfully and replied, "Yeah, why would I want to do that?"

"Well, with the extra fish you could buy a bigger net and catch even more fish," said Felipe.

"And what would I want to do that for?"

"Then you could save up enough money to get a bigger boat and go out into the deep waters where the really big fish are."

"And then...?" asked Juan.

By this point his friend was getting frustrated, "Don't you get it? With all the money you make, you wouldn't have to work so hard. You'd be able to relax and enjoy your life."

Juan leaned back, put his dark, calloused feet on the gunwale and with a satisfied, toothy grin answered, "I'm already enjoying my life."

Felipe, driven by unconcious feelings of inadequacy, had bought into the matrix's endless quest for "more." Juan, on the other hand, operating from the Law of Original Wholeness, understood the meaning of "enough."

In our mercantile society, we often conflate money with value. In a marketplace, the value of goods and services is determined by what one is willing to pay for them. But to apply the same logic to such things as health, love, parenting, or a meaningful life is to reduce these things to a commodity, an object that can be bought and sold, and in the transaction, we risk losing our humanity.

Conflating money with value leads to uncomfortable questions such as: What is a human life worth? Should health care be a right or a privilege? What's more valuable, raising your child or pursuing your career? These are ethical questions that cannot be measured in dollars alone.

Work is more than a way of earning a living. It is a way of earning a life. Through our work, we connect with the world and it is through this social interaction that we find meaning and purpose. But that's not to say that meaning is conferred by the external world. It is up to you to decide what is meaningful, what is of value. Meaning, like love, is sourced from within, but we need an external form through which to express it. Or as my father used to say, "You may have a deep well, but you need a scoop to get the water out."

I once received some advice from the father of a high school girlfriend, who said, "If you love what you do, you'll do it well and the money will follow." He had a successful career putting up high-tension wires across the country and enjoyed every minute of it. But he didn't quite get it right; the money may not follow. What surely does is the satisfaction of living an authentic life rich with meaning, purpose, and freedom. When young people seek advice about finding a career, I tell them, "*Where your talents intersect with the needs of your community, therein lies your vocation.*"

The *äsis* experience

While relationships and work are the arms of the Vitruvian Man and represent the ways we reach out to the world, the *äsis* "limb" is appropriately at the head because it simultaneously informs and depends upon the other essentials. The *äsis* experience is intensely personal. As discussed in Chapter 18, it is not a matter of intellectual belief as much as an attitude, a way of standing (being) in the world where the vital centers of pelvis, heart, and head are awakened and attuned to resonate with the higher frequencies, enabling a connection to a Source beyond words.

Each of us connects to Source in our own way. "What is the Source?" you may ask. The simple answer is, I don't know. It's a mystery, yet one that is intimately related to consciousness. As noted in Chapter 8, we can't comprehend our consciousness directly, but we can observe its effects and intuit its existence from the intelligence that we see all around us in other creatures, forests, mountains, rivers, sky, and ocean.

For me, the *äsis* experience boils down to a daily practice, both formal and informal, of remembering who I am before words, images, or personal identity. Over the years, my practice has taken different forms. When I was a young child, I would spend hours watching ants scurrying about in the cracks on our stone back porch or lose myself playing neighborhood games and sports. Later in life, I gazed at the stars at night and studied martial arts, meditation, yoga, dance, music, and more recently, swimming and cycling. Each of these activities provides its own particular lens to illuminate the Self. I practice informally throughout the day, merging with ordinary experiences—looking at a spring bud, washing dishes, lying down for a nap, or chopping vegetables. As Rumi wrote, "There are hundreds of ways to kneel and kiss the ground."[24]

Of all my practices, the most enduring and profound has been sitting meditation. It's said there are four levels: in the beginning one meditates to relax and quiet the inner clamor; at the second level, one meditates to be more effective in the world; at the third level, one meditates to achieve spiritual insight and enlightenment; and at the fourth and highest level, one meditates for no reason at all.

Doing something for no reason turns out to be extremely radical. Practically everything we do in life is for a reason, a desire to improve, achieve, or get something. Because desire is a function of the ego, doing something for no reason loosens the ego's grip. Meditation is a practice of doing and non-doing (balancing desire and surrender), of letting go and dying to the moment to be reborn in service to life. Like drip irrigation, the results come slowly, but penetrate deep to the roots.

Note that *äsis* knowledge is not the same thing as having technical skills like fixing a car or tuning a piano. When it comes to consciousness, we are all on a level playing field. While there are those who may have more experience in self-awareness and can provide helpful guidance, their consciousness is in no way superior. A spiritual teacher can't fix anything. At most, she or he can act as a guide or catalyst to help you deepen your relationship to yourself and find the guru within, as the Hindus say, or as the Gnostics put it, discover the god within (theosis).

Working with a spiritual teacher can be useful, but be aware, they are of two sorts: scripturalists and practitioners. The scripturalist recites the words of the mystic who has returned from the mountain top. Their authority rests on their interpretative skill and intellectual acumen. The practitioner attempts to climb the mountain to see for themselves. Their authority rests on their personal experience. It's easy to distinguish between the two. Over time, the scripturalist accumulates more and more words, writing commentaries on the commentaries and embroidering the embroidery, until they have created so many layers of complexity that only they possess the special knowledge to interpret them. They become the high priests, the Brahmans, the clerics. In contrast, the practitioner over time says less and less until, at last, they have nothing to say at all. The scripturalist is drawn to the institution; the practitioner is drawn to the mountain top. Hence, Laozi's maxim: "Those who know don't talk. Those who talk don't know."[25]

Of the two, the path of the practitioner is the more reliable because it has built-in feedback. I might think I am an enlightened yogi, given my deep study of Patanjali's Yoga Sutras, but if I begin to tremble and panic after holding a deep forward bend for fifteen breaths, well, I'm just not there yet. However, just because I can twist myself into a pretzel or sit motionless for hours doesn't mean I am enlightened. It is not *what* we do, but *how* we do—the quality of awareness we bring to our intentions and actions.

As with other areas of life, *caveat emptor* (let the buyer beware). It's worth remembering an old Zen saying, *if you meet the Buddha on the path kill him*. Obviously, if you kill him prematurely, you will have missed an opportunity to study with a great teacher, but if in the end you don't kill him and free yourself of his opinions and dogma, you will have missed the point entirely—to grasp the truth through your own direct experience and allow it to change how you live your life.

The *āsis* quest proceeds along two trajectories, and spiritual traditions tend to emphasize one or the other. The Zen direction aims toward the cosmos, like looking up at the starry night sky and coming to peace with the insignificance of all that we do on our tiny speck of a planet. Accordingly, Zen emphasizes the emptiness of *sunyata*, zero (the Buddha sitting in meditation). The other direction, which is more characteristic of Indian Hindu spirituality, is to fully embrace our humanness in relationship to the divine and emphasize the fullness of *sunyata* in its infinite form, the reciprocal of zero (the god with multiple heads and a hundred arms). A spiritually mature person explores both directions fully and can move between them with equal aplomb, as appropriate.

▲▲▲▲▲▲▲

In brief:

The six essentials of a good life are nutrition, exercise, sleep, relationship, work, and *äsis* connection. When these are brought into harmonious balance, we're in the sweet spot. The goal of a successful career is unidimensional and measured in comparison to your peers. The goal of a successful life is multidimensional and measured in comparison only to yourself. You are free to decide what constitutes a good life. In my estimation, the acid test is the degree to which you have achieved freedom (have found your sweet spot)—not outwardly, but inwardly. Achieving a measure of freedom means becoming a virtuoso of your life and a true Vitruvian Human.

Considerations:

- Now that you have read about the six essentials of a good life, how might you practice them?

- Consider studying a physical art like dance or yoga, learning how to cook, exploring dream work, developing a healthy social life, finding meaningful and engaging work, and cultivating an *äsis* practice.

- Allow your formal practice to support your informal practice.

- Trust the truth of your inner experience.

CHAPTER 28

Renewable Pleasure for a Sustainable World

▲ 7. The Law of Renewable Pleasure

> *Because we all share this planet earth,*
> *we have to learn to live in harmony and peace*
> *with each other and with nature.*
> *This is not just a dream,*
> *but a necessity.*
> —Dalai Lama XIV

IN THIS FINAL CHAPTER, WE'LL LOOK AT HOW UNDERSTANDING PLEASURE CAN HELP us solve the planetary crises that face us, and along the way, dispel a few more outdated myths. Geologically speaking, we have entered the brave new world of the Anthropocene, the epoch where human activity directly affects the earth's climate and environment.[1] Many biologists believe we are already in the throes of a sixth mass extinction that could wipe out 90 percent of all species living today.[2] When confronted with such huge problems as overpopulation, climate change, environmental pollution, and nuclear annihilation, it's easy to feel overwhelmed and sink into despair or turn away in denial. After all, what can I, as just one person, do? And what on earth does any of this have to do with feeling good? The answer is a lot, as the following story illustrates:

One dreary Chicago winter morning, I was waiting for a local commuter bus at the Lincoln Park stop. The muffled sound of cars plowing through furrows of thick, gray slush from the previous night's snowfall softened the hard, urban edge. The air, the asphalt, the buildings, even the condensing breath of the commuters bundled in their thick jackets and scarves were heavy with grayness. I was halfway through my first year of medical school, and the workload was getting to me. The novelty had given way to endless days of lectures and cramming lists of facts. I was pitying my grim fate when the bus heaved to a stop and the folding doors opened with a pneumatic blast.

Ernie, a heavyset black bus driver, greeted me, as he did everyone, with a broad smile and a rich, baritone drawl, "Welcome to the Happy Bus! Come on in and take a ride. You're looking mighty fine this glorious morning!" Refusing to be bowed by the banality of his job or the bleak weather, he brightened everyone's day with his light banter and infectious laugh and roused me from my self-pity. He was conducting his own mobile ministry, preaching the gospel of joy for no other reason than to celebrate the extraordinary miracle of being alive. Ernie was *en-thused* (filled with God), a beacon of possibility in an expressive wasteland. My father used to say, "Some men are sources of light; others shine in their reflection." Ernie was certainly a source. He understood one of the deep secrets of renewable pleasure: *The surest way to get love is to give love.* Renewable pleasure is the pleasure we freely give to one another and is what makes us uniquely human in the best sense of the word. And as we shall see, renewable pleasure holds a critical key to our collective survival.

Technology can't save us from ourselves

Because we are the cause of our current predicament, it requires a distinctly human solution. Unfortunately, we are in denial of this simple truth. Like a sick person looking for a new drug to ease their symptoms and avoid having to change how they live, we are focused on discovering the next technological breakthrough so we can go on living as usual, but a bit "greener." Making it through the narrowing evolutionary bottleneck is going to take a lot more than quantum computing, gene splicing, and putting out the recycle bin once a week.

We have a perverse proclivity to use our mad genius for good and for ill. We can light a city with a nuclear reactor and destroy it with a thermonuclear bomb. We have eliminated the scourge of small pox and weaponize super viruses. We invent software and corrupt it with malware. We create the World Wide Web and use it to commit crimes. Technology can't save us from ourselves. If we don't radically transform our human heart and the way we live together on the planet, the Anthropocene will likely be one of the shortest "scenes" in the geological record.

The threats that face us are the symptoms of a much deeper problem, and it's not overpopulation. If it were simply a matter of population, all 7 billion of us could stand shoulder to shoulder within the 500 square miles of Los Angeles or fit more comfortably in an area the size of Texas in an urban sprawl the density of New York City.[3]

The problem is not how many of us there are, but how *much* each one of us wants and *what* we want. *The problem is our voracious appetite!* In 2015, global human consumption required the resources of 1.7 earths (on a renewable basis). Yet, only a small proportion of the human population overconsumes. The richest 20 percent of households account for three-quarters of the world's income and consume nearly 80 percent of the natural resources.[4] To put this in perspective, 80 percent of the world's population lives on less than $10 a day, and half (three billion people) lives on less than $2.50 a day.[5] As a result, a staggering 30,000 to 60,000 people die each and every day from hunger alone.[6]

While the standard of living for humanity as a whole has increased dramatically—even the wealthiest kings of old could not travel faster than a horse or call someone on a cell phone—very little has changed on a relative basis. A small privileged elite continues to consume the lion's share, supported by vast legions of Third World wage-serfs in what amounts to a kind of global neofeudalism. Even billionaires (the 0.1 percent) are beginning to talk about the evils of wealth disparity, not out of guilt but for fear of peasants storming the gates of their mansions.[7] It's already happening on an international scale, as throngs of desperate immigrants risk the dangerous passage north across the Mediterranean Sea and through Central America to enter the First World.

Who are the privileged elites of the world? They are us. According to a 2018 Credit Suisse report, if you have a net worth of $100,000 (investments, home, and car, minus debts), then you are among the wealthiest 10 percent of people on the planet. A net worth of $900,000 will place you in the top 1 percent (who own 47 percent of all household wealth).[8] Of course, you may not feel exceptionally wealthy in comparison (and contrast) to your neighbors, but that's because nearly one out of three Americans are members of the richest 10 percent, more than any other nation. This is significant because if every person on the planet consumed as much as an average American, it would require the resources of four earths.[9]

Yet, despite the glaring inequity between the rich and the poor, at the first Earth Summit in Rio de Janeiro in 1992, President H. W. Bush declared, "The American way of life is non-negotiable,"[10] a sentiment Barack Obama reaffirmed seventeen years later during his inaugural address: "We will not apologize for our way of life, nor waiver in its defense."[11] Translation: "We will consume as much as we want, and no one can stop us."

But what if we could enjoy the benefits of a modest First World life with plentiful food, clean water, shelter, security, health care, education, and community without the waste of overconsumption and the toxic anxiety of fear? What if we could have our cake and eat it too, sustainably? At a personal level, it comes down to this: Would you be willing to "live simply so that others may simply live," as Mahatma Gandhi put it?[12] Moral twinges aside, if your goal is to truly enjoy an *aah*some life, then the answer is a resounding *yes*! Living a simple Epicurean life is by far the more pleasing choice, especially when you factor in the tremendous value of renewable pleasure.

▲ The Law of Renewable Pleasure

Renewable pleasure encompasses several meanings, from the simple to the simply profound. As a general concept, it gives us a way to think about pleasure objectively, free of cultural bias, as we would any other natural resource. Seen from this perspective through the lens of the Pleasure Prism, *pleasure is an essential resource as vital to our health and well-being as fresh air and clean water.*

We encountered a simplified version of renewable pleasure in Chapter 15. Recall that authentic pleasures have a robust cycle of active, passive, and neutral pleasure that naturally engages us at multiple levels (physical, emotional, mental, and *āsis*), require minimal equipment, and provide enjoyment proportional to the personal effort expended. From here, it is but a small step to consider the ecological footprint of the pleasures we enjoy—the amount of the earth's surface required to supply the resources and dispose of the waste in a sustainable way. For example, walking on the beach is a high-quality, authentic pleasure that leaves a small ecological footprint and is eminently renewable, but if you have to fly a thousand miles to get there, it is much less so. Assessing the ecological footprint of the pleasures we enjoy is a useful way of thinking about renewable pleasure.

As a natural resource, we can ask: Where is renewable pleasure found? What is its intrinsic value? Who should control access and distribution? And most importantly, how can it be best used to benefit humanity? We will approach these questions from the indigenous wisdom tradition of the forest people as expressed by Native American faith keeper Oren Lyons, "You must not think of yourself or your family, not even of your generation ... make your decisions on behalf of the seven generations coming, so that they may enjoy what you have today."[13] As a link in the sacred chain of being, each of us bears the weight of responsibility of the generations who came before and of those who will follow. This brings us to renewable pleasure in the profound sense.

Where is the highest quality renewable pleasure found? Within the human heart.

Renewable pleasure is unique as a natural resource because we are the source of it. Each one of us is a potential wellspring of pleasure for ourselves and one another: through the offering of our body we give physical pleasure; through the offering of our care we give love; through the offering of our interest, we bestow meaning and purpose; and through the offering of our gratitude and magnanimity, we ennoble the human spirit. Since we ourselves are the source of these pleasures, they are abundantly renewable. And as Ernie the bus driver so ably demonstrated, the more pleasure we share, the more we have. Just as wind creates more wind and solar fusion generates more fusion, pleasure begets itself. Joy and happiness, meaning and purpose are infectious, which is why we like to be around such people. An unlimited supply of renewable pleasure is potentially available to us all.

What is its intrinsic value? Immeasurable.

At the end of our life, it is not how much money we've made, the places we've been, or the material possessions we've amassed that matters. What matters the most and touches us most deeply are the caring relationships we have shared. Consider how much of your striving to succeed is motivated by the belief that material success is necessary to attract the love and acceptance you long for. There's a reason. As herd animals, the good life *(eudaimonia)* is good only in and through relationship with others. It's been said, "Everything is love or a cry for love." Indeed, it is through Love that we perfect ourselves and experience our greatest fulfillment. Ultimately, human-sourced, renewable pleasure is the highest quality pleasure we seek.

If this makes sense to you, then you might be wondering, if we are the source of renewable pleasure and it's something we all need, why don't we just give it to one another?[14] What's stopping us? Which raises the last two questions.

Who should control access and distribution? All of us.

Like fresh air and clean water, renewable pleasure is part of the human commons. The freedom to seek pleasure and to give pleasure is entirely natural and among the inalienable human rights memorialized in the Declaration of Independence as "the pursuit of happiness." But here's where things get radical in the original Latin sense of the word (*radix*, meaning "root," "fundamental"). If we were to exchange pleasure freely among ourselves, it would threaten the power structure of the matrix. Why, if love were free, we might put a flower in our hair and beat our swords into ploughshares. After all, why go off to war, exploit others, or work ourselves to the bone to get ahead if we already have everything we need? We might "turn on, tune in, and drop out,"[15] as the notorious apostle of the New Age, Timothy Leary, urged a crowd of 30,000 hippies in San Francisco's Golden Gate Park to do in 1967. Leary was a flawed messenger, but as a combatant in the war on consciousness, his message has merit: *turn on* your awareness, wake up to the miracle of the reality that surrounds you (and turn off the numbing 24/7 media feed); *tune in* to your deep inner wisdom and authentically engage the world; and *drop out* of the cradle-to-grave expectations of the matrix and express yourself fearlessly and creatively. The war on consciousness to control the pleasure narrative and human behavior has been going on for millennia. The only difference now is we're running out of natural resources and are therefore running out of time.

How can renewable pleasure best be used to benefit humanity? To bring us together as one family—one species with a common origin, aspiration, and destiny.

There's an ancient Chinese parable about a group of well-dressed people sitting at a round table with a sumptuous assortment of delicacies arranged in the center. The table is so large that they must use extra-long chopsticks to reach the food. After plucking a delicious morsel, however, they discover their arms aren't long enough to place the food in their own mouths. They are in Hell. Heaven is when they learn to feed each other.

As this story suggests, *the way to control the human appetite is to satisfy it, and the only thing that can truly satisfy it is high-quality renewable pleasure*—the very thing we all yearn for.

For the first time in history, we possess the technology to provide for the basic physical needs of every human being on the planet. We have the ability to create heaven on earth *materially*, but to do so, we must first create peace on earth *spiritually*. This will require the wisdom and political will to feed each other the love, kindness, belonging, and respect we all deserve and need to thrive.

The obstacle of fear

The only thing stopping us is fear. You may recall that Epicurus came to the same conclusion and identified fear of death and fear of the gods as the greatest sources of anxiety (Chapter 5). We have seen how fear causes us to contract against the life-stream and withdraw into an ego-walled fortress of dualistic judgments, cutting us off from the Garden and causing us to feel alienated and alone, to distrust and lock our doors and our hearts. Indeed, *fear is the root cause of crime, deceit, jealousy, greed, exploitation, and war.* Because our political, economic, legal, and military institutions are based on fear, they perpetuate, with Orwellian logic, the very problems they would solve.

Of course, it is natural to be fearful if you don't know where your next meal is coming from and a cloud of dust on the horizon could be an advancing band of marauders. But if you are fortunate enough to be a ten-percenter living in the midst of plenty and still fear you haven't enough money, that's as pitiable as a millionaire who feels poor in the company of billionaires. Clinging to a fear-centric operating system is not only inappropriate, it is sickening. The fear of insufficiency and inadequacy—that there is not enough, that we are not enough, that this moment is not enough—prevents us from truly enjoying the bounty of our good fortune. It drives the kind of toxic greed and malignant overconsumption that is destroying us and our planet. Like a snake that swallows its own tail, we have become consumers consumed by our own desire, where the more we have, the more we want, the more we spend.

Psychologist Abraham Maslow observed that there is a hierarchy of need and once our basic survival and safety are secured, we long for love and belonging, esteem, and self-actualization (the higher frequencies of the Pleasure Prism). However, as mentioned earlier, the matrix has conditioned us to believe that to fulfill these higher biological needs, we must prove ourselves worthy through the acquisition of wealth and the trappings of "success." By this sleight of hand, our need for love, respect, and community has been hijacked by the fear of inadequacy and commoditized into the pursuit of empty (symbolic) pleasures. Driven by the need to fill our emotional emptiness, we accumulate ever more stuff (preferably well-known brand name stuff) to demonstrate our worthiness and status within the herd. But driving a Porsche doesn't make one a Porsche among men and wearing Prada high heels doesn't make one a Prada model after all. The true measure of your wealth is how much you'd be worth if you lost all your money.

We're told competition is innate in our human nature—an expression of natural selection and the survival of the fittest. That's why we flock to sporting events,[16] our elite universities select the most ambitious (aggressive) students, and talent rises to the top. It's just "the Law of the Jungle—as old and as true as the sky," as Kipling writes.[17] But this social Darwinist narrative turns out to be yet another myth created by the matrix to justify the status quo.

"Survival of the fittest" is a phrase philosopher Herbert Spencer coined after studying Darwin's theory of evolution, which Darwin later adopted. Darwin's understanding of fitness, however, was far more nuanced. In *The Descent of Man*, he tells us that a tribe whose members "were always ready to aid one another, and to sacrifice themselves for the common good, would be victorious over most other tribes; and this would be natural selection."[18] Although competition is a part of our human nature, it is a relatively small part. We are, after all, social animals who live in close quarters and value sharing love and friendship. We have a natural capacity to care for one another. As human beings, we possess a range of behaviors from the most sublime to the most despicable. Which aspect of our character is brought forth, as Aristotle noted, depends on the ethical training we receive from the society in which we live. In other words, much of the fear we experience in our competition for "scarce" resources is self-engineered.

Our true identity

Evolution is driven by cooperation far more than by competition. We see this in the microbial world where different bacterial strains freely exchange genetic information, join forces in biofilms and colonies, and merge into each other to form the mitochondria and other key structures of the first eukaryotic cells. As evolutionary biologist Lynn Margulis has argued, complex organisms like us are the result of billions of years of symbiotic microbial evolution.[19] In fact, humans have recently been reclassified as a superorganism because there is ten times more bacterial DNA in and on our body than there is human DNA.[20] We are like a coral reef, a human and microbe cooperative, working together for the benefit of the collective. Distinguishing where we end and our microbiome begins is no longer meaningful or relevant. The same can be said for the air we breathe, the water we drink, the soil we farm, the oceans we fish, and the forests we cut. "No man is an island, Entire of itself,"[21] as John Donne put it. To care for the biosphere is to care for ourselves.

Our true identity is that we don't have one! Our very existence depends on one another as surely as a bee depends on the hive or an ant on the colony, and this dependency holds at every scale of our existence. In the words of the Buddha, "This arises, that becomes." You can't have this without that. Everything is interconnected—nothing is separate, nothing stands alone.[22] At its core, the emptiness of *sunyata* is the nonexistence of an individual self. To be precise, we are not even a thing but an activity, a whirlpool in a river of consciousness that spins for some 75 to 90 years and then vanishes.

In a world with hydrogen bombs that can wipe out all of human life in a nuclear winter, an Ebola virus that can travel from Kinshasa to London in a few hours, and pollution that can be carried in the ocean currents and jet stream, the notion of political boundaries and the us-against-them way of thinking is passé. If we do not evolve to our next incarnation of *Homo spiritualis*, we will go extinct like the other 99 percent of species that once existed on the planet. And make no mistake about it, there is no get-out-of-jail-for-free card for any of us. If the science of ecology has taught us anything, it is that all of life is inextricably linked. We are all in this together, rich and poor alike.

Yet, it is precisely because we lack an independent self that our personal actions are so powerful. As a holon—a semi-autonomous cell within the body politic—how you live your life is both *the problem* and *the solution*. Remember, in a holarchy, a change at one dimension is a change at every dimension. Just as your pleasure habits largely determine your personal health, when multiplied billions of times over, how we collectively seek pleasure determines the health of our species and biosphere. We create the world for each other. *By learning how to authentically and renewably enjoy yourself, you are, in a very real and powerful way, doing your part to save the world.* Welcome to the Happy Bus.

Renewable Pleasure for All

Imagine, for a moment, what life would be like if we learned to cultivate, refine, and distribute renewable pleasure freely throughout society. Imagine if we were raised feeling valued and loved instead of inadequate and fearful. Imagine if we didn't have to impress others to be accepted.

Growing up with love, we would know better how to value and care for each other, which would generate a virtuous cycle of renewable pleasure for everyone. The mindless consumerism, overeating, overdrinking, drugging, and media consumption we use to dull the pain of our dissatisfaction would lessen, giving us more time and energy to do the things that actually nurture us and the people we love. Imagine if human relationships were valued more than material gain and if the Gross National Happiness was deemed more important than the Gross Domestic Product. Imagine if all our decisions and national policy were made in the best interest of children, all the children of the world and the seven generations to come. Imagine if people were enlisted in armies to construct rather than destruct.

We could task our social scientists, anthropologists, and psychologists to research the best practices of human relationship, and then with our artists and educators, undertake pilot projects in experimental schools and communities to develop them. Once perfected, we could disseminate these practices throughout society. This is not some naïve, utopian vision. It is our only real choice: we can choose fear and go extinct, or we can choose Love and thrive.

▲▲▲▲▲▲▲

I have a special relationship with a place I call meditation rock that, for many years, I have been going to for inspiration. It sits on one shoulder of a massive granite notch above Boulder, where you can look east across the Great Plains to the horizon, west to the snow-covered Continental Divide, and north and south along the Front Range almost to Wyoming.

In the notch, an old ponderosa pine has made a difficult home. The trunk is perfectly straight, but where it rises above the notch, it bends and twists in a graceful *pas de trois* with the sunlight and the wind like a giant *bonsai* tree. Some limbs as big around as my thigh have broken off. I imagine that when the limb no longer served the needs of the tree, the tree withdrew its sap, causing the branch to become brittle and snap off—a sacrifice for the greater whole. In the same way, when a person or a species no longer serves a useful function, its energy is withdrawn and it breaks off from the tree of life.

One day, sitting on my stone perch, I witnessed a most courageous display of desire and surrender. At first, it looked like a small leaf about the size of a silver dollar strangely suspended in a light breeze. Then it began to slowly move forward directly into the wind, and I realized it was a small moth determined to fly through the notch. I watched in amazement as the free edge of its wings fluttered, surrendering to the breeze, slipping through the tiny micro-eddies of turbulence like a salmon swimming upstream. If you've ever tried to swim against the stream, you know how incredibly difficult it is.

Sometimes I feel like that small moth buffeted in a cultural wind of fear, greed, and ignorance. But if I remain in touch with my true intentions and stay present, I can align myself in the turbulence and humbly move forward. I can feel pessimistic about what is likely to happen and at the same time be optimistic about what is possible.

We are standing together, you and I, on the razor's edge of an evolutionary Pleasure-Pain Threshold. It is exhilarating and terrifying. The potential to create heaven and the potential to create hell have never been closer. It's up to us how we choose to relate to each other. The way forward, I suggest, is to step back from the brink toward the sweet spot and awaken from the suicidal matrix that we have collectively dreamed into existence. It is time to reclaim our human dignity. It is time to reclaim our birthright of renewable pleasure. It is time to fulfill our evolutionary destiny for the benefit of our children, ourselves, and the world.

May the Pure Light
within you
Guide your way home.

Afterword

As you view the world through your new "prism" glasses, you may notice things appear more vivid. You may find yourself delighting in simple activities, smiling more easily, and enjoying a refreshing sense of lightness. You are becoming coherent, and this is what it feels like to source renewable pleasure. And as you share your good feelings with others, your inner light will radiate in ever-widening circles, creating a resonant field that ignites and attracts the light of others.

Awakening from the matrix doesn't happen overnight. It is not an event but a process. To help you deepen and embody what you are learning, please visit my website at jiagottliebmd.com where you will find: a companion *aah ... The Pleasure Workbook*; a quiz to assess your PQ (Pleasure Quotient); information about workshops and events; and an "Ask Dr. Jia" link to answer your questions.

As a book lives in the hands of those who read it, please share *aah ... The Pleasure Book* with your family, gift a copy to a friend, and tell your social media tribe. Together, with your help, we can gather a community of like-minded individuals to radically change how we inhabit our precious planet for the benefit of all.

See you at jiagottliebmd.com

APPENDIX

The Amadeus Equation

BERTRAND RUSSELL CONSIDERED MATHEMATICS TO BE ONE OF THE HIGHEST FORMS of poetry because, like a poem, a mathematical equation communicates meaning in the sparest terms and must be read slowly. I offer the Amadeus Equation as a kind of haiku to describe the essential physics of pleasure:

$$P = \frac{\Delta I}{\Delta T} \times \frac{1}{|D-S|}$$

where P is pleasure, ΔI is the change in sensual intensity, ΔT is the time duration, D is desire, S is surrender, and the value of I is in the pleasant range of the Sensual Continuum (below the Pleasure-Pain Threshold).

The first term ($\Delta I / \Delta T$) indicates that a big change in intensity over a short period of time can yield a lot of pleasure, as for example the rush of a rapid shift of consciousness. Conversely, when the intensity increases gradually over a long period of time (slow pleasure), the quantity $\Delta I / \Delta T$ is small and may be easily overlooked as in the case of neutral pleasure.

The second term requires a little more unpacking. As desire and surrender come into balance, D – S approaches zero and the term, $1/|D-S|$ (read 1 over the absolute value of desire minus surrender), expands to infinity and becomes a zero-larity—the Big Nothing that contains everything discussed in Chapter 17.

Thus, even a low intensity pleasure ($\Delta I / \Delta T$ just above zero), when approached with balanced desire and surrender, can deliver a huge amount of pleasure because the product of a small number multiplied by an infinite number is also infinite. This was the secret of Epicurus's *ataraxia* (equanimity).

The same, of course, holds true with high-intensity pleasure, when $\Delta I / \Delta T$ is large, as in the case of extreme active and passive pleasures. In other words, whenever desire and surrender come into balance, the three gateways to Paradise (ecstasy, equanimity, and bliss) swing open, the small self is blown away, and only the Big Self remains to revel in the Garden. In this way, the Amadeus Equation can serve as a handy algorithm for an *aah*some life.

Acknowledgments

This book could not have been written without the help of many people—especially my mother and father, who did the hard work of raising an immigrant family, and my older brother George, Annapolis graduate and truth seeker, who broke trail and pointed me in the right direction early in life. Though they are no longer with us, their contribution is very much alive in these pages.

Many thanks to Lee Thomas and the Writers Without Borders in Chiang Mai, Thailand, for providing a safe cove at a critical stage in my writing. To my editor, Jennifer Phelps, I owe special gratitude for her keen insights and gentle guidance in bringing the manuscript to a finished form. I was most fortunate to work with Kersti Frigell, whose illustrations and artistic direction, along with Amy Clay's original art, and Sue Campbell's elegant book design expressed visually what I struggled to say in words.

The enthusiastic support of my friends has been a perpetual source of encouragement. I am especially grateful to Sina Simantob for sheltering me in my time of brokenness, to Mark Mitchell for his creative brilliance, and to Lorraine Moller for her unpretentious greatness. I wish to thank Robyn Lawrence for her helpful writing advice, Doug Dupler for his careful proofreading, and Magdalena Rzyska for her generosity of spirit and unflagging kindness.

I have tried to be accurate in my accounts but respect that others may have a different experience and interpretation of events. My intention is to express my truth, not to offend. While I supplied the writing effort and am responsible for any shortcomings, the wisdom was imbibed from the Pierian springs, and I bow deeply with humble gratitude to all my guides, all my mentors, and all my helpers for leading me to its sacred waters.

Chapter Notes

Chapter 1 Why Pleasure

1. To learn more about the World Happiness Scale or Cantril Scale, see http://news.gallup.com/poll/122453/Understanding-Gallup-Uses-Cantril-Scale.aspx?utm_source=link_newsv9&utm_campaign=item_206468&utm_medium=copy.
2. Martin E. P. Seligman, "Happiness is Not Enough," *Flourish: A New Theory of Positive Psychology*, University of Pennsylvania, April 2011, https://www.authentichappiness.sas.upenn.edu/newsletters/flourishnewsletters/newtheory
3. E.S. Ford, M.M. Bergmann, J. Kröger, A. Schienkiewitz, C. Weikert, and H. Boeing, "Healthy Living is the Best Revenge: Findings from the European Prospective Investigation Into Cancer and Nutrition-Potsdam Study," *Archives of Internal Medicine* 169, no. 15 (Aug 2009): 1355-62, https://jamanetwork.com/journals/jamainternalmedicine/fullarticle/1108507.
4. In an actual prism, red bends the least and blue the most, which is reversed in our model for heuristic purposes.
5. Alexander Pope, "A Little Learning," https://www.poetsgraves.co.uk/Classic%20Poems/Pope/a_little_learning.htm.

Chapter 2 Welcome to the Pleasure Matrix

1. Emily Pronin, quoted in Graham Lawton, "The Grand Delusion: Blind to Bias," NewScientist, May 11, 2011, https://www.newscientist.com/article/mg21028122-200-the-grand-delusion-blind-to-bias/.
2. To read more about the cognitive bias codex, see https://commons.wikimedia.org/wiki/File:Cognitive_bias_codex_en.svg.
3. The early Hebrews were also polytheists. It was only after the Babylonian captivity in the sixth century BCE—when they came into contact with Zoroastrians who believed in one god (Ahura Mazda) above all others—that monotheism entered Jewish theology.
4. Genesis 1.26-27
5. G. Ballard, "Chief Seattle," *California Indian Education*, http://www.californiaindianeducation.org/famous_indian_chiefs/chief_seattle/

Chapter 3 The Origin of Original Sin

1. To read more about Clarence Darrow, see https://en.wikiquote.org/wiki/Clarence_Darrow.
2. Augustine, *Confessions*, 2nd edition, trans. F.J. Sheed, ed. Michael P. Foley (Indianapolis: Hackett Publishing, 2006), 37.
3. Augustine, Confessions, 152.
4. Romans 13:13-14

5. *The Confessions of Saint Augustine*, Book VIII, Paragraphs 28 and 29 as quoted in "Augustine of Hippo," https://en.wikipedia.org/wiki/Augustine_of_Hippo.
6. Augustine, *The Anti-Pelagian Writings of St. Augustine of Hippo*, trans. Benjamin B. Warfield, Robert Ernest Wallis, and Peter Holmes (Charleston: Createspace, 2019), 317.
7. Ed Rehmus, "The Cream of Christ," *The Ecphorizer*, 54, (February 1996), https://www.ecphorizer.com/EPS/site_page.php?issue=75&page=1148.
8. Romans 7:19.
9. Phyllis Chesler, "Why are Jihadis so Obsessed With Porn?" *New York Post*, February 17, 2015, https://nypost.com/2015/02/17/why-are-jihadis-so-obsessed-with-porn/; Bahar Gholipour, "Religious People Say They Don't Watch Porn. Internet Data Says Otherwise," *Huffington Post*, July 6, 2016, https://www.huffpost.com/entry/research-porn-religion-study_n_577d1bc6e4b09b4c43c1bfbe; David J. Ley, "Porn vs. Religion," *Psychology Today*, June 8, 2016, https://www.psychologytoday.com/us/blog/women-who-stray/201606/porn-vs-religion.

Chapter 4 the Ethics of Pleasure

1. Although this quote is often attributed to Aristotle, it is actually philosopher Will Durant's summary of Aristotle's words. See https://www.brainyquote.com/quotes/will_durant_145967.
2. For more quotes from Marcus Tullius Cicero, see https://allauthor.com/quotes/124591/./
3. Aristotle, *Nicomachean Ethics*, trans. W.D. Ross, Book 1/Section 7, http://classics.mit.edu/Aristotle/nicomachaen.1.i.html.
4. Aristotle, *Nicomachean Ethics*, quoted in Greek Texts & Translations, http://perseus.uchicago.edu/perseus-cgi/citequery3.pl?dbname=GreekFeb2011&getid=1&query=Arist.%20Eth.%20Nic.%201098a.

Chapter 5 An Epicurean Conspiracy

1. Epicurus, *Selected Fragments #221*, trans. Peter Saint-Andre, June 4, 2013, http://monadnock.net/epicurus/fragments.html.
2. Epicurus, from *On Goals*, The Ethics of Epicurus (webpage), http://hume.ucdavis.edu/mattey/phi143/epieth.htm.
3. Epicurus quote. *On Goals*.
4. Epicurus, *Letter to Menoikos* 127, trans. Peter Saint-Andre, November 21, 2011, http://monadnock.net/epicurus/letter.html
5. Epicurus, Menoeceus 131-132, EpicurusWiki, June 11, 2008, http://wiki.epicurism.info/Menoeceus_131-132/.
6. Epicurus, Menoeceus 131-132.
7. Epicurus, Menoeceus 127-128, EpicurusWiki, June 9, 2008, http://wiki.epicurism.info/Menoeceus_127-128/.

8. Epicurus, *On Goals* 1.37-38, in *The Epicurus Reader: Selected Writings and Testimonia*, trans. and ed. Brad Inwood and Lloyd P. Gerson (Indianapolis: Hackett Publishing, 1994), 60.

9. For more Laozi quotes, see https://www.brainyquote.com/quotes/lao_tzu_393061.

10. Epicurus, *Letter to Menoeceus* 124-25, in *The Epicurus Reader: Selected Writings and Testimonia*, trans. and ed. Brad Inwood and Lloyd P. Gerson (Indianapolis: Hackett Publishing, 1994), 29.

11. This quote is based on the "Vatican Collection of Epicurean Sayings #14," in *Hellenistic Philosophy*, 2nd edition, trans. and ed. Brad Inwood and Lloyd P. Gerson (Indianapolis: Hackett Publishing, 1997), 36.

12. See https://www.goodreads.com/quotes/8199-is-god-willing-to-prevent-evil-but-not-able-then.

13. Epicurus, *Letter to Menoikos* 123, trans. Peter Saint-Andre, November 21, 2011, http://monadnock.net/epicurus/letter.html

14. The indeterminacy of atoms, Epicurus argued, was the basis for free will. See Maureen Corrigan, "'The Swerve': Ideas that Rooted the Renaissance," *Fresh Air*, NPR, September 20, 2011, http://www.npr.org/2011/09/20/140463632/the-swerve-ideas-that-rooted-the-renaissance.

15. Jeremy Bentham, "A Fragment on Government," 2nd para., *Constitution Society*, https://www.constitution.org/jb/frag_gov.htm.

16. From Thomas Jefferson's letter to his private secretary William Short in 1819. See http://www.csun.edu/~hcfll004/jefflet.html.

17. To read Jefferson's 1810 letter to William Baldwin, see https://founders.archives.gov/documents/Jefferson/03-02-02-0124-0002#D26338ID2.

18. To read Jefferson's 1814 letter to Horatio Spafford, see https://founders.archives.gov/documents/Jefferson/03-07-02-0167.

19. To read Jefferson's 1810 letter to Samuel Kercheval Monticello, see http://www.let.rug.nl/usa/presidents/thomas-jefferson/letters-of-thomas-jefferson/jefl199.php.

20. United States Conference of Catholic Bishops, *The Nature and Scope of Sexual Abuse of Minors by Catholic Priests and Deacons in the United States 1950-2002*, February 2004, http://www.usccb.org/issues-and-action/child-and-youth-protection/upload/The-Nature-and-Scope-of-Sexual-Abuse-of-Minors-by-Catholic-Priests-and-Deacons-in-the-United-States-1950-2002.pdf.

21. Mary Louise Kelly, "What Allows Sex Abuse to Proliferate Within the Catholic Church," *All Things Considered*, NPR, August 16, 2018, https://www.npr.org/2018/08/16/639371736/what-allows-sex-abuse-to-proliferate-within-the-catholic-church

Chapter 6 The Anatomy of Pleasure

1. Charles E. Moan and Robert G. Heath, "Septal Stimulation for the Initiation of Heterosexual Behavior in a Homosexual Male," *Journal of Behavioral Therapy and Experimental Psychiatry* 3, no. 1 (March 1972): 23-30.

2. Paul D. MacLean, *The Triune Brain in Evolution* (New York: Plenum Press, 1990), 23.

3 MacLean, *The Triune Brain*, 23.

Chapter 7 Your Sphinx Brain

1. For more quotes from Archilochus, see https://www.goodreads.com/quotes/387614-we-don-t-rise-to-the-level-of-our-expectations-we.
2. For a wonderful discussion on habit, see William James, The Principles of Psychology (New York: Henry Holt and Company, 1890), http://psychclassics.yorku.ca/James/Principles/prin4.htm.
3. Nikhil Swaminathan, "Girl Talk: Are Women Really Better at Language?" *Scientific American*, March 5, 2008, http://www.scientificamerican.com/article/are-women-really-better-with-language/.
4. Jeff Thompson, "Is Nonverbal Communication a Numbers Game?" *Psychology Today*, September 30, 2011, https://www.psychologytoday.com/us/blog/beyond-words/201109/is-nonverbal-communication-numbers-game.

Chapter 8 The Pleasure Prism and Light-body

1. For more quotes from William Wordsworth, see https://www.azquotes.com/quote/435808.
2. Viktor E. Frankl, *Man's Search for Meaning* (Boston: Beacon Press, 1959).

Chapter 9 Real Compared to What

1. Anaïs Nin, *Seduction of the Minotaur* (Chicago: The Swallow Press, 1961), 124.
2. Rhett Herman, "How Fast is the Earth Moving?" *Scientific American*, October 26, 1998, http://www.scientificamerican.com/article.cfm?id=how-fast-is-the-earth-mov.
3. Federico Rios, "Coming of Age in the Amazon Jungle," Matador Network, https://matadornetwork.com/read/coming-age-amazon-jungle/.
4. Nikos Kazantzakis, *Zorba the Greek* (New York: Simon & Schuster, 1952), 65.
5. Kazantzakis, *Zorba the Greek*, 35.

Chapter 10, 11 (no notes)

Chapter 12 Go with the Flow

1. *Misogi* is not to be done lightly. It is best to approach such levels of intensity with an attitude of sacred humility. One New Year's day in Lake Tahoe, I had gone a little too far, and as I waded back to shore my leg muscles began to grow heavy and unresponsive, which could have turned into a serious problem.
2. William Blake, "Eternity," *Poets.org*, https://www.poets.org/poetsorg/poem/eternity.
3. One of the most reliable ways to grow and increase your Pleasure Capacity is to keep your heart open in the midst of emotional pain.

Chapter 13 The Evolution of Desire

1. For more quotes from Lord Acton, see https://acton.org/research/lord-acton-quote-archive.
2. This quote has been attributed to several Greek writers; see https://en.wikiquote.org/wiki/Euripides#Misattributed.
3. Elaine Pagels, *The Gnostic Gospels* (New York: Vintage Books, 1979), pp. xiii-xxiii. See http://gnosis.org/naghamm/Pagels-Gnostic-Gospels.html.
4. Martin Luther King Jr., "Letter from a Birmingham Jail [King, Jr.]," African Studies Center, University of Pennsylvania, https://www.africa.upenn.edu/Articles_Gen/Letter_Birmingham.html.
5. Daniel Kahneman and Angus Deaton, "High Income Improves Evaluation of Life but Not Emotional Well-Being," *PNAS* 107, no. 38 (September 21, 2010): 16489-16493, https://www.princeton.edu/~deaton/downloads/deaton_kahneman_high_income_improves_evaluation_August2010.pdf.
6. Zameena Mejia, "Billionaire Warren Buffett: Doubling Your Net Worth Won't Make You Happier," *CNBC*, February 27, 2018, https://www.cnbc.com/2018/02/27/warren-buffett-doubling-your-net-worth-wont-make-you-happier.html.
7. See https://www.brainyquote.com/quotes/epicurus_119455.
8. See also Kim Bhasin, "15 Facts About Coca-Cola That Will Blow Your Mind," *Business Insider*, June 9, 2011, https://www.businessinsider.com/facts-about-coca-cola-2011-6#coca-cola-spends-more-money-on-advertising-than-microsoft-and-apple-combined-11.
9. Office on Smoking and Health, "Economic Trends in Tobacco," Centers for Disease Control and Prevention, July 23, 2019, http://www.cdc.gov/tobacco/data_statistics/fact_sheets/economics/econ_facts/.
10. Epicurus, *Letter to Menoikos* 123, trans. Peter Saint-Andre, November 21, 2011, http://monadnock.net/epicurus/letter.html.
11. Epicurus, "Vatican saying 45," Society of Friends of Epicurus, November 24, 2018, http://societyofepicurus.com/vatican-sayings-brief-study-guide/.

Chapter 14 Supersize Me

1. Mihaly Csikszentmihalyi, *Flow: The Psychology of Optimal Experience* (New York: HarperCollins, 1990), 17.
2. Jake Christensen, "This History of the Big Gulp," *Iowa State Daily*, February 24, 2015, http://www.iowastatedaily.com/dct/the-history-of-the-big-gulp/article_8b67a7de-bbb2-11e4-ad36-c7d887961666.html.
3. "What Goes Up Must Come Down: A Brief History of the Codpiece," University of Cambridge, Research, April 30, 2015, https://www.cam.ac.uk/research/features/what-goes-up-must-come-down-a-brief-history-of-the-codpiece.
4. "US Plastic Surgery Statistics: Chins, Buttocks and Breasts Up, Ears Down," *The Guardian*, Datablog, http://www.guardian.co.uk/news/datablog/2011/jul/22/plastic-surgery-medicine.

5 Keiper Lauren, "Best Face Forward: Chin Implants Surge in Popularity," *Reuters*, May 3, 2012, https://www.reuters.com/article/chinimplants/best-face-forward-chin-implants-surge-in-popularity-idUSL4E8G18JS20120503.

6 Coco Khan, "Skin-Lightening Creams are Dangerous—Yet Business is Booming. Can the Trade Be Stopped?" *The Guardian*, April 23, 2018, https://www.theguardian.com/world/2018/apr/23/skin-lightening-creams-are-dangerous-yet-business-is-booming-can-the-trade-be-stopped.

7 Jill Viglione, Lance Hannon, and Robert DeFina, "The Impact of Light Skin on Prison Time for Black Female Offenders," *The Social Science Journal* 48, no. 1 (January 2011): 250-258, https://www.sciencedirect.com/science/article/abs/pii/S0362331910000923.

8 Katie Richards, "Study: Ad Industry Accounted for 19 Percent of U.S. GDP in 2014," *AdWeek* 4, November 17, 2015, https://www.adweek.com/brand-marketing/study-ad-industry-contributed-nearly-20-percent-toward-us-gdp-2014-168164/.

Chapter 15 The Pleasure Cycle

1 Epicurus, Menoeceus 128-130, EpicurusWiki, June 11, 2008, http://wiki.epicurism.info/Menoeceus_128-130/.

2 Ambrose Bierce, *The Devil's Dictionary* (eBook), July 26, 2008, https://www.gutenberg.org/files/972/972-h/972-h.htm.

3 Alan Watts, "Future of Communications," *The Library*, https://www.organism.earth/library/document/121. (Humans try to opt out of the eating society by making themselves thoroughly inedible through embalming.)

4 Coca-Cola was originally sold as a patent medicine in 1886 containing extracts of cocaine and kola nuts (caffeine) from which it got its name.

5 Henry Blodget, "Chart of the Day: American Per-Capita Sugar Consumption Hits 100 Pounds Per Year," *Business Insider*, February 19, 2012, https://www.businessinsider.com/chart-american-sugar-consumption-2012-2.

6 "San," Kruger National Park, Siyabona Africa, http://www.krugerpark.co.za/africa_bushmen.html.

7 To see what a natural human being is physically capable of, check out the extraordinary 1925 documentary *Grass*. https://www.fandor.com/films/grass

8 Julie McCarthy, "The Most Captivating Voice in the World," *All Things Considered*, NPR, March 17, 2007, https://www.npr.org/templates/story/story.php?storyId=8976813.

Chapter 16 Surrender: the Artless Art

1 Alfred Lord Tennyson, "Ulysses," Poetry Foundation, https://www.poetryfoundation.org/poems/45392/ulysses. Tennyson's line inspired the Outward Bound motto: "To serve, to strive, and not to yield."

2 Laozi, *Tao Te Ching*, Verse 78.

3   While this quote is often attributed to John Lennon from his song, "Beautiful Boy," it can be traced back even further. See https://quoteinvestigator.com/2012/05/06/other-plans/.

4   Dogen, Mystic Poets, https://onetruename.com/dogen.htm.

5   If you shine a light through two narrow slits onto a fluorescent screen detector, it registers a series of bright bands similar to two stones simultaneously dropped into a pond of water create an interference pattern of intersecting waves. But if you install a detector to observe which slit the individual photon passes through, the interference pattern is replaced by two bands as you would expect of tiny billiard balls. For more information, see "Physics in a Minute: The Double Slit Experiment," +*Plus Magazine*, February 5, 2017, https://plus.maths.org/content/physics-minute-double-slit-experiment-0.

6   For a short explanation of quantum field theory, see Fermilab, "Quantum Field Theory" (video), YouTube, January 14, 2016, https://www.youtube.com/watch?v=FBeALt3rxEA.

7   For more quotes from Ajahn Chah, see https://www.azquotes.com/quote/520561.

Chapter 17 Paradise Now

1   For the origin of this Aristotle quote, see https://en.wikiquote.org/wiki/Aristotle.

2   Nicholas of Cusa quoted in Martin Lings and Clinton Minnaar, eds., *The Underlying Religion: An Introduction to the Perennial Philosophy* (Bloomington, IN: World Wisdom, 2007), 189.

3   For more quotes from Niels Bohr, see https://www.goodreads.com/quotes/27461-there-are-trivial-truths-and-there-are-great-truths-the.

4   Additional Niels Bohr quotes can be found at https://www.goodreads.com/author/quotes/821936.Niels_Bohr.

5   Richard B. Clark, trans., "Seng-Ts'an: The Mind of Absolute Trust," http://www.selfdiscoveryportal.com/cmSengTsan.htm.

6   John Manoogian III, "Cognitive Bias Codex," *Wikimedia Commons*, April 12, 2017, https://commons.wikimedia.org/wiki/File:Cognitive_Bias_Codex_-_180%2B_biases,_designed_by_John_Manoogian_III_(jm3).jpg.

7   Tobias Danzig quoted in Dick Teresi, "Zero," *The Atlantic*, July 1997, https://www.theatlantic.com/magazine/archive/1997/07/zero/376900/.

8   Patanjali's Yoga Sutra, Chapter 2:46, https://www.ashtangayoga.info/philosophy/source-texts-and-mantra/yoga-sutra/chapter-2/.

9   The entire activity of the universe can be understood as a movement toward thermal equilibrium.

10 Matthew 18:3

Chapter 18 The 3 Gateways to Paradise

1   From "The Stranger Song" by Leonard Cohen, who I met once at a retreat as we had the same Zen teacher: Sasaki Roshi. *On Songs of Leonard Cohen* (New York: Columbia Studio E, 1967). See https://genius.com/Leonard-cohen-the-stranger-song-lyrics.

Chapter Notes

2. Static Eternal, "Kobe Bryant Explains 'Being in the Zone'" (video), YouTube, August 19, 2013, http://www.youtube.com/watch?v=wl49zc8g3DY.

3. In Japanese, *Ki-ai* means to harmonize (*ai*) the life-stream (*ki*), similar to the martial art Aikido "the way" (*do*) of harmonizing *ki*.

4. *Amrita* is another name for *soma*, the mysterious elixir that is praised with over a hundred hymns in the Rig Veda.

5. See this extraordinary video clip of an infant bathing: Le Bain de Sonia, "Thalasso Bain Bebe par Sonia Rochel" (video), YouTube, October 14, 2011, http://www.youtube.com/watch?v=OPSAgs-exfQ].

6. William Strauss and Neil Howe, *The Fourth Turning: An American Prophecy* (New York: Broadway Books, 1997), 50.

7. Epicurus, "Vatican Saying 69," *Vatican Sayings*, http://epicurus.net/en/vatican.html.

8. The kinesthetic nervous system is an ancient part of the nervous system that controls spatial awareness through a network of muscle, tendon, and joint stretch receptors.

Chapter 19 It's a Fractal Thing

1. Epicurus, *Selected Fragments* #182, trans. Peter Saint-Andre, June 4, 2013, http://monadnock.net/epicurus/fragments.html.

2. For more quotes from Li Po, see https://www.goodreads.com/author/quotes/4058.Li_Bai.

3. Angelus Silesius, "God, Whose Love and Joy Are Present Everywhere," *Poem Hunter.org*, July 23, 2016, https://www.poemhunter.com/poem/god-whose-love-and-joy-are-present-everywhere/.

4. This poem from Kabir, a 15th century Islamic, Indian Saint appears in Stephen Mitchell, ed., *The Enlightened Heart: An Anthology of Sacred Poetry* (New York: HarperCollins, 1993), 70.

Chapter 20 Make Relationship

1. Rebecca Lake, "How Long do Average U.S. Marriages Last?" *The Balance*, June 24, 2019, https://www.thebalance.com/how-long-do-average-u-s-marriages-last-4590261.

2. My grandfather was a watchmaker, my father an engineer, and my brother and I majored in physics.

3. McDonald's, "Your Right to Know," FAQs, https://www.mcdonalds.com/gb/en-gb/help/faq/18940-how-long-does-it-take-to-cook-a-burger-on-the-grill.html.

4. This statistic is based on 392 videotaped office visits in an elderly care clinic. See Ming Tai-Seale, Thomas G McGuire, and Weimin Zhang, "Time Allocation in Primary Care Office Visits," *Health Services Research* 42, no. 5 (October 2007): 1871-1894. https://www.ncbi.nlm.nih.gov/pmc/articles/PMC2254573/.

5. Bruce Y. Lee, "11 Seconds: How Long Your Doctor Listens Before Interrupting You," *Forbes*, July 22, 2018, https://www.forbes.com/sites/brucelee/2018/07/22/how-long-you-can-talk-before-your-doctor-interrupts-you/#7b49ce391443.

6   The sci-fi film *In Time* explores the broader implications of this idea. View the Trailer at: https://www.youtube.com/watch?v=lv6xAJqU9DM.

7   300 years ago, before the scripturalists took over, monasteries were going concerns where monks withdrew from worldly affairs to undertake a life of prayer. A common practice was the Prayer of Recollection (from the Latin: *re-* again + *col-* gather + *lect-* to bind), virtually identical in meaning to *samadhi* (*sam-* together + *a-* toward + *dhi-* to put).

8   Jalal al-Din Rumi, "A Great Wagon," *The Essential Rumi*, trans. Coleman Barks (New York: HarperCollins, 2010).

Chapter 21 The Myth of Discipline

1   Rebecca Lake, "23 Gym Membership Statistics That Will Astound You," *CreditDonkey*, December 29, 2014, https://www.creditdonkey.com/gym-membership-statistics.html.

2   K.A. Gudzune, R.S. Doshi, A.K. Mehta, Z.W. Chaudhry, D.K. Jacobs, R.M. Vakil, C.J. Lee, S.N. Bleich, and J.M. Clark, "Efficacy of Commercial Weight Loss Programs: An Updated Systematic Review," *Annals of Internal Medicine* 162, no. 7 (April 2015): 501-512. https://www.ncbi.nlm.nih.gov/pmc/articles/PMC4446719/.

3   A popular meme base on the book *Nothing Tastes Better Than A Healthy Thin Feels: The Spiritually Empowered Way to Weight Loss Success* by Alice Johnson (Bloomington, IN: Trafford Publishing, 2004).

4   K.A. Ericsson, R.T. Krampe, and C. Tesch-Romer, "The Role of Deliberate Practice in the Acquisition of Expert Performance," *Psychological Review* 100, no. 3 (1993): 363-406.

5   M. Admin, "Mozart Wasn't Born a Musical Genius," *KnowledgeNuts*, May 27, 2014, http://knowledgenuts.com/2014/05/27/mozart-wasnt-born-a-musical-genius/.

6   Heather Hodson, "Amy Chua: 'I'm Going to Take All Your Stuffed Animals and Burn Them!" *The Guardian*, January 14, 2011, https://www.theguardian.com/lifeandstyle/2011/jan/15/amy-chua-tiger-mother-interview.

7   Joan Anderman, "Yo-Yo Ma and the Mind Game of Music," *The New York Times*, October 10, 2013, https://www.nytimes.com/2013/10/10/booming/yo-yo-ma-and-the-mind-game-of-music.html.

8   Andre Agassi, Open: An Autobiography (New York: Random House, 2009), 3.

Chapter 22 (no notes)

Chapter 23 Freedom from Addiction

1   Office of Adolescent Health, "Adolescents and Tobacco: Risk and Protective Factors," *HHS.gov*, http://www.hhs.gov/ash/oah/adolescent-health-topics/substance-abuse/tobacco/risk-and-protective-factors.html.

2   Enoch Gordis, "Youth Drinking: Risk Factors and Consequences," *National Institute on Alcohol Abuse and Alcoholism*, no. 37 (July 1997). https://pubs.niaaa.nih.gov/publications/aa37.htm.

3 Institute of Medicine, *Ending the Tobacco Problem: A Blueprint for the Nation* (Washington, DC: The National Academies Press, 2007). https://www.nap.edu/read/11795/chapter/4.

4 For an excellent review of the reward system neuroanatomy, check out this YouTube video: https://www.youtube.com/watch?v=StxdPsmx744.

5 Rita Z. Goldstein and Nora D. Volkow, "Dysfunction of the Prefrontal Cortex in Addiction: Neuroimaging Findings and Clinical Implications," *Nature Reviews Neuroscience* 12, (2011): 652–669. http://www.nature.com/nrn/journal/v12/n11/full/nrn3119.html.

Chapter 24 Erotica

1 Oliver H. Turnbull, Victoria E. Lovett, Jackie Chaldecott, and Marilyn D. Lucas, "Reports of Intimate Touch: Erogenous Zones and Somatosensory Cortical Organization," *ScienceDirect* (2013): 1-9. http://turnbull-lab.bangor.ac.uk/documents/TurnbullErogenousCortex2013.pdf.

2 HealthyWay Staff Writer, "8 Disturbing Historical Practices that Prove 'Beauty Is Pain,'" *HealthyWay*, March 20, 2017, http://www.healthyway.com/content/disturbing-historical-practices-that-prove-beauty-is-pain.

3 Kissinger as quoted in *The New York Times* (28 October 1973) See https://en.wikiquote.org/wiki/Henry_Kissinger#Quotes_about_Kissinger.

4 R.O. Deaner, A.V. Khera, M.L. Platt, "Monkeys Pay Per View: Adaptive Valuation of Social Images by Rhesus Macaques," *Current Biology* 15, no. 6 (March 29, 2005): 543-8. https://www.ncbi.nlm.nih.gov/pubmed/15797023.

5 Christopher Hudson, "Genghis Kahn: The Daddy of All Lovers," *Daily Mail*, May 22, 2007, http://www.dailymail.co.uk/news/article-456789/Genghis-Khan-The-daddy-lovers.html.

6 Nicholas Farrell, *Mussolini: A New Life* (Amazon Digital Services, 2018).

7 TEDx Talks, "The Great Porn Experiment/Gary Wilson/TedxGlasgow" (video), YouTube, May 16, 2012, https://www.youtube.com/watch?v=wSF82AwSDiU.

Chapter 25 Orgasm 1.0

1 For more quotes from Marlene Dietrich, see https://www.brainyquote.com/quotes/marlene_dietrich_127131.

2 Marcel D. Waldinger, Paul Quinn, Maria Dilleen, Rajiv Mundayat, Dave H. Schweiter, and Mitradev Boolell, "Original Research—Ejaculation Disorders: A Multinational Population Survey of Intravaginal Ejaculation Latency Time," *The Journal of Sexual Medicine* 2, no. 4 (July 2005): 492-497. http://www.jsm.jsexmed.org/article/S1743-6095(15)31189-9/fulltext.

3 Premature ejaculation. https://www.nature.com/articles/3901507

4 C. Carson and K. Gunn, "Premature Ejaculation: Definition and Prevalence," *International Journal of Impotence Research* 18, (Sept 5, 2006): S5-S13. https://doi.org/10.1038/sj.ijir.3901507.

5. Alfred C. Kinsey, Wardell B. Pomeroy, Clyde E. Martin, and Paul H. Gebhard, *Sexual Behavior in the Human Female* (Indianapolis: Indiana University Press, 1981), 163-173. Originally published 1953.

6. Forty-five percent of females who reported having masturbated indicated that they could reach orgasm within three minutes (Kinsey, *Female*, p. 163).

7. Linda P. Rouse, *Marital and Sexual Lifestyles in the Unites States: Attitudes, Behaviors, and Relationships in Social Context*, (New York: Routledge, 2011), 137.

8. Check out this amusing YouTube video with over nine million views: https://www.youtube.com/watch?v=Vc8tPTVBRSc

9. Shere Hite, *The Hite Report: A Nationwide Study of Female Sexuality* (New York, NY: Seven Stories Press, 2004), 125.

Chapter 26 Orgasm 2.0

1. Martin Booe, "Kundalini Yoga Dangers," *LiveStrong.com*, January 31, 2018, https://www.livestrong.com/article/149739-kundalini-yoga-dangers/.

2. Pancham Sinh, trans., *Hatha Yoga Pradipika* (Chapter 2, Verse 15), https://www.sacred-texts.com/hin/hyp/hyp04.htm#page_13.

3. Whatever amazing experiences you may encounter in your inner explorations (pleasant or unpleasant), accept them fully and then drop them with an attitude of "so what." That way, the gifts you receive will remain as a quiet knowing, and you will be open and available to the next experience, whatever it may be. To read more, see Michael J. Formica, "Cutting Through Spiritual Materialism," *Psychology Today*, December 2, 2008, https://www.psychologytoday.com/us/blog/enlightened-living/200812/cutting-through-spiritual-materialism.

4. J. Allard, W.A. Truitt, K.E. McKenna, L.M. Coolen, "Spinal Cord Control of Ejaculation," *World Journal of Urology* 23, no. 2 (June 2005): 119-26. https://www.ncbi.nlm.nih.gov/pubmed/15947961.

Chapter 27 Living in the Sweet Spot

1. Da Vinci notes, "If you open your legs enough that your head is lowered by one-fourteenth of your height and raise your hands enough that your extended fingers touch the line of the top of your head, know that the centre of the extended limbs will be the navel and the space between the legs will be an equilateral triangle." See Walter Isaacson, *Leonardo Da Vinci* (New York: Simon & Schuster, 2017), 155.

2. Stephen Strauss, "Clara M. Davis and the Wisdom of Letting Children Choose Their Own Diets," *Canadian Medical Association Journal* 175, no. 10 (November 7, 2006): 1199-1201. https://www.ncbi.nlm.nih.gov/pmc/articles/PMC1626509/.

3. Federation of American Societies for Experimental Biology (FASEB), "Highly Processed Foods Dominate U.S. Grocery Purchases," *ScienceDaily*, March 29, 2015, www.sciencedaily.com/releases/2015/03/150329141017.htm.

4. P.B. Laursen, "Training for Intense Exercise Performance: High-Intensity or High-Volume Training?" *Scandinavian Journal of Medicine & Science* 20, no. s2 (Sept 14, 2010). https://onlinelibrary.wiley.com/doi/full/10.1111/j.1600-0838.2010.01184.x.

5   See National Sleep Foundation, "How Much Sleep Do We Really Need?" https://www.sleepfoundation.org/articles/how-much-sleep-do-we-really-need. (Note that teenagers need 8-10 hours of sleep.)

6   Thomas M. Heffron, "Insomnia Awareness Day Facts and Stats," *Sleep Education*, March 10, 2014, http://www.sleepeducation.org/news/2014/03/10/insomnia-awareness-day-facts-and-stats.

7   A. Roger Ekirch, *At Day's Close: Night in Times Past* (New York: W.W. Norton, 2005).

8   Valerie Coulman, "You Snooze, You Lose? Not Necessarily…" *Joy Magazine*, August 15, 2007, https://saramednick.com/htmls/press/media/JoyMag_Aug2007.pdf.

9   T.C. Erren, P. Falaturi, P. Morfeld, P. Knauth, R.J. Reiter, and C. Piekarski, "Shift Work and Cancer: The Evidence and the Challenge," *Deutsches Ärzteblatt International* 107, no. 38 (Sept 24, 2010): 657-662. https://www.ncbi.nlm.nih.gov/pmc/articles/PMC2954516/.

10 Natural killer cells are part of our more ancient, innate immune system, which is responsible for removing cells damaged by viral infections and precancerous changes to the genome.

11 Arialdi M. Miniño, "Mortality Among Teenagers Aged 12-19 Years: United States, 1999-2006," *National Center for Health Statistics Data Brief*, no. 37 (May 2010). https://www.cdc.gov/nchs/products/databriefs/db37.htm.

12 Mathew Walker, *Why We Sleep: Unlocking the Power of Sleep and Dreams* (New York: Scribner, 2017).

13 Mathew Walker, *Why We Sleep*

14 Mathew Walker, *Why We Sleep*

15 Kat Duff, *The Secret Life of Sleep* (New York: Atria Books, 2014), 43.

16 For more quotes from Zhuangzi, see https://www.brainyquote.com/quotes/zhuangzi_393083.

17 Carl G. Jung, *The Structure and Dynamics of the Psyche, Collected Works* Vol. 8 (Princeton, NJ: Princeton University Press, 1972), para. 507.

18 Levititticus 16:8, 16:10, 16:26

19 Jung, *Collected Works* Vol. 8, Para. 519

20 Thich Nhat Hahn, "Interrelationship" as recited at a psychotherapist conference, Granby, CO.

21 Wallace Stegner, *All the Little Live Things* (New York: Penguin, 1991), 8.

22 Amy Adkins, "Employee Engagement in U.S. Stagnant in 2015," *Gallup*, January 13, 2016, http://www.gallup.com/poll/188144/employee-engagement-stagnant-2015.aspx.

23 Mary Oliver, "The Summer Day (poem 133)," from Poetry 180: A Poem a Day for American High Schools, hosted by Billy Collins, Library of Congress, https://www.loc.gov/poetry/180/133.html.

24 Jalal al-Din Rumi, *The Book of Love: Poems of Ecstasy and Longing*, trans. Coleman Barks (New York: HarperCollins, 2003), 123.

25 Lao-Tzu, "Fifty-Six," *Tao Te Ching*, trans. S. Mitchell, http://thetaoteching.com/taoteching56.html.

Chapter 28 Renewable Pleasure for a Sustainable World

1 David Biello, "Did the Anthropocene Begin in 1950 or 50,000 Years Ago?" *Scientific American*, April 2, 2015, https://www.scientificamerican.com/article/did-the-anthropocene-begin-in-1950-or-50-000-years-ago/.

2 Daniel Simberloff, "Roundtable: A Modern Mass Extinction?" *Evolution*, WGBH/NOVA Science Unit and Clear Blue Sky Productions, https://www.pbs.org/wgbh/evolution/extinction/massext/statement_04.html.

3 Population Research Institute, "Overpopulation: The Making of a Myth," https://overpopulationisamyth.com/episode-1-overpopulation-the-making-of-a-myth/.

4 World Centric, "Social & Economic Injustice," http://www.worldcentric.org/conscious-living/social-and-economic-injustice.

5 Anup Shah, "Poverty Facts and Stats," *Global Issues*, January 7, 2013, http://www.globalissues.org/article/26/poverty-facts-and-stats.

6 To read more statistics about hunger deaths, see http://www.worldcentric.org/conscious-living/social-and-economic-injustice.

7 Dominic Rushe, "The Kings of Capitalism are Finally Worried About the Growing Gap Between Rich and Poor," *The Guardian*, April 24, 2019, https://www.theguardian.com/commentisfree/2019/apr/24/ray-dalio-jamie-dimon-kings-of-capitalism-concerned?CMP=Share_iOSApp_Other.

8 Kathleen Elkins, "How Much Money You Need to be Among the Richest 10 Percent of People Worldwide," *Make It*, CNBC, November 7, 2018, https://www.cnbc.com/2018/11/07/how-much-money-you-need-to-be-in-the-richest-10-percent-worldwide.html. To calculate your relative financial wealth, see http://www.globalrichlist.com/wealth.

9 Charlotte McDonald, "How Many Earths Do We Need?" *BBC News*, June 15, 2015, https://www.bbc.com/news/magazine-33133712.

10 George H.W. Bush quoted in Erik Lindberg, "Apres Moi Le Deluge," *Resilience*, April 7, 2014, https://www.resilience.org/stories/2014-04-07/apres-moi-le-deluge/.

11 "Obama's Inaugural Speech," CNN Politics, January 20, 2009, http://www.cnn.com/2009/POLITICS/01/20/obama.politics/.

12 For more quotes from Mahatma Gandhi, see https://www.goodreads.com/quotes/286133-live-simply-so-that-others-may-simply-live.

13 Oren Lyons (Seneca faith keeper, Onondaga and Seneca Nations) quoted in "Seven Generations—the Role of Chief," *Warrior*, PBS, https://www.pbs.org/warrior/content/timeline/opendoor/roleOfChief.html.

14 Umair Haque, "If the Point of Capitalism is to Escape Capitalism, Then What's the Point of Capitalism?" *Medium*, September 7, 2018, https://eand.co/if-the-point-of-capitalism-is-to-escape-capitalism-then-whats-the-point-of-capitalism-bedd1b2447d.

15 To hear Timothy Leary speak to "turn on, tune in, and drop out," check out this short YouTube video: https://www.youtube.com/watch?v=LTCxINKT7l4. For a modern take, see Paul Rosenberg, "Turn On Tune In Drop Out—A Modern Interpretation," *Free-Man's Perspective*, June 18, 2013, https://www.freemansperspective.com/turn-on-tune-in-drop-out/.

16 The popularity of competitive sports and the Super Bowl extravaganza is the result of a concerted marketing effort that began after the Civil War. Pro football struggled for years with little popularity. See Pro Football Hall of Fame, "Birth of Pro Football," https://www.profootballhof.com/football-history/birth-of-pro-football/.

17 Rudyard Kipling, "The Law of the Jungle," in *Rudyard Kipling's Verse: Inclusive Edition* 1885-1918 (New York: Doubleday, 1922), https://www.bartleby.com/364/316.html.

18 Charles Darwin, *The Descent of Man*, quoted in John van Wyhe, ed., *The Complete Work of Charles Darwin Online*, http://darwin-online.org.uk/. Also, see Pyotr Kropotkin, a Russian naturalist and contemporary of Darwin. During his research in Siberia, he looked for signs of competition but instead found overwhelming evidence of mutual aid. He discusses the evolutionary role of cooperation in his book, Mutual Aid, which forms the basis of his anarchist philosophy..

19 Lynn Margulis and Dorion Sagan, *What is Life?* (New York: Simon & Schuster, 1995), 115.

20 Melinda Wenner, "Humans Carry More Bacterial Cells than Human Ones," Scientific American, November 30, 2007, https://www.scientificamerican.com/article/strange-but-true-humans-carry-more-bacterial-cells-than-human-ones/ ; R.D. Sleator, "The Human Superorganism—of Microbes and Men," *Medical Hypotheses* 74, no. 2 (February 2010): 214-215. https://www.ncbi.nlm.nih.gov/pubmed/19836146.

21 John Donne, "No Man Is an Island," *Poem Hunter.org*, May 30, 2013, https://www.poemhunter.com/poem/no-man-is-an-island/.

22 Christina Feldman, "Dependent Origination," *Insight Journal*, (Spring 1999): 37-41. https://www.buddhistinquiry.org/article/dependent-origination/.

GLOSSARY

Abbreviations:
Chin: Chinese
Ger: German
Grk: Greek
Lat: Latin
Jp: Japanese
San: Sanskrit

A

aah-**centric**—A life based on the pursuit of feeling good—the good life.

*aah*some—An *äsis*-inspired sense of awe.

amygdala—Aggression-fear center located in the limbic brain (almond shaped).

anahata chakra—San. heart center associated with balance, serenity, and *nada*, "the unstruck" primordial sound that fills the cosmos (the sound of silence); location of the equanimity center.

anandamaya kosha—San. energetic bliss body or sheath (from *ananda*, "bliss"); the Light-body.

arête—Grk. excellence, skill, virtue.

asana—San. a specific yoga posture.

äsis—Highest level of (spiritual) pleasure; the clear, white light of consciousness.

äsis **center**—Energy center located a hands-breadth above the crown of the head (see *sahasrara chakra*).

ataraxia— Grk. Epicurus's highest pleasure of equanimity and peace of mind (from *a*, "not" and *tarassein*, "disturbed").

atman—San. essence; breath of an individual soul.

Glossary

artificial pleasure—Technology-enhanced pleasures with an unhealthy Pleasure Cycle, based on satisfying empty desires with a narrow spectrum, and a large ecological footprint.

authentic pleasure—Simple pleasures with a healthy Pleasure Cycle, based on satisfying real needs with a full spectrum, and a small ecological footprint.

B

bliss center—Located above the soft palate at the back of the throat (see *talu chakra*).

body-stream—Flow of physical sensations through the body.

Brahman—San. ultimate reality underlying all phenomena; the Tao; the Source.

brainstem—Neural chassis is comprised of the midbrain, hindbrain, and upper spinal cord.

body-tube—refers to the head and torso through which our life-stream flows.

Buddha—San. honorific title meaning "one who has awakened" (from *budh*, "to awaken").

C

chakra—San. center of *pranic* energy in the body (see *prana*).

consciousness—Non-personal awareness (see witness).

Continuum of Authenticity— Range of pleasure quality from artificial (junk) pleasures to authentic (organic) pleasures.

cortical brain—Cerebral cortex, the most recent division of the triune brain, appearing in primates and associated with abstract reasoning and judgment.

Cyrenaic—Grk. hedonistic school of philosophy advocating sensual pleasures (400 BCE).

D

daemon — Grk. embodiment of spirit associated with one's genius; a genie.

desire center — Located in the Ventral Tegmental Area (VTA, "underside of the roof") in the midbrain of the neural chassis.

E

ecstasy center — Located two centimeters in front of the lumbo-sacral junction in the pelvis at the physical center of gravity in the upright position (see *muladhara chakra*).

epistemology — Study of truth-making (from Grk. *episteme*, "knowledge"). How we know what we know.

equanimity center — Located at the juncture where the heart rests upon the dome of the respiratory diaphragm (see *anahata chakra*).

ethics — Development of one's character shaped by virtue (see *arête* above).

eudaimonia — Grk. good spirited (from *eu*, "good" and *daemon*, "spirit"); fulfillment assessed at the end of one's life; the good life.

F

fractal — Self-similar geometrical patterns at different scales (from Lat. *fractus*, "broken," "fractured").

G

ganglia — Collection of neurons forming knots of tissue often in a net (plexus).

H

hippocampus — Memory center located in the limbic brain (seahorse shaped).

holarchy — Hierarchy of holons.

holon—"Organizational fractal" where each functional unit is simultaneously a semi-autonomous whole and part of a larger whole like nesting Russian dolls.

Homo spiritualis—Next step in human evolution.

K

katana—the keen edge of a Samurai blade that like exquisite beauty, has the power to give life and take life.

kinesthetic—ancient part of nervous system concerned with spatial (proprioceptive) awareness (see *vedana*).

koan—Jp. paradoxical question posed by a Zen master to a student that transcends logic and requires an intuitive, nondualistic answer.

kundalini—San. primal "serpent" energy coiled three and a half times at the base of the spine.

L

life-stream—Life force comprised of the body-stream and mind-stream which propagates through the medium of consciousness. Synonymous with: Lat. *spiritus*, San. *prana*, Chin. *qi*, Jp. *ki*, French *élan vitale*, Grk. *pneuma*, Hebrew *ruach*, Hawaiian *ha* (as in *aloha*).

Light-body—Subtle energy body (see *anandamaya kosha*).

limbic brain—Second division of the triune brain, appearing in early mammals and associated with emotion, memory, and the pleasure center.

M

mind-stream—Flow of thoughts through the mind.

muladhara chakra—San. root center (from *mula*, "root" and *adhara*, "base") anatomically related to the physical center of gravity and the pelvic floor, levator ani muscles; location of ecstasy center.

N

nucleus accumbens—Pleasure center located in the limbic brain adjacent to (recumbent on) the forebrain septum.

O

ontology—Study of the nature of being.

Original Inadequacy—the abiding feeling of insufficiency and lacking in all things.

Original Wholeness—Primal state of completeness in which we are born.

P

phenomenology—Study of what can be perceived directly with one's own senses.

Pleasure Capacity—Amount of pleasurable intensity one can experience before becoming uncomfortable.

pleasure center—Located in the nucleus accumbens of the limbic brain (see above).

Pleasure Cycle—The integrated rising and falling wave of active, passive, and neutral pleasures.

Pleasure-Pain Threshold—Point on the Sensual Continuum at which the intensity of an experience changes from pleasure into pain.

Pleasure Prism—Refers to the triune brain which "refracts" pleasurable experiences into three primary colors (frequencies): red (physical); green (emotional); and blue (mental)—and when properly balanced, combine to form the clear white light of *āsis* pleasure.

pleasure-time graph—Plot of the intensity of pleasure as a function of time.

prana—San. vital life force (see life-stream).

prefrontal cortex—Area of cerebral cortex located behind the forehead concerned with abstract thought, planning, judgment, and coordinating thoughts and actions; makes up the personality.

R

Renewable Pleasure—1. human-derived pleasure. 2. a natural resource. 3. a form of authentic pleasure (see above).

S

sahasrara chakra— San. crown center of thousand-petaled lotus blossom; location of *äsis* center.

samadhi— San. the spiritual merging of subject and object into a state of Original Wholeness (from *sam*, "together," *a*, toward" and *dhi*, "to put").

samsara—San. realm of endless drifting, wandering, mundane existence and metaphysical cycle of death and rebirth.

Sensual Continuum—Range of perceived sensual intensity.

Seven Immutable Laws of Pleasure—1. Original Wholeness; 2. Colors; 3. Contrast and Comparison; 4. Thresholds; 5. Cycles; 6. Desire and Surrender; 7. Renewable Pleasure.

schadenfreude—taking pleasure in others' misfortune.

shakuhachi—Jp. end blown, five-holed, bamboo flute (1.8 *shaku* in length).

shushumna—San. central energy axis of the body.

summum bonum—Grk. highest, ultimate good.

sunyata—San. emptiness; empty of an independent self; zero; the nothing that contains everything.

T

Taiji—Chin. *yin* and *yang* symbol of complementary, cosmic principles: *Yin* is earth, matter, substantial, slow to change, soft, passive, surrender; *yang* is heaven, spirit, light, quick, hard, active, desire.

talu chakra—San. palate center from *talu,* "palate"; location of bliss center (see above).

U

umwelt—Ger. an organism's unique perception of and relationship to its environment.

V

vedana—San. sense of body position through internal, kinesthetic touch (proprioception).

Ventral Tegmental Area (VTA)—desire, motivational center located in the underside of the midbrain roof; produces dopamine in the nucleus accumbens (pleasure center).

W

witness—non-personal observation (pure consciousness) through which we experience all of life.

Z

zero—Most powerful number in the universe; the balancing point where paradox resolves; the nothing that contains infinity (see *sunyata* above).

Image Credits

Frontispiece: The Preasure Prism, Kristi Frigell (page 2)
Part 1: Amy Clay (page 13)
Figure 1: Kersti Frigell (page 32)
Figure 2: Photographer unknown, Albin Polasek modeling *Man Carving His Own Destiny*, c. 1918, gelatin silver print, Collection of the Albin Polasek Foundation, Winter Park, Florida (page 51)
Part 2: Amy Clay (page 73)
Figure 3: James Olds and Peter Milner, 1954. (page 76)
Figure 4: Kersti Frigell (page 78)
Figure 5: Kersti Frigell (page 81)
Figure 6: Wikimedia.org, Metropolitan Museum of Art (page 85)
Figure 7: Kersti Frigell (pages 2 and 99)
Figure 8: Kersti Frigell (page 106)
Part 3: Amy Clay (page 109)
Figure 9: Kersti Frigell (page 128)
Figure 10: Kersti Frigell (page 137)
Figure 11: Kersti Frigell (page 140)
Figure 12: Wikipedia.org (page 159)
Figure 13: Kersti Frigell (page 167)
Figure 14: Kersti Frigell (page 169)
Figure 15: Kersti Frigell (page 170)
Figure 16: Kersti Frigell (page 173)
Figure 17: Kersti Frigell (page 175)
Figure 18: Kersti Frigell (page 177)
Figure 19: Kersti Frigell (page 179)
Figure 20: Wikipedia.org (page 185)
Part 4: Amy Clay (page 193)
Figure 21: Kersti Frigell (page 210)
Figure 22: Kersti Frigell (page 215)
Figure 23: Kersti Frigell (page 217)

Figure 24: Kersti Frigell (page 218)
Figure 25: Pixabay.com (page224)
Figure 26: Free-Images.com, Pixabay.com (page 225)
Figure 27: Kersti Frigell (page 227)
Part 5: Amy Clay (page 235)
Figure 28: Wikipedia.org (page 274)
Figure 29: Kersti Frigell (page 288)
Figure 30: Kersto Frigell (page 289)
Figure 31: Leonado DaVinci/Kersti Frigell (page 296)

Index

A

absolute refractory period 287, 288
active pleasure 166, 181, 209, 211–213, 220
acupuncture 137
Adam 31–33, 40
addiction 81–83, 261–267, 302
adolescence 117–119, 262, 277, 301
advertising and marketing 150, 157, 160–162
afterlife 65–66, 71
agape 242, 272
Agassi, Andre 250
agnosticism 38
alcohol 121–123, 169
Allegory of the Cave 55
Alzheimer's disease 302
Amadeus Equation 325
amygdala 81, 82, 85, 285
anandamaya kosha 106
anesthesia 128, 130
anger 304
animal studies 75–76, 158, 276
Anthropocene 311
anxiety, pleasure 124–125
appetite
  controlling by satisfying 22, 317
  sustainability and 313
archery 290–291
arête 51. *See also* virtue
Aristotle 51–55, 61
art and mastery 253–255
artificial pleasure 171, 173–175, 177–178, 180, 267
Ashani 9–11, 196–198, 238–239, 259
äsis
  alignment of field 217–219
  balanced life 295, 307–310
  creating from small moments 228
  daily practice 307–308
  described 102–103, 107
  drugs and 261
  equanimity in 216
  experiencing 107
  mantra 219, 221
  paradise and 198
  re-cognition in 230
ataraxia 63, 166, 170, 181, 216
atheism 38, 69
Atman 105
attachment 139–140, 258
Saint Augustine 33, 39–41, 43, 54, 272
Authentic Happiness 17
authority of teachers 308
awareness
  vs. consciousness 104
  of desires 144–155
  perception and 128
Axial Age 28, 35, 187

B

baby steps 256–259, 263

balance 51, 295–306
baptism 42
BDSM (Bondage and Discipline, Sadism and Masochism) 34
beauty 54, 56, 225–226, 234
Bentham, Jeremy 67
be present 238–239, 244, 245, 286
bias 28
Bible 28–34
A Billion Wicked Thoughts (Ogas and Gaddam) 277
black holes 203
Blake, William 140
bliss
  alignment in *äsis* field 217–219
  bliss center 214, 220
  defined 209
  mixed with ecstasy and equanimity 219
  orgasm and 285
blue, mental pleasures in Pleasure Prism 21, 80, 101–102, 108, 297
body
  alignment in *äsis* field 217–219
  attuning 219–220
  bliss center 214–215, 220
  body-tube and flow 135–139
  center of emotional pleasures 101, 108
  center of mental pleasures 102, 108
  center of reptilian pleasures 98, 108
  continuum of intensity 131
  ecstasy center 212–213
  equanimity center 216
  erogenous zones 273–277
  microbiome 320
  understanding of 96, 105–107
body-stream 100, 108, 135
Bohr, Niels 185, 198–199
Bondage and Discipline, Sadism and Masochism (BDSM) 34
Book of Genesis 30–38
boredom 116, 120
Brahman 105
brain
  addiction and 81–83
  desire and 80–84, 143
  embryological development 78–79
  evolution of 21, 77, 90, 143
  mammalian 21, 79, 80–84, 90–92, 99–101, 108
  neurobiology of pleasure 75–84
  perception and 113–114
  primate 21, 77, 79, 80–84, 92–93, 101–102, 108
  reptilian 21, 79, 84, 87–89, 97–99, 108, 143
  reward system 80–84, 264, 265, 284
brainstem. *See* neural chassis
breath 10, 131, 212, 299
Bryant, Kobe 212
Burning Man 43
Bush, George H. W. 314

C

capacity for pleasure. *See* Pleasure Capacity
Catholic Church 41–42, 64–65, 68, 136, 201–202, 248

chakras 98–99, 101, 102, 103
Chinese medicine
   äsis and 103
   emotional pleasure and 101
   life-stream in 136
   mental pleasures and 102
   meridians 105
   pelvis and 99
   persistent genital arousal syndrome 289
   yin/yang of body 210
Christianity. *See also* Catholic Church
   discipline in 248
   Judeo-Christian culture 28–34
   Original Sin 39–46
   suppression of Epicurus 64–65
circadian rhythms 301
clitoris 274, 282
clockmind 239–241, 245
clocks. *See* clockmind
clothing 159–160, 274–276
cold water training 133–135
collective unconscious 146
color. *See also* Law of Colors
   blue for mental pleasures 21, 80, 101–102, 108, 297
   green for emotional pleasures 21, 99–101, 108, 297
   red for physical pleasures 20, 97–99, 108, 297
   white for spiritual pleasures 21, 102–103, 108, 297
comfort trap 177–178
coming of age rituals 117–119
comparison. *See* Law of Contrast and Comparison
competition 319, 320
consciousness
   vs. awareness 104
   doorways to 114
   intelligence and 208
   light as 106
   shift in 168
   surrender and 184
   war on 70, 71, 317
Constantine 64
constriction 134, 137, 139–144
consumption 313, 314, 318, 321
Continuum of Authenticity 173
contradictories
   micro-pleasures and 228
   of paradise 198–199
   in Pleasure Cycle 211
contrast. *See* Law of Contrast and Comparison
cooperation 319–320
Council of Nicea 64
creative suffering 139
crown chakra 103, 108
crystal radio 207–208, 217, 218
Csikszentmihalyi, Mihaly 157, 211
cultural operating system 27. *See also* matrix
cycles. *See* Law of Cycles
Cyrenaics 62

D

daemon 42, 55
Darwin, Charles 319
daughters
   contrast and comparison example 116
   dedication 9–11
   estrangement from 153, 154
   meditation with 196–198
   technology and 161
da Vinci, Leonardo 295–296
death
   coming of age rituals and 117–119
   fear of 65–66, 134, 191, 318
   in sensual continuum 128
Declaration of Independence 69, 316
delayed gratification 170–171, 181
denial, as ineffective 144–147
Descartes, René 136
The Descent of Man (Darwin) 319
desire. *See also* Law of Desire and Surrender
   advertising and marketing of 160–162
   Amadeus Equation 325
   baby steps 258
   balancing point 200–204
   brain and 80–84, 143, 265
   decoupling from pleasure 81–82
   denial as ineffective 144–147
   empty desires 148
   fractal waves 226
   in meditation 308
   needs vs. wants 147–153
   in orgasm 285
   vs. pleasure 143
   supernormal 158
   types of 148
   as wanting 143
   as *yang* 211
diaphragm 216, 219
discipline 247–251
Divine Feminine 30
Dogen 184
dopamine 80–84, 143, 264, 265
dreaming 302–303
drug use 168, 264–266, 302

E

earth 33, 99
ecstasy
   alignment in *äsis* field 217–219
   center 211–213, 220
   defined 209
   flow and 212, 230
   mixed with bliss and equanimity 219
   orgasm and 285
education and virtue 52–53
effort and authentic pleasure 173–175
egalitarianism 69
ego
   balancing point 200–204
   disconnection 231
   self and 185–186, 230
   sex and 290
   surrender and 185–187
ejaculation
   female 283

mechanism of 291
premature 281, 284
resolution phase and 287
elites 313–314
emotional pleasures 21, 80, 99–101, 108, 243, 297
emotions
acknowledging 304
continuum of intensity 131
describing 99–100
evolution of 91
flow and 139
increasing emotional capacity 244
use of 91–92
empty desires 148
empty pleasures 216
endorphins 293
energy 208
enlightenment 229, 231
Epicurus 59–67
on desire 148, 149, 151
on empty pleasures 216
on fear of death 65–66
on fear of gods 65, 66
influence of 56, 67–70
misinterpretation of 59–60
on net pleasure 169–170
on scaling pleasure 228
suppression of 64–65
epilepsy 285
equanimity 209, 210, 215–216, 217–219, 220
equanimity center 215–216, 220
erections, in paralyzed men 292

Ericsson, Anders 249, 250
erogenous zones 273–277, 279
eros 272
erotica 271, 271–278
Esalen 44–45
ethics/ethos 49–56, 51, 227
eudaimonia 55–56, 238, 316
Eve 31–33
evil 31–33, 66
evolution
brain 21, 77, 90, 143
cooperation 319–320
emotions 91
gender differences in approach to sex 278
excitement phase 284
exercise 178, 248, 295, 299–300
extinction 311

F
Fall of Man 31–33
fear
as central to matrix 46
constriction and 134
of death 65–66, 134, 191, 318
of gods 65, 318
of insufficiency 318–320
love and 243
Original Sin and 54
sustainability and 318–319
female ejaculation 283
fertility cults 40
fixed action patterns 158

flow 134, 135–139, 141, 178–180, 211, 230
fluid dynamics 179
food 16, 80, 172, 295, 298–299
foot binding 275
foot fetishism 273
forebrain 78. *See also* triune brain
foreplay 283
fractals 223–231
St. Francis of Assisi 248
Frankl, Victor 102
Freeman, Richard 95, 121
free will 41, 42
Freud, Sigmund 303
friendship 63

G
games 91
Garden of Eden 31–33, 198, 318. *See also* Paradise
generosity 52
Genesis 30–33
genius 56
giftedness 249–251
Gnosticism 65
gods, fear of 65, 66, 318
gratification, delayed 170–171, 181
Greek philosophy 28, 49–56, 59–67. *See also* Epicurus
green, emotional pleasures in Pleasure Prism 21, 99–101, 108, 297
grey matter 79, 80
Gross National Happiness 321
G-spot 283

guilt 32, 41, 42, 43, 46, 249, 266

H
habit/habituation 52, 87, 115, 149, 216
Haggard, Ted 144, 266
happiness
  cultural differences 100
  in Declaration of Independence 69, 316
  defining 16–17
  in Greek philosophy 55–56, 61
  mammalian brain and 80
  money and 148
  vs. pleasure 16
  research 16–17
  vs. satisfaction 100
  sweet spot 295–306
Hawaiian islanders 274–275
health 18–20, 45, 125, 150, 178, 220
heart 101, 108, 216, 219, 220, 299
hedonism 61–62
Heisenberg's Uncertainty Principle 67
hindbrain 78
hippocampus 81, 82
holarchy 227, 233, 321
holons 227, 228
Homo spiritualis 21, 102, 320
homunculus 273
The Human Sexual Response (Masters and Johnson) 284

I
identity 125, 186, 320–321
impotence 277

imprinting 158, 161
information 208
inhibitory function 83
inner child 197, 205
inner conflict 84
insomnia 300
intelligence 208-209
interbeing 146
intimacy, increasing capacity for 244, 245

J
James, William 89
Japan 69, 275, 277
Jefferson, Thomas 68, 69
Jesus 145
Jhana 9-11, 44
Jois, Pattabhi 95-96, 107
Judaism 29, 41
judgment 199, 205, 228
Jung, Carl 146, 303, 304

K
Kabir 233, 234
Kalahari Bushmen 175-176
The Kalevala 50
Kazantzakis, Nikos 118
Khan, Genghis 276
ki. See life-stream
King, Martin Luther, Jr. 146
Kinsey Reports 282
koan 190-191
koshas 106
kundalini 99, 289

L
laminar flow 179
Laozi 64, 183, 309
Law of Attraction 101
Law of Colors 23, 97-103, 297
Law of Contrast and Comparison 23,
 113-119, 149, 158, 297, 299
Law of Cycles 23, 166-168, 173, 261, 283, 297
Law of Desire and Surrender 23, 209-211,
 255, 258, 290-293, 297
Law of Original Wholeness 23, 63-64, 70,
 146, 198, 242, 267, 297, 298, 306
Law of Renewable Pleasure 23, 315-321
Law of Thresholds 23, 129-131, 257, 297
Leary, Timothy 317
life force 97, 101
life-stream 135-139
Light-body 106, 217-219, 220
Lilly, John C. 76
limbic brain. *See* mammalian brain
Li Po 229
Lorenz, Konrad 158
love
 conditional 239
 eros 272
 mammalian brain and 80
 mastery and 253-255
 relationships and 239-244
 as renewable pleasure 312, 321
 true 242-244
 unconditional 241-242

M

MacLean, Paul 77, 78, 84, 92
magnanimity 53–54
make relationship 237–244
mammalian brain 21, 77, 79, 90–92, 99–101, 108
Man Carving his Own Destiny 51
Mandelbrot, Benoit 224, 225
mantra, *äsis* as 219, 221
Margulis, Lynn 320
Marx, Karl 239
Maslow, Abraham 211, 318
massage 129–130
master-slave matrix 34
Masters, William 284
mastery 253–255
masturbation 282
mathematics 325
matrix
    erotica and 274–285
    as fear-centric 46
    happiness and money 150, 153
    history 28–33
    identity and 186
    Original Sin 39
    success and 318
    understanding 27–35
The Matrix (1999) 55
matter 208
Ma, Yo Yo 250
McDonald's 157, 240
medicine, corporatization of 240–241
meditation
    as *äsis* practice 308
    with baby 196–198
    criticism of 146
    levels of 308
    sesshin 187–192
    surrender and 187–189
men
    association with spirit 33
    gender differences in approach to sex 278
    gender differences in orgasm 282
    patriarchy 30–33
    pornography use 277, 282
    resolution phase 287–288
    sexual response 282
mental pleasures 21, 80, 101–102, 108, 297
meridians 105, 136
mesocortical pathway 80–81, 83
mesolimbic pathway 80–81, 83
microbiome 320
midbrain 78
Milner, Peter 75–76
mind-stream
    body-tube and 135
    confusion vs. calm in 114
    term 100
mirror neurons 180
Moller, Lorraine 249
money 148–150, 306–307
monotheism 29–33, 66
morality vs. virtue 52
Mother Nature 197
motion, perception of 113

motorcycle accidents 118–119
Mozart, Wolfgang Amadeus 249
muladhara chakra 98
multiple orgasms 286, 287–293
muscle tone and plateau phase 284
muscular strength 299–300
Mussolini, Benito 276

N

nadis 105, 136
napping 301
nature
　balance in 203
　fractals 224–225
　Mother Nature 197
needs
　hierarchy of 318
　vs. wants 147–153
negative-hedonism 62
neocortex 80, 92–93
net pleasure 168–170, 283
neural chassis 78–79
neural plasticity 264
neurobiology
　of addiction 265
　of pleasure 75–84
neurons
　mirror neurons 180
　perception and 113
neutral pleasure 209, 220. *See also ataraxia*
Nicholas of Cusa 198
Nicomachean Ethics 51

nicotine 263
Nietzsche, Friedrich 56
nucleus accumbens 75–76, 265, 284, 285
nutrition 295, 298–299

O

Obama, Barack 314
obedience, cult of 68
obesity 150, 298
objectification 239–242
objective reality 196
Olds, James 75–76
organic foods 299
orgasm
　as convulsion 285
　gender differences in 282
　intensity and path 290
　multiple 286, 287–293
　Pleasure Cycle 284
　surrender and 187
　understanding 281–285
　valley 291, 292
Original Inadequacy 44–46
Original Sin 33, 39–46, 54, 272
Original Wholeness. *See* Law of Original Wholeness
Orwell, George 60
oxytocin 293

P

pain
　comfort trap 177–178
　Epicurus on 61, 62

importance of 17
opposite of 19, 62, 127, 130, 177
receptors 20
palate. *See* soft palate
Paradise. *See* Garden of Eden
   balancing point 200–204
   concept 198–199
paradox 198–199, 202, 211
parental investment 278
passive pleasure 166, 181, 209, 214–215, 220
Patanjali 204
patriarchy 30–33
Saint Paul 43
peaking 292. *See also* valley orgasm
pederasty 276
pelvic floor muscles 213
pelvis 98–99, 213, 219, 220, 285
penis 273, 282
perception
   Law of Thresholds and 129–131
   level of awareness and 128
   of time 229
   understanding 111–118
perfume 161
persistent genital arousal syndrome 289
physical pleasures 20, 80, 97–99, 106, 108, 297
piercings 275
plastic surgery 160
plateau phase 284
Plato 55
play 91

pleasure. *See also* Pleasure Prism; Pleasure-Pain Threshold; Pleasure Cycle
   active pleasure 181, 209, 211–213, 220
   Amadeus Equation 325
   artificial pleasure 171, 173–175, 177–178, 180, 267
   as shift in consciousness 168
   decoupling from desire 81–82
   defined 20, 62
   vs. desire 143
   emotional pleasures 21, 80, 99–101, 108, 243, 297
   Epicurus on 60–61
   vs. happiness 16
   importance of 15, 17–23
   mental pleasures 21, 80, 101–102, 108, 297
   as misunderstood 15–17
   net pleasure 168–170, 283
   neutral pleasure 209, 220
   opposite of 19, 62, 130
   passive pleasure 181, 209, 214–215, 220
   as path-dependent 168, 211, 290
   physical pleasures 20, 80, 97–99, 106, 108, 297
   renewable pleasure 21–23, 311–321
   spiritual pleasures 21, 102–103, 108, 297
pleasure anxiety 124–125
Pleasure Capacity 124–125, 130–132
Pleasure Cycle
   authentic pleasure and 171
   exercise and 299
   increasing emotional capacity 244

in Law of Desire and Surrender 209–211
orgasm and 284–286
pleasure as a wave 165–168
positivity and 305
Pleasure-Pain Threshold
  authentic pleasures and 176
  balancing flow with 137, 140
  in cold training 134
  comfort trap and 177
  development of concept 125
  discipline and 248, 249, 251
  love and 243, 244, 245
  maximizing capacity with 130–132
  multiple orgasms and 291
  needs and 147
  smoothness and 179
  sustainability and 323
  understanding 129–131
  valley orgasms and 292
  visual erotica and 275
Pleasure Prism
  blending in 106
  continuum of intensity 131
  described 20–21, 97–103
  equanimity and 216
  Light-body and 106–107
  scaling pleasure 228
  summary 107
pleasure-time graph 168–170, 283
pneuma 135
Polasek, Albin 51
politics and ritual 91
Polynesian societies 274, 277

polytheism 30
pornography
  author's first experience with 271–272
  gender differences in 277, 282
  religiosity and 43
positive thinking 101
posture 219
power
  as aphrodisiac 276
  balance and 204
  connection to body 35
  misuse of 34–35, 145
  relationships and 243
prana. *See* life-stream
prefrontal cortex 81, 83, 122, 266, 285
premature ejaculation 281, 284
present, being 238–239, 244, 245, 286
priapism 289
primate brain 21, 79, 80–84, 92–93, 101–102, 108
Principle of Eternal Recurrence 56
The Problem of Evil 66
prodigies 249–251
projection 303–304
prolactin 293

Q

qi. *See* life-stream
quantum mechanics 67, 185, 186, 199
question-and-answer game 9–11

R

radio 207–208, 217, 218

Ramachandran, V. S. 273
red, physical pleasures in Pleasure
    Prism 20, 80, 97–99, 108, 297
relationships
    in balanced life 295, 303–304
    being present 238–239, 244, 245
    make relationship 237–244
    objectification in 241–242
    renewable pleasures and 316
    similars/dissimilars 243
    sustainability and 321
    true love 242–244
relaxation 214
renewable pleasure 21–23, 311–321
repetition
    addiction and 263
    religion and 89
    reptilian brain and 89, 97–98
reptilian brain 21, 77, 79, 80, 84, 87–89,
    97–99, 108, 143
res cogitans 136
res extensa 136
resisting pleasure 139–140
resolution 284, 287–288
resonance 217–219
reward mechanism of brain 80–84, 264,
    265, 284
rhinencephalon 76
rhythm 98, 212
Rinzai Zen 231
rituals 89, 97–98, 117–119, 161
Roshi, Sasaki 189–191
ruach 135

Russell, Bertrand 325

S

sadhu 243
samsara 150
San people 175–176
satisfaction vs. happiness 100
Satya 9–11, 63, 116, 138
scaling pleasure 228–229, 234
scarification 275
Schrödinger's cat 199
Schrödinger Wave Equation 166
Chief Seattle 227
self
    addiction and 266–267
    art and 256
    evolution of sense of self 93
    falling in love and 242
    sense of self as illusion 93
    surrender and 184–186
    vanishing of 229–231, 234
self-conflict 42–46
self-intimacy 244
self-mastery 51–52
Seligman, Martin 17
Sengcan 199, 266
sense organs and perception 114
Sensual Continuum 127–132, 179, 325
sesshin 187–192
Seven Immutable Laws of Pleasure 23, 297.
    See also specific laws
sex
    equated with pleasure 16

erotica and 271–278
    gender differences in approaches 278
    reptilian brain and 80
shadow 303
shakuhachi 257–258
shame 32, 41, 43, 46, 249, 266, 268
sheaths 106
Simpson, Joe 256
singularity 203
sixth mass extinction 311
skin-lightening products 160, 275
sleep 129, 295, 300–302
smell brain 76
smoking 18, 262–264, 265, 267
smoothness 178–180
social media 76
Socrates 55
soft palate 102, 108, 214, 219, 220
Soto Zen 231
Source 52, 198, 233, 295, 307
Spencer, Herbert 319
sphinx 85, 86, 213
spinal cord 78
spirit. *See also* life-stream
    association with the masculine 33
    continuum of intensity 131
    mind-body split 136
    as pure 136
spiritual pleasures 21, 102–103, 108, 297
spiritual teachers 308–310
spiritus 135
stress and addiction 265
stress-reduction program 123

stroke 186
subconscious
    desire and 144
    majority of behavior as 93
    reptilian and mammalian brain as 84
subjective reality 196
suffering 60, 138–139
sukham 204
sunyata 214, 309, 320
supernormal desire 158
supernormal stimulus 158, 162, 276
superorganisms 320
supersizing 157–162
surrender. *See also* Law of Desire and
        Surrender
    Amadeus Equation 325
    baby steps and 258
    balancing point and 200–204
    bliss and 214–215
    cold water training and 135
    discipline and 252
    ectasy center and 211
    in fractal wave 226
    in meditation 308
    in orgasm 285
    understanding 183–191
    as *yin* 211
survival of the fittest 319
sustainability 21–26, 101, 311–320
sweatshop experience 88–89
sweet spot 295–306

T

Taiji symbol 210–211
talu chakra 102
tattoos 275
Taylor, Frank 49–50, 54
technology 148, 161, 174, 176, 312–313, 317
Theory of Complementarity 185
Thich Nhat Hahn 146, 304
thinking
   bliss and 214
   continuum of intensity 131
   contrast and comparison in 114
   orgasm and 283
   positive 101
   primate brain and 92–93
   surrender and 186
   suspending 114
Tibetan Buddhism rituals 89
ticks 111
time
   in Amadeus Equation 325
   perception of 229
   pleasure-time graph 168–170
   primate brain and 92
Tinbergen, Nikolaas 158
Touching the Void (Simpson) 257
training 171, 189
Tree of Knowledge of Good and Evil 31–33
triune brain
   defined 79
   embryological development 78
   evolution of 77, 79–80
   in history 84

   Pleasure Prism and 21
   pleasure types and 80
The Triune Brain in Evolution (MacLean) 92
truth
   addiction and 269
   in Declaration of Independence 69
   flow and 139
   mammalian brian and 92
   paradoxical nature of 199
   as virtue 52
turbulence 179

U

umwelt 112, 127, 196, 303
unconscious
   collective 146
   desire and 144
   making conscious 84
   reptilian and mammalian brain as 84
Utilitarianism 68

V

valley orgasm 291–293, 292
van der Post, Laurens 175
Ventral Tegmental Area (VTA) 80–84, 115, 265, 284, 285
Venus of Willendorf 159
virtue 51–54, 145
Vitruvian Man 295–296
VO2 max 299
von Uexküll, Jacob 112

W

WAC 298
wanting
  desire as 143
  wants vs. needs 147–153
war on consciousness 70, 71, 317
waves
  as fractal 226
  pleasure as 165–168
  resonance 218
  Schrödinger Wave Equation 166
wealth and happiness 148–152
Weininger, Ben 237–238
Western civilization
  concept of one 202
  cultural matrix 28–34
  needs vs. wants 147
white, spiritual pleasures in Pleasure Prism 21, 102–103, 108, 297
wholeness. See Law of Original Wholeness
will. See free will
Williams, Serena 98
witness
  described 104–105
  inner conflict and 84
  life-stream 135
women
  association with earth 33
  Divine Feminine 30
  gender differences in approach to sex 278
  gender differences in orgasm 282
  objectification of 33

Original Sin 44
patriarchy and 30–33
pornography use 277, 282
resolution phase 288
sexual response in 282–283
work 102, 295, 305–306
workbook 324
World Happiness Report 16
World Shakuhachi Festival 258

X

Xin Xin Ming 199

Y

yang
  äsis and 103
  desire as 211
  in *Taiji* symbol 210–211
Yates, Simon 256
yawning 214–215
yin
  of pelvis 99
  surrender as 211
  in *Taiji* symbol 210–211
yoga 95–96, 107, 137, 204, 214

Z

zero 11, 200–204, 297, 309
zone 212. See also flow
Zorba the Greek (Kazantzakis) 118

www.ingramcontent.com/pod-product-compliance
Lightning Source LLC
Chambersburg PA
CBHW031055080526
44587CB00011B/697